PRAISE FOR *HOW COVID CRASHED THE SYSTEM*

"Global pandemics are always disruptive, but they also represent wonderful opportunities to learn by taking advantage of the crisis invoked. The authors have delivered an excellent analysis on how the current pandemic created several learning opportunities because of the multitude of failures within the US health care system that became widely evident. This analysis of a broken, multi-level system is profoundly insightful and worth the read all by itself. However, the authors take it a step further by also providing a series of superb recommendations on how best to move the current US health care system forward to an improved future state for the betterment of the American population. All who are interested in learning more on how to significantly improve American health care should read this well-crafted and highly articulate treatise."

—**Peter Angood, MD**, president and CEO, American
Association for Physician Leadership

"This book does an unparalleled job of explaining what went wrong as it relates to Covid and health care delivery. It will take dedication to the principles of responsible innovation to ensure that we do not repeat the same mistakes."

—**Hemant Taneja**, managing partner, General Catalyst

"As the authors lay out so well, the pandemic may have uncovered many deficiencies in the American health care system, but through the sharing of their insights, they also reveal the very blueprint for a better system for tomorrow, not just to battle future pandemics but also to improve health overall."

—**Jaewon Ryu, MD, JD**, president and CEO, Geisinger Health

"David B. Nash presents an expert's view of how a pandemic exposed a systemically fragmented health care system. He reveals how the pandemic further uncovered the counterproductive hierarchical culture within healthcare, the urgency to train professionals across the patient care continuum to function as teams, the undeniable shift toward active patient management of their health and health care, and the crucial need to embrace technological innovations and to make health care accessible to all by fostering equality in public health policies."

—**H. Richard Haverstick Jr.**, interim president,
TJU and CEO, Jefferson Health

"This is a fascinating, well-researched, and gripping account of one of the most important stories of our time: how the Covid-19 pandemic defeated America's health defenses and caused so much preventable loss. But while that analysis is crystal clear, the book's positive insights may be even more important, because *How Covid Crashed the System* shows an inspiring path to improve our nation's health and make us all safer from the next pandemic."

—**Leana Wen, MD**, research professor of health policy
and management, George Washington University
Milken Institute School of Public Health

"Weaving together compelling real stories with detailed background history, David Nash and Charles Wohlforth have created a wonderful, yet brutal, exposé of the deficits in American health care that led to poor performance in the face of the Covid pandemic. They offer powerful insights into the changes we need to make now so we can avoid repeating these mistakes in the future."

—**Jerry Penso, MD, MBA**, president and CEO,
American Medical Group Association

How Covid Crashed the System

A Guide to Fixing American Health Care

David B. Nash, MD, and
Charles Wohlforth

ROWMAN & LITTLEFIELD
Lanham • Boulder • New York • London

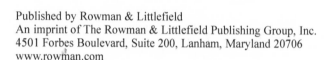

Published by Rowman & Littlefield
An imprint of The Rowman & Littlefield Publishing Group, Inc.
4501 Forbes Boulevard, Suite 200, Lanham, Maryland 20706
www.rowman.com

86-90 Paul Street, London EC2A 4NE

British Library Cataloguing in Publication Information Available

Library of Congress Cataloging-in-Publication Data

Names: Nash, David B., author. | Wohlforth, Charles P., author.
Title: How Covid crashed the system : a guide to fixing American health care /
  David B. Nash and Charles Wohlforth.
Description: Lanham : Rowman & Littlefield, [2022] | Includes bibliographical
  references and index. | Summary: "An influential, big-picture thinker and a
  science writer investigate why America's health care system failed so tragically
  during the Covid pandemic and how the forces unleashed by the crisis could be
  just the medicine for its long-term cure"— Provided by publisher.
Identifiers: LCCN 2022004606 (print) | LCCN 2022004607 (ebook) | ISBN
  9781538164259 (cloth : alk. paper) | ISBN 9781538164266 (epub)
Subjects: MESH: COVID-19—economics | Delivery of Health Care—
  organization & administration | United States
Classification: LCC RA644.C67 (print) | LCC RA644.C67 (ebook) | NLM WC
  506.7 | DDC 362.1962/414—dc23/eng/20220525
LC record available at https://lccn.loc.gov/2022004606
LC ebook record available at https://lccn.loc.gov/2022004607

To the thousands of health care workers who gave their lives caring for patients and the hope we can build a system that makes such sacrifices unnecessary ever again

Contents

Contents

Acknowledgments

As coauthors, we decided to investigate the root causes of America's Covid crash before the pandemic was half over, and our research and writing continued amid the events the book describes, ending in December 2021. We could not have attempted this audacious mission without the help of many people who helped with day-to-day tasks, provided critical insights and descriptions, and reviewed pages for errors. We thank all of those who made our work possible, especially David's remarkable wife and daughter, Drs. Esther and Rachel Nash, who also appear in the book. Charles also especially thanks his wife, Sarah Rowland, for her patience and loving support.

Dr. Sandro Galea was extraordinarily gracious and responsive in providing his introduction to the book, which perfectly frames and highlights our subject. Dr. Stephen Klasko was David's colleague and mentor through an extraordinary period of growth and innovation at Thomas Jefferson University and its health system. We are deeply grateful for his insightful foreword. David is also thankful for decades of support from Dr Mark Tykocinski, the provost of Thomas Jefferson University.

David's brilliant student, Zach Goldberg, performed essential research and provided editorial comments. David's assistants, Victoria McMonagle and Elizabeth DeBonis, were critical parts of the team from beginning to end. Literary agent Sara Camilli and Rowman &

Littlefield editor Suzanne Straszak-Silva guided the work from concept to print.

An extraordinary list of doctors and other experts on the health sys-
tem helped develop our thinking and bring the book to life, including
Dr. Theresa Andrasfay, Dr. David Ansell, Dr. Nick Bloom, Dr. Sandra
Brooks, Dr. Christopher Cannavino, Dr. Marty Cetron, Dr. Mary
Cooper, Timmy Del Vecchio, Dr. Karen DeSalvo, Michael Dowling, Dr.
Lisa Eyler, Julie Freeman, Michael Fronstin, Dr. Jonathan Gleason, Dr.
Oren Guttman, Dr. Judd Hollander, Marty Lupinetti, Dr. Bruce Meyer,
Dr. William Mobley, John Nance, Dr. Alex Navarro, Dr. Lawrence
Prybil, Dr. Jaewon Ryu, Dr. Byron Scott, Dr. Steven Scheinman, Dr.
Mark Schuster, Dr. Olga Shvetsova, Dr. Leana Wen, Dr. Leah Windsor,
and Jeff Zucker. We are also grateful for the corrections many of them
provided, although we are responsible for any remaining errors.

Foreword

Dr. David Nash has been a prophet in the area of population health, first by creating and serving as dean of the first college of population health in an American medical college, and then by working with health care leaders around the country to actualize the necessary changes toward a transformed health care delivery system. In this book, authors Nash and Wohlforth highlight both the problem that demands that transformation and the solution itself.

The problem: Health care policy over the last twenty years has been about how we give more people access to a fundamentally broken, fragmented, expensive, inequitable, and occasionally unsafe health care delivery system, with mere "hope" the system will transform itself. In many ways, this book contains the answer, by looking outside the health care world to other complex sectors of the economy with seemingly impossible safety and quality issues that were able to creatively construct highly reliable organizations. The lesson of airline safety, for example, is one of leadership: it is, in fact, possible to change complex systems. This book is the equivalent of an airline safety review. The authors have laid out, piece by piece, the components of the failure of the health care system in response to Covid-19, especially the unique failure of in the United States.

And at each stage, they remind us: Complex failure starts at the top. It starts with misplaced values and with hubris. In fact, as history shows repeatedly, the failure of experts is much more damaging than the failures of incompetents. We weed out incompetence quickly, but we allow "experts" to lead whole systems into danger.

Start with values. How? The core of values is ethics. Ethics is not a list of rules; it is a process of asking the big questions—first, before we create programs and products that could injure people even inadvertently.

In my vision of health care for 2032, I see a new dashboard for keeping people well, allowing them to thrive, based on technology that is only now emerging. As David Nash has repeatedly said, precision medicine will be the core of population health—allowing us to show you your own pre-disease markers, your own strategy for thriving. And by using technology to shift health care delivery to the home, we will unleash new tools for strengthening family dynamics and community resiliency. I believe we're on the cusp of a once-in-a-lifetime transformation of health care as it becomes digital and mobile.

Now imagine it's January 2, 2032. A mutant strain of an RNA-encapsulated virus has been afflicting people in Australia. Of course, people old enough to remember the dark days of early 2020 and the Covid-19 crisis immediately panic, especially health care workers (at least for a second), and then they smile. Because they know health care has evolved from a broken, fragmented, expensive, inequitable "sick care" system to a "health assurance" system in which most of their care happens at home.

In 2032, most of your health care data is continuously streamed to the cloud, and AI "bots" are constantly analyzing it for any changes, so the early symptoms of this new virus are immediately identified and anyone throughout the world who exhibits them is immediately notified and asked to socially isolate. If needed, their employer is notified and asked for an excused absence. Software immediately communicates through the internet of things to your home 3D printer, which begins to create masks for you and your family. Those who are having panic attacks remembering the Covid-19 crisis immediately communicate with their "bot psychiatrist" and, if necessary, promptly receive drone-delivered treatment.

This picture is a far cry from what we witnessed throughout the country during the Covid crisis. While not enough can be said in praise of the front-line health care heroes at Jefferson Health—the system I had the honor to lead—and throughout the country, data was scarce and not analyzed in a coordinated fashion. There were different strategies in different states and, in some cases, different counties of the same state. Jefferson Health went from fifty telehealth visits a day to three thousand, but many health systems did not have the bandwidth to accomplish broad virtual care. And, speaking of bandwidth, most public schools shut down for months as cities such as Philadelphia had a large percentage of their population without broadband or computers at home.

The dirty not-so-secret secret of health care as it existed when the pandemic hit was that almost everybody made more money when more people were sick. It was hard to get big institutions excited about changing something when their revenue depended on them not changing it. So, the health care industry had failed to transform itself.

Consumers, business owners, and all rational observers could see how health care escaped the consumer revolution, as they watched hospitals fail and insurers experience record profits during the Covid crisis. Underserved and minority populations suffered because we had failed to address social determinants. Things we took for granted in other areas of life were difficult in health care (even telehealth was viewed as a "new technology"!). The pandemic made clearly visible the failure of entrepreneurs and the traditional health care ecosystem to disrupt health care. Most providers were not ready to increase their telehealth bandwidth, most physicians and nurses had not been trained in virtual visits, the worlds of electronic medical records and new technology were fragmented, and there was no natural repository for data or mutually agreed-upon population health analytics.

At the Davos World Economic Forum in 2020, the CEO of a banking conglomerate said to me, "Twenty years ago, the two groups that had escaped the consumer revolution were banking and health care. Now you are alone!" It's true. During the crisis no one had to worry about groups of people congregating at banks to make deposits, because everything that should have happened in health care had already happened in banking—the data was continuous, owned by the consumer, and almost all transactions could be done at home. Think about how differently the pandemic would have been if we had continuous data coming in from patients through their wearables and other sources with temperature, respiratory rate, and other variables. Or if 3D printers were as ubiquitous as cell phones.

Looking back from 2032, we can imagine great progress made in the delivery of health, a transformation that would not have been as dramatic if not for the Covid crisis. In some respect, future lives may be saved because the pandemic was a jolt and lightning rod for American health care to have an extreme makeover and for the "sick" system to finally get well.

But this transformation can itself have side effects, like every other transformation. We have to be resolute in pursuing the goal of "responsible innovation." Just look at the great revolutions of the past: If we'd known that the oil-based industrial revolution would have led to a century of wars to control oil, could we have changed course? If we'd known that the corn-based agricultural revolution would spur obesity, could we have prevented the rise in obesity and its concomitant diseases? If we'd known that the social media revolution would not just give us pictures of grandchildren but also provide the power spew hate and affect elections, would we have erected guardrails?

This is what leadership is all about: raising the big questions and identifying the many ways to answer them. There is no question that the time is now for radical collaboration, radical communication, and radical construction of a transformed health care delivery system. That transformation must be grounded in values, in responding to ethical questions, and in reversing inequity.

When I ask groups to list the ideal health care system ten years from now, that's what I hear: holistic, family centered, community supportive, and universal.

I believe the globe faces two linked existential crises: climate change and health disparities. Both of these worked together to make the pandemic a disaster. They both require urgent action that does what this book proposes: be clear about the causes and be bold about the values it will take to make change. Nash and Wohlforth set out a clear path as to how we can move forward, taking lessons from population health, social determinants, and predictive analytics and moving them from philosophic and academic exercises into the mainstream of clinical care, payment models, and medical education.

And so I leave you with what I believe is the core message of this book: the courage to change. Standing together, we can do anything.

Stephen K. Klasko, MD, MBA
Executive in Residence, General Catalyst
Distinguished Fellow, World Economic Forum
Retired, President, Thomas Jefferson University, and CEO, Jefferson Health

Introduction

Should a book on health mostly be about doctors, nurses, and hospitals? Most Americans would have assumed that was true a few years ago, before the Covid pandemic. Medical professionals were expected to take care of us, our illnesses, and our injuries, and, as our final hours approached, their miracle drugs and high technology would provide hope against the inevitable end of each of us. The United States provided the world's most advanced and innovative care and drugs—the best money could buy, absorbing almost 18 percent of our national economic output. The world's other wealthy nations spent, on average, less than half as much. Although they generally offered universal health coverage, they could not boast the cutting-edge technology found in American hospitals, our individual hedge against death.[1]

Then Covid arrived on our shores, and we saw doctors, nurses, and hospitals overwhelmed, with terrible scenes in New York of refrigerator trucks of corpses parked outside morgues. Doctors couldn't stop the pandemic. It spread across the country in repeated waves, with deaths counted in mounting hundreds of thousands. Even after US pharmaceutical companies created extremely effective vaccines, ready to use just seven months after the pandemic was declared, waves of preventable illness continued, with more Americans dead in the second year, 2021, than in the first.[2] Other countries suffered greatly, too, but the grim scoreboard of mortality persistently showed the United States near the top, worse than every comparable wealthy country, even though those others had spent so much less on medicine in the years leading up to the catastrophe.[3]

As these words are written, we have passed three-quarters of a million dead in the United States. The enormity of the loss is impossible to fully grasp. But every American should now be able to see that our outsized spending on medical care did not protect us. In fact, those of us in public health had long recognized that Americans as a population suffered poor health compared to our sister countries, with higher infant mortality, worse incidence of chronic diseases such as diabetes and asthma, and shorter lifespans, despite our expensive, advanced medicine. Covid exploited our poor health. And it exploited our misguided sense of what health is about.[4]

Only a relatively small percentage of our health outcomes are determined by health care. Doctors know this, because we see so many patients whose illnesses are caused by conditions of their lives and can be resolved only by changes made outside the clinic. Stereotypically, we might think of the cardiac patient who refuses to exercise or stop smoking, but much more insidious and impactful are life situations that people cannot change, based on where and how they live, their income, and the color of their skin. For example, a woman shows up in the emergency room with uncontrolled diabetes. Doctors stabilize her and send her home. But she cannot afford medications to manage the disease and has no access to healthy foods that could prevent it. She will be back. Her health will worsen. Everyone involved knows it.

The conditions where we live, work, and learn—the most important factors for our well-being—are called the social determinants of health. Doctors and medical schools began taking them into account well before the pandemic, largely out of a sense of futility with the old way of caring for patients. We will learn in this book (in chapter 7) about ideas such as the Food Farmacy at Geisinger Health in Pennsylvania, where doctors send patients home with a prescription for healthy food and cooking lessons, paid for out of the enormous savings created by supporting good health rather than fixing sick people. A great idea, since feeding a person costs so much less than caring for her diabetes. But shouldn't everyone have access to good food? How would our nation's health outcomes look then?

Covid demonstrated that providing care for the sick—and even giving them food—is not enough. Our health inequities went much deeper. They created a sickly society that could not fight the virus. As I write in my book, *The Contagion Next Time*, extraordinary disparities emerged rapidly as the numbers of deaths exploded in communities of color.[5] Poor neighborhoods had trapped these people with polluted air, crowded living conditions, unsafe streets, unhealthy food, and little access to health care. The residents suffered poor health, making them vulnerable, and had nowhere to avoid the virus in dense housing and with low-paid jobs that forced extensive contact with the public.

In the post-vaccine phase of the pandemic, inequities continued to aid the spread of the disease. Vaccination of Black and Brown people lagged in part because many did not trust the medical establishment—a lack of trust that was well deserved, as we will learn in chapter 4. But hesitancy to get the vaccine was only one factor. Many low-income Americans were not hesitant, but they faced barriers in language, education, and transportation and lacked connection to mainstream information sources. Rumors filled that void.

We all suffered due to these inequities, even the well off, as the pandemic wore on for so long, affecting every aspect of our lives. No one was immune from the damage caused when Covid exploited our national ill health. The pandemic made it clear that health does not belong to us as individuals. Our communities and society must be healthy to ensure a healthy life for each of us. And creating a healthy society requires far different tools than those that doctors and nurses use in the hospital. Inequity in American society begins with the educational system, which boosts those who are born ahead and leaves behind children who need help the most. The workings of a poorly regulated market-driven economy affect health, too. Increasingly unequal incomes in our country correlated over the last two decades with our declining health statistics.[6] Structural racism reinforces these inequities, as the Covid death rates force us to finally acknowledge.

Health care, it turns out, would be better known as sick care. In our country, it comprises the unproductive but profitable business of selling medical services as a commodity. The health system, by contrast, is much larger. It includes the many levers we have to support wellness outside the walls of hospitals, including the tools of public health and also the strategies of public policy to create a healthier, more just society. The health system should include the provision of health as a public good that belongs to everyone. To reach that goal, our conception of the health system must become broader and more inclusive, including all the conditions of our society and environment that can benefit of our collective wellness.

To answer my opening question, clearly, a book about health must be about more than doctors, nurses, and hospitals. Nash and Wohlforth, in this investigation of the pandemic (and the fatal flaws it exposed), rightly take such a wide-view approach. Their investigation is systemic, seeking the root causes of our collective failure. Those root causes go deep, into American culture, race, the social determinants of health, and public health. It is fitting that they do not reach an examination of hospitals until the chapter 6, because the health system is so much larger than the medical industry. The health system is the entire complex of our life conditions that determine our health. In the wake of this unimaginable tragedy, we must look closely and critically at this system as a whole and find the path to a healthier and more resilient society.

Sandro Galea, MD, DrPH
Dean and Robert A. Knox Professor
Boston University School of Public Health

PART I

What Went Wrong

Chapter 1

Our Investigation

This is an investigation, but we are not looking for a culprit. Amid the Covid pandemic, villains are abundant and unhidden—and heroes, too. Faced by a test as great and deadly as a war, humanity once again has produced its wondrous extremes: of selfishness and ignorance, of courage and ingenuity, of death and endurance. The stories will be retold for ages. Our investigation goes deeper.

Think of an aircraft lying disintegrated and cratered in a farmer's field, just outside the fencing beyond the runway. Fires are out and ambulances have departed. At the airport, the bright lights of news cameras glare on scenes of grief. Out in the scorched field, a crew of investigators in black baseball caps is alone, picking through the pieces, searching the fragments for clues. A plane roars overhead, departing from the airport. The work here in the field is to keep those above safe and to protect everyone on airplanes everywhere. Blame won't save lives now. Preventing errors may.

The American health care system crashed as surely as the most magnificent of technological machines that has ever fallen from the sky. The novel coronavirus posed a deadly threat, but it should have been manageable, and for some nations, it was. But against the United States, with the world's most expensive and scientifically advanced medical system, the virus won. America recorded more Covid deaths than any other nation.[1] Short of death, Covid also caused long-term illnesses, bankrupt businesses, blocked educations, the mentally devastating isolation of two years of repeated lockdowns and social disruptions, and bitter divisions about vaccination and public health measures. More than thirty-six hundred US health care workers lost their lives taking

7

care of Covid patients in the first year, a fourteenfold increase over deaths in an ordinary year.[2]

Why?

Why did the United States fare uniquely poorly among developed nations? Why did the 18 percent of gross domestic product we spend on health care fail to protect us? It's as if the US military, mightier than the forces of all other nations combined, suddenly was routed by a mainland invader. And our spending on the military is "only" 3 percent of GDP, not 18 percent.[3]

A partial, obvious explanation for the Covid failure could be that hospitals were never intended to handle the millions of sick people suddenly arriving at their doors. But the health system reaches far beyond hospital doors. Why did Americans get sick in such great numbers?

Our investigation will answer that question. We will look deeply into this complex system. And, as in any investigation of a complex system that failed, we will find more than one answer. An airliner's crash always requires more than one mistake. So says our friend, the pilot and author John Nance, who first taught David about the National Transportation Safety Board model of investigations. "This is the lesson that we learned in aviation safety in the late '70s and early '80s," he said. "Every single solitary contributing cause must be addressed or you will see it as part of a causal chain in another accident."[4]

Airline crashes almost never happen anymore. In the 1970s, aviation also was considered safe, but if the rate of accidents back then were happening now, with skies many times busier, we would be seeing the equivalent of a jumbo jet of passengers dying every other day, Nance told us. Instead, years pass without a single death. That improvement happened because the NTSB investigated crashes looking for every cause—and without looking for anyone to blame.

"Blame has absolutely nothing to say to us about how to prevent things in the future," Nance said. "That's an ethical thing, but it is definitely not for repairing, through understanding causation, what needs to be corrected."

David has frequently taken these ideas into investigations of medical errors. In 2005, he was at his daughter's field hockey game when Connecticut's health commissioner called to ask him to investigate three recent deaths at the Connecticut Children's Medical Center in Hartford. A child had died overnight because an emergency room doctor misread an X-ray and failed to order a needed test. A victim of a car crash with an injured heart could have been saved by emergency surgery but died because no one looked at his X-ray for ninety-nine minutes. A visiting seven-year-old boy was allowed to wander alone into the room of an unrelated, severely disabled baby and dropped her on the floor. The baby died.

In an understaffed, overtaxed, undertrained emergency room with an inexperienced, interim head, the doctors' errors were understandable. No one could blame the seven-year-old. But when David visited the hospital board's chair, he immediately saw a deeper cause. The chairman—who was a banker, very smooth, with a beautiful office—said he was not responsible. David informed him that he was wrong. Legal precedent going back to 1961 made the board responsible for the quality of patient care. But more important than the law, the leaders hadn't created a culture of patient safety. "Members of the Board of Directors of CCMC do not have a clear strategic-level commitment to quality measurement and safety improvement," David wrote in his report (which was then leaked to the local newspaper).[5]

To understand that conclusion, set aside how you think of investigations. TV detectives sleuth for clues to narrow responsibility for a crime to a single person at a discrete moment. Investigating a flawed system—whether in aviation, medicine, or any other complex human enterprise—is more like diagnosing an ill patient. The system has produced an error or a close call, so we know something is not right, but errors are unintentional, so knowing of the error alone does not, by itself, reveal the cause. Errors point to a cause, like the symptoms of a disease. A symptom is not the same as the disease, and a disease is not the same as the infectious agent that caused it, and the ability of that agent to produce the disease also is influenced by the environment and perhaps other issues that weakened the body's defenses.

Errors can never be reduced to zero. To err is human. But some complex systems have reduced accidents to near zero, including commercial aviation, by interposing layers of safeguards. A pilot makes a mistake, but the copilot catches it. Or the copilot also misses the mistake, but a checklist helps, or a computer. Each layer has some holes, like a slice of Swiss cheese, but with enough layers in place, the probability drops to near zero that the holes in all the layers will line up and allow an error to slip through. Investigating errors in a complex system is more complicated than finding a culprit because the goal is larger: to find systemic vulnerability and fix it. Where are the missing layers or the oversized holes?[6]

When David entered that emergency room in Connecticut, he didn't see confusion, or disorder, or improper health care. He didn't ask primarily about the three fatal errors or the sequence of events in those particular incidents. His questions were diagnostic, using techniques developed in aviation and, over the last twenty years, by pioneers in performance improvement and population health, fields in which David has worked for decades. Since we are planning to use this framework to investigate the Covid disaster—the biggest medical error in history— it's worth explaining the process step by step.

In an emergency room, junior doctors frequently have expert attending physicians they can call on at home, who are paid to be available for those questions. Sometimes doctors get in trouble and need advice or simply lack the expert knowledge of a specialist. David asked each young pediatrician in the emergency department what he or she would do when uncertain. Would they call? He got eye-rolling. Follow-up question: Calling should be routine; why not call for help? "Well, Doctor So-and-So reams you out when you call." Another senior doctor just wouldn't pick up the phone.

That answered diagnostic question one: What was the authority gradient? The idea of the authority gradient goes back to a 1977 aviation disaster in Spain's Canary Islands, the deadliest crash in history. The extremely experienced, high-ranking pilot of a KLM 747 attempted to take off in a fog without getting clearance and hit another 747 taxiing on the runway. Cockpit tapes of the KLM crew—who all died—indicated that the copilot and flight engineer had recognized the pilot's mistake but were too intimidated by his superior authority to forcefully point out his error. The lesson for health care: flattening the authority gradient and creating collaborative teams in hospitals can help stop errors.[7]

David's next diagnostic question checked for loners among the doctors in the ER. Often, full-time doctors in an emergency department have a cowboy attitude—highly confident in their own abilities, moving rapidly and skillfully in a crisis, and without the burden of follow-up contact with their patients. A certain personality type gravitates to the work. Other doctors rotate into the department and can bring a more collaborative style, different skill sets, and a greater willingness to reach out for help. But at the hospital in Connecticut, a few conversations made it clear that the cowboys ran the show and set the standard. Loners might not make more errors than the rest of us, but the errors they do make are less likely to be caught by colleagues before doing harm.

The third diagnostic question was for the nurses. David asked—pulling each aside in quiet moments—whether, when seeing something that was clearly wrong, they felt empowered to say "stop" and call a halt to a procedure, as if pulling an emergency brake or "stopping the line" in manufacturing. They looked at David as if he were from another planet. Impossible! That response isn't unusual in a hospital with patient safety problems—which is the great majority of hospitals. Numerous examples have been documented of nurses staying silent even when they knew a surgeon was operating on the wrong part of a patient's body, something that still happens hundreds of times a year in the United States.[8] A toxic culture makes it impossible to challenge an exalted doctor.

A baby was dropped, an X-ray misread, a patient overlooked—but the real problem at the hospital in Connecticut was cultural. And it permeated the organization, all the way up to the board chair, with his refusal to take responsibility.

This is the final and most important question for a medical error investigation: Is the culture just? That is, does it treat everyone equally, respect the contributions of all members of the team, and avoid assigning blame to individuals for failures of the system? In that Connecticut hospital, the culture was unjust, and patients suffered. Is America's health care culture just? That question is among the most important for investigating why we failed the Covid challenge.

THE SYSTEM'S DESIGN

"Every system is perfectly designed to get the results it gets." Dr. Paul Batalden's quote has spread far and wide, but it still fits best within the movement for health care quality, where he originally intended it to apply.[9] On one level, the truth of the saying is self-evident, but when thinking of health care systems, it is profound. If you are unsatisfied with the output of a system, you must address its design to get different results. Given the disastrous performance of the American health care system during the Covid pandemic, the need for a redesign is obvious, but we must first acknowledge a possible reservation about the applicability of Batalden's quote: Who would say US health care had been "designed" in the first place?

America's health care system includes university, for-profit and community hospitals, HMOs, surgery centers, clinics, nursing homes, long-term care facilities, community health centers, and school nurse offices; doctors, dentists, nurses, midwives, psychotherapists, physical therapists, chiropractors, acupuncturists, and faith healers; insurance companies, union trusts, self-insurance schemes, employer HR departments, Medicare, Medicaid, Obamacare marketplaces, bill collectors, and community fundraisers for ill friends; pharmaceutical companies, pharmacies, pharmacy benefit managers, nutritional supplement dealers, and medical marijuana dispensaries; federal and state regulators, professional societies, patient advocates, nongovernmental organizations, and religious orders; national research institutes, academic labs, life-science startups, disease-based organizations, and internet quacks; national, state, and local public health authorities, workplace wellness programs, nutritionists, school food programs, and morning jogging groups; medical schools, health journalists, and the opinionated trainer at the gym. It may be the most complex and expensive human system on Earth.

No one controls the system. No one likes it. The system emerged over time from disparate pieces to meet various needs and desires, but it grew in unplanned, unproductive ways. It is probably too fragile, intricate, and deeply embedded with powerful, interlocking forces for a total, top-down redesign. Rather than thinking of design, a healing metaphor might fit better. This malformed system is sick—some of its pathologies have been evident for a long time—but we can diagnose what ails it and prescribe thoughtful changes that work their way curatively through the entire, colossal organism. Indeed, we will argue in these pages that the American health care system is capable of a kind of homeostasis—buffeted by Covid, it is beginning to heal itself in promising ways. The tragic, abject failure of Covid broke the inertia holding back positive change with a therapeutic shock.

The US health care system failed during Covid because it is the wrong system for our needs. We investigate the disaster throughout part I of this book. Like other medical errors, this failure involved many layers. The holes in the Swiss cheese lined up to allow a catastrophe to pass through, killing (at this writing) eight hundred thousand Americans.[10] We should never forget the extraordinary contributions of heroic individuals, the many thousands of health care workers—nurses, doctors, and even medical students—who risked or even gave their lives caring for patients, and the brilliant scientists who created vaccines in record time. But they were ill served by a system that called on them for superhuman contributions to fight illnesses that never needed to happen. Our investigation of the system is a tribute to them. We believe in a health care system that doesn't require heroes.

Health care workers made their stand at overwhelmed hospitals, but why did so many Covid victims arrive at the hospital in the first place? The answer is fascinating, complex, and far reaching—we will explore it in detail in the chapters ahead. As Sandro Galea explained in the introduction, the circle bounding the health system is much larger than hospital walls or even the periphery of health care. Consider the epidemic of lifestyle diseases he mentioned, especially type 2 diabetes, which is caused largely by diet and is a major risk factor for severe Covid. Treatment for type 2 diabetes is many times more expensive than the healthy food required to prevent it, and some health plans and medical systems have started saving money by giving patients groceries and cooking lessons as well as prescriptions for medicine—making everyday nutrition formally part of the health care system (as we document in chapter 7). But what about providing healthy food *before* people get diabetes? Many Americans live in urban food deserts where good, fresh food is out of reach. Addressing that lack would be less expensive and more effective than our current medical strategy against diabetes and just as much a part of our system of health. Instead, the virus preyed on people with diabetes living in food deserts—and exposed a fatal flaw in our health system.

In each of the next chapters of part I, we will look at a part of this system. In chapter 2, we consider preparation and leadership, with the understanding that we knew what we needed to know to handle the pandemic better. In chapter 3, we investigate the cultural context underlying our health system, which deeply influenced pandemic response, to learn how we should design a successful system to be built on this ground. In chapter 4, we explore the racial inequities that Covid exposed, along with how the social determinants of health dominated the pandemic's outcome. In chapter 5, we dig into the failure of the public health system and its much greater potential. At the end of part I, in chapter 6, we reach the hospitals, and we will see how the structure of the health care system affected their ability to cope.

Some readers may believe we should investigate only the first topic—the failure in leadership—and that we don't need to consider systemic problems to understand the pandemic disaster. Certainly, if Covid were an American plane crash, our grossly negligent pilot, President Donald Trump, could not be absolved of flying the plane into the ground. His own White House Covid coordinator later blamed the weak initial response for most of the deaths.[11] By that reckoning, hundreds of thousands of Americans would be alive today but for Trump's downplaying of the danger of the virus and politicizing the public health measures needed to control it—all apparently done in a warped sense of self-interest. But, in fact, the United States was culturally primed for his message of doubt and division. Our defenses were weak and our resources wrongly deployed. Given the system as it existed when the virus reached our shores, a better president could not have prevented disaster.

Part of the agony of the pandemic was watching the suffering and knowing how an effective public health system could have avoided so much of it. Public health as a science did not fail, but public health as a practice was too weak, both because its institutions had been starved of financial support and because our cultural fabric had ripped, disabling the translation of public health directives into collective behavior. Public health interventions are humankind's most effective life savers, adding far more years to Americans' longevity than medical care, and for a small fraction of the cost.[12] The holes in our public health defenses are among the most important failures we must analyze in our systemic investigation of what went wrong.

American culture itself was a fundamental difficulty—American federalism, individualism, and exceptionalism. American federalism contributed to an uncoordinated and ineffective national response. States at times competed for scarce personal protective equipment. Governors adhering to public health guidance had to restrict travel from states with leaders whose refusal to require masks or limit gatherings caused outbreaks. American individualism gave political fuel to that refusal and further undercut public health. Somehow, unsafe practices became statements of liberty and identity. American exceptionalism allowed many to believe this situation was normal, making them blind to Covid solutions that were working elsewhere in the world. That ignorance helped protect failed US leaders from accountability.

Americans' culture of poor health also contributed to the disaster. All physicians are familiar with entitled patients who refuse to change their daily activities to protect their health, instead counting on expensive medical interventions to save them later, such as the heart patient who won't diet or exercise but expects emergency surgery for blocked arteries. Trump's own Covid infection was a microcosm of this phenomenon. After refusing to wear a mask or avoid crowds, he inevitably caught the virus, spread it to others around him, and received world-class treatment and experimental medications from a team of top doctors. Returning to the White House, Trump bragged of "beating" Covid, while the outbreak he had fueled swept through scores of White House officials, housekeepers, and Secret Service agents.[13]

Trump's behavior vividly illustrates a wider issue: the inefficiency, expense, and illogic of spending on medical care while neglecting prevention. The US medical system itself contributes to the problem with perverse financial incentives that reward costly hospital care while discouraging the low-cost measures that could slow the flow of patients upstream of the hospital doors. The culture contributes as well. Obesity and diabetes—key risk factors for severe Covid disease—correlate strongly in the United States with poverty, food insecurity, and the sedentary lifestyles led by poor people living in dangerous neighborhoods and areas lacking low-cost recreational facilities.[14]

Why is poverty endemic in many areas of the United States? Our investigation of the Covid disaster necessarily leads to the problem of systemic racism. Communities of color not only suffered from more frequent Covid infections but also often received inferior care, as we document in chapter 4. Old age in America also strongly correlates with poverty and with Covid death. To find the root causes of what happened, we will attempt to untangle these connections. Our idea of the health system includes the social system that largely determines our well-being and longevity.

What is just culture in this context? The meaning is only slightly different in society at large compared to the emergency room, where professional equality supports good care through teamwork. In the hospital, a toxic culture of inequality threatens patient safety; in America's cities and towns, inequality helped drive the pandemic. The virus spread fastest among those without ready access to primary care, who lacked safe housing, or who were insecure in their income. We believe in building an America where everyone has the opportunity and basic needs for a fulfilling life: education, health care, healthy sustenance, and safe shelter. We are privileged white men who want to live in a just society. But even for those who don't care about justice for its own sake, our investigation of the Covid disaster reveals a threat to the self-interest of the privileged. Our health care system requires a fundamental level of justice and equality in society in order to effectively respond to a pandemic.

After we take our investigation through public health, culture, and the social determinants of health in our initial chapters, we will bring our inquiry to the system of doctors and hospitals that comprise America's high-tech medical establishment—the pilots and the airplane itself. The system was already broken and serving America poorly, but its fractured pieces became especially deadly in the pandemic. Where smaller, rural hospitals were overwhelmed, transfers to large hospitals sometimes required many phone calls, with days of delay for clumsy logistics and receiving hospitals' checks of insurance coverage. Some people died because of that delay. Large hospital systems coordinated facilities better, but they failed for another reason: financial decisions. Some hospital systems operating with Wall Street oversight were crippled by just-in-time inventory and other penny-pinching efficiencies that left staff vulnerable and without surge capacity when they needed it. Our investigation will look at these issues, as well as hospital systems that performed well. Their successes offer essential clues.

In most cases, the pandemic turned hospital finances upside down, with revealing (but totally unexpected) results. Even in areas of the country with plenty of hospital capacity, patients stayed away during the first phase of the pandemic, avoiding care for serious conditions that normally cannot be put off, such as strokes and heart attacks. Non-Covid admissions dropped by almost half in April 2020, with Covid cases offsetting only a small portion of the decline.[15] Without those revenue-generating patients, hospitals lost money, creating the bizarre situation of "hero" staff being laid off soon after their heroic acts were completed. In hard-hit areas, substantially more people died at home during that initial spike, showing they avoided care they needed.[16]

After the pandemic cooled in June and July 2020, however, the regular flow of patients still failed to return to normal nationally, remaining depressed by 16 percent and staying there for some time, including for serious heart and lung conditions, infections, and mental illnesses. Where were the patients? And what had happened to their health without getting the medical care they presumably required?[17]

As the summer wore on, hospitals and health officials begged patients to come back to see their doctors and receive care, fearing a huge surge of secondary deaths from untreated illnesses, which we call the untold burden. But something extraordinary occurred. That secondary surge didn't materialize. Patients stayed away, care was not given—and not much happened. It was a deep mystery. Without more research, doctors can only speculate why so many patients didn't show up for care. Did they all die at home, a continuing untold burden? Evidence suggests not. Visits for dermatology and alcohol use did return to normal levels, so some patients, at least, did not avoid care during those months. Some researchers supposed that Americans' health improved thanks to mask wearing and a slowing of the economy—with less air pollution and less general activity—making hospital visits less necessary. To some degree, that explanation may be right, and it demonstrates how public health stops the upstream flow of illness leading to the hospital. Making Americans healthier is fundamentally good and saves billions of dollars on medical care.[18]

But it's also likely that some of the missing medical care was simply never needed in the first place. Research tells us 25 percent of medical spending is wasted.[19] For example, the literature says a third of all heart stents inserted in patients are of no value to them.[20] In the traditional model of medicine in the United States, doctors and hospitals make more money for seeing more sick patients and doing more procedures on them. The financial incentive—and the unconscious bias that money engenders—results in diagnoses that require the procedures that doctors are trained to perform and that earn the most money. Fear of Covid kept patients away from the hospital, diagnoses requiring care went down, and the evidence suggests that many of those patients did fine. Staying away apparently shielded people from medical care they didn't need and from the attendant risk of medical error. Such errors cause 10 percent of deaths, the third leading cause of death in the United States (until Covid beat that number), according to the most credible estimate.[21] In effect, Covid kept some patients out of a medical system that would have done them harm.

We are able cite these chilling statistics because the problems have been documented for a long time. Yet progress to improve patient safety has been patchy and slow. America has been aware of medical waste and excessive cost for generations without solving the problem. We wouldn't write this book just to repeat old news about these issues. But Covid has changed the landscape. It has allowed us to see the shape of the problems in a new way and to see brand new hope for solutions.

All by itself, Covid probably wrung some unneeded medical care from the system. But its larger impact will be on the future. The shock of the pandemic is powering a transformation. Tragedy is driving change. That hope infuses our investigation for root causes. We find positive signs that Americans will become safer and healthier in the future and that medical providers will be more fulfilled working in a system that makes sense.

HOW INVESTIGATION LEADS
TO POSITIVE CHANGE

Charles worked for many years as a science writer and investigative journalist, writing exposés about health care as well as other subjects. A sense of service inspires most journalists, with the belief that uncovering problems and telling human stories helps improve and connect society. The work doesn't offer many other rewards beyond the satisfaction of curiosity and the hope of making a positive difference. Good journalists earn their unpopularity by delivering bad news and difficult truths.

David's career has been more explicitly about helping. As an internist, practicing until just recently, he cared for individual patients, but from early on he focused more on improving the quality and safety of medical care for everyone. It's a role that requires a willingness to anger powerful people and make statements that colleagues don't want to hear, because improvement means looking squarely at the reasons for errors and failures. When he was offered the job of founding dean of the Jefferson College of Population Health, a student asked whether the administration did it to shut him up. If so, that was unsuccessful.

In this book, we plan to call on our skills of investigation and analysis, and also on our connection to the personal stories and human images that make these lessons real. Our approach is rooted in our experience. We believe issues matter because of people, and the more personal our analysis, the closer to solutions it will take us. We are fortunate to have many key figures in the Covid story near at hand, in David's extraordinary contact list of the nation's health leaders. And we also have connections with ordinary people who fought on the front lines of the pandemic. You will meet them and learn their names, and we hope you will feel the urgency and sympathy that we do for the predicaments the system created for them. Finally, we won't avoid putting our own emotions on the page. The tragedy of the pandemic still haunts us, as it does so many others, and we take our drive to write from feelings of outrage and helplessness as so many died.

Among the most difficult meetings of David's professional career were ones that happened during his nine years on the board of Main Line Health, a four-hospital system in Philadelphia. As chair of the Quality and Safety Committee, he invited grieving families to meet with the board and hospital leadership to talk about medical errors that had taken their loved ones. The board twice held retreats for these meetings. David and clinical leaders first explained to board laypeople what had gone wrong and what investigation showed about the systemic failure that allowed an error to hurt a patient. Then the family would come into the room and tell the story as they experienced it, down to the heartbreaking loss of a family member, while board members, doctors, and administrators listened respectfully and attentively.

That was the hardest part. Many doctors have experienced something similar now; others have seen films and presentations by grieving family members. So often, the errors are embarrassingly and infuriatingly simple. Usually, they include the failure of providers to listen to family members or colleagues of lesser status. At root, the commonalities in these errors outweigh the differences, but each family is different and their experience uniquely poignant and painful. Finally, when they had their say, the board would apologize and explain what was being done to prevent the errors from happening again.

Two decades ago, hospitals that hurt patients routinely denied making errors, froze out grieving families, and prepared to be sued. That brutal and dishonest process still happens far too often. What we have learned, however, is that families usually go to court for something other than money. They need respectful apologies and substantive changes to prevent recurrence of the error that hurt their loved one. The process of investigation, disclosure, and improvement creates meaning out of their loss. Pennsylvania law now supports us in conducting honest, open investigations into the roots of errors and disclosing what we did wrong as part of the process of fixing systems of care. When we hold those meetings, the system heals and families begin to heal, too. Truth is medicine for both.

With this book, we hope to tell a grieving nation what went wrong in the pandemic and how our medical system can improve. We would bring meaning to our collective loss by looking honestly at our flaws and showing a path to change.

Part I is the investigation. Part II describes the path to healing.

We begin part II with the hospital story, in chapter 7. The financial disruptions of Covid are pushing providers away from the old fee-for-service model to adopt new ways of doing business. For many months, hospital and clinic revenues dwindled because patients stayed away. Meanwhile, insurance companies, managed care organizations, and other payers banked health care premiums from members but paid few claims, because the flow of procedures had slowed. Now those cash-rich payers are in a position to buy the distressed providers, creating organizations we call "payviders." These unified entities will collect premiums in return for health rather than paying à la carte fees for individual procedures. When Americans buy all their health care from a single source—a payvider or managed care organization—providers become responsible for health rather than billings, which eliminates the incentive to perform unnecessary procedures.

The pandemic also has forced a fresh approach to medical education, as we will learn in chapter 8. We will need doctors trained in new ways for the new health care organizations where they will work. Medical schools also are scrambling to catch up to the technology that exploded into wide use during the pandemic. Doctors and insurance companies had resisted telemedicine; everyone is using it now, empowering patients, and we won't be going back. Technology also will allow health care providers to monitor a patient's condition during the day, every day, overcoming some of the cultural barriers to our well-being—topics in chapter 9.

Employers' roles are changing, too. They became unwilling public health experts during the pandemic. They have always held the purse-strings for the US health care system. Now they also will become a key to addressing the inequities that hurt our collective health, as we discuss in chapter 10.

Finally, in chapter 11, we will return to our overriding concern for the just culture that enables safe, high-quality health care, as well as the just culture that can promote health for our entire society. Americans have spoken in the streets and at the ballot box for social justice. Covid and the need to change health outcomes can help advance that movement.

The scale of needed change is almost unimaginable. Before the pandemic, we could see the right direction, but moving the vast edifice of the health system forward happened only in limited, decade-long increments of change. Insiders alone cared about the wonky domain of "health care reform," while most Americans treated the unreasonable costs and mediocre results of the system with resignation, like bad weather.

Covid changed that. Many events that were barely imaginable before 2020 have now happened. The health system lies in smoking rubble where it crashed, like an airliner that fell from the sky. The disaster took innumerable precious lives. Standing in the wreckage, we must not shy away from the work of examining the causes of the crash and following them where they lead. We owe that to the dead, as well as the survivors. We will try to bring meaning to this loss.

Chapter 2

Failures of Leadership

Neither of us saw it coming. We both believed the United States would be a rock against the pandemic, not a basin for its flash flood of illness. Charles, a writer without medical training, viewed the approaching wave with concern, but not fear. On March 1, 2020, he noted that China seemed to be turning the corner on its epidemic after eight weeks, so the United States should do at least as well and be over Covid by summer—a prediction that would be off by well over a year but wasn't far out of the uninformed mainstream. David, however, is a doctor and a health policy expert who had studied and written about the flaws in the US health care system for thirty years. His optimism is harder to explain. He understood the many faults in the system that would ultimately prove fatal to so many Americans, but his hope, anxiety, and wishful thinking told him that if Asian and Arab nations had prevailed against the previous viral threats of SARS and MERS, then surely the towering technical edifice of American medicine could handle Covid.

How do we explain the pairing of overconfidence and persistent failure, those paradoxically joined qualities endemic in American health care? As privileged members of our powerful nation, we enjoyed the satisfaction of US exceptionalism and technological superiority, only to feel the shock of pride inverted as we learned our country was not only unready for Covid but also uniquely weak in its response. Doctors who make fatal errors in the hospital can feel similar overconfidence. They, like the two of us, often enjoy meaningful work, rewarded by success, praise, and status, gaining a protective shell against criticism or darker realities. But we're in the autopsy room now, where the truth cannot be obscured. The Covid disaster is evident in statistics, through two years of high rates of infection and death, and also in devastating

23

social impacts, including a mental health epidemic and a breakdown of civic cohesion. Even two years after the pandemic started, with so much known about prevention, and with effective vaccines abundant, American hospitals have continued to be overwhelmed and forced to ration care.[1]

These markers of failure, like the broken pieces of a crashed airplane, expose the hubris that led to the downfall of American health care—relying on heroic healing rather than prevention and public health, ignoring racial and income inequalities that determine health, and elevating profit above more meaningful goals, a bias that yielded a brittle system and misallocated resources. These peculiarly American attributes contributed to catastrophe. Now disaster should open all of our eyes.

All that said, we also had another, better reason for misplaced optimism about the American response to the pandemic. American doctors and scientists had anticipated the pandemic and planned for it. Many people saw the danger coming and raised the alarm. Numerous health care leaders reacted appropriately and in time. Everything that science and medicine needed to know was known for a strong response that could have protected a substantial portion of those who died. When the virus arrived, Americans would mobilize unparalleled wealth, skill, and technology. Nurses and doctors would perform courageously, selflessly, and to the best of their ability. Why did we collectively fail? As in a classic dramatic tragedy, internal flaws brought down American health care, not external forces. A well-armed hero fell without ever raising his shield. Our goal is to understand the internal flaw that brought down the tragic hero of American medicine—the systemic faults that contributed to the national disaster and disgrace of eight hundred thousand dead, and counting.[2]

As we will see in the next chapter, American culture itself contributed to our vulnerability, and we need to understand that weakness as a critical element in how the health system failed. Embedded with those issues, in the chapter after the next, we consider our country's racial inequities and the social determinants of health, which constituted perhaps the deadliest systemic flaw in the Covid catastrophe. Following and connected to those concerns, we will then examine the disempowered American public health system, which was too weak to defend us. The health system comprises each of these elements.

We are investigating America's Covid failure in the model of an NTSB aviation accident probe, concentrating on the system, not the performance of individuals. As we explained in the previous chapter, these analytical tools allow an investigation to find systemic flaws—the kind of flaws that can cause bad outcomes regardless of who is in charge. Before going into the cultural, racial, and public health roots of the disaster, however, in this chapter we will also consider the leadership errors that contributed to the crash. To begin our investigation, we will inventory what was known to prevent the disaster—the pieces that leaders had in hand to respond effectively. And we will look at parts of the system that *did* work successfully. The remarkable foresight of some doctors created the opportunity for America to protect many of its citizens. Evaluating what they did right highlights the gaps and failures that led to an overall disaster and makes the astounding larger failure of leadership even more bitter. We already knew what we needed to know for a far more effective response that would have saved lives and left our country more intact today.

In this chapter, we consider what we knew and what our leaders did with that knowledge.

WHAT WE ALREADY KNEW

Another historic shock inspired contemporary pandemic planning in the United States—another event that knocked America off its pedestal. On September 11, 2001, America lost its sense of invulnerability as the world's lone superpower when terrorists attacked the World Trade Center and Pentagon with commercial airliners. We suddenly perceived our fragile global network of connections and constant movement. Within weeks, mail containing anthrax spores began arriving at news outlets and congressional offices, killing five people and widening 9/11 fears to include biological attack. The Bush administration responded with investments in biodefense, work that also included preparation for a naturally arising pandemic—a fresh concern in the early 2000s after the H1N5 Avian flu and the SARS viruses arose in Asia with scary outbreaks that fortunately failed to catch fire as global infections.

One Bush era project, funded by the Defense Threat Reduction Agency in the US Department of Defense, asked whether sequestering military units on a ship or otherwise isolated from the world would protect them from a potential widespread infection. It was a difficult question to answer, because the premise could only be tested in the midst of a pandemic. Many public health experts believed in the early 2000s that isolation and lockdowns would not work because they couldn't happen quickly or completely enough to stop a contagion, according to historian Alex Navarro, assistant director at the Center for the History of Medicine at the University of Michigan. None of the experts had lived through a truly catastrophic global pandemic, but what they believed about the last, worst worldwide infection—the 1918 pandemic—was not promising.

Today, as veterans of the Covid pandemic, most of us know something about the 1918 influenza pandemic, but around the time of 9/11 it was a niche historical topic, not often taught in medical school. The so-called Spanish flu outbreak got started in the last year of World War I, during the spring of 1918, with a highly contagious virus that at first killed few victims. In August of that year, the virus mutated into a form that caused a killer respiratory disease, including taking healthy, young people. Over the next two years, some fifty million people died globally, about ten times the reported Covid death toll (as of this writing), while 675,000 died of the flu in the United States—a number roughly similar to our Covid toll (although US population today is more than three times greater).[3]

Despite the passage of almost a century, medicine still had a lot to learn. In the 1990s, medical researchers sequenced the 1918 H1N1 virus in tissue samples recovered from a military repository and from corpses buried in permanently frozen ground in Alaska—from the Iñupiat village of Brevig Mission, where 85 percent of the adult population had died in five days in November 1918.[4] To answer the Defense Department's question, Navarro and other historians at Michigan read old newspapers and medical records from seven communities, including Princeton University and Bryn Mawr College, as well as Yerba Buena Island, California, and Gunnison, Colorado. People in each had sequestered themselves from the virus to some extent and used other non-pharmaceutical interventions (NPIs), such as social distancing and masking, which might have helped.

In 1918, as in 2020, NPIs were controversial and became politically divisive. President Woodrow Wilson prioritized the war effort.

Communities lent popular support to lockdowns early in the pandemic, when business owners thought they would only need to be closed for a few weeks, but opposition rose as time passed and the economic damage accumulated, Navarro said. Afterward, a scientific consensus developed that social distancing and the other NPIs had not worked, because they were widely used and yet many people died. A definitive retrospective book in 1926 reflected that point of view, with the authority of the American Medical Association.[5] Even during the 2000s work for the Defense Department, the Michigan scholars encountered skepticism. "Some very prominent epidemiologists basically said we're barking up the wrong tree, it's just stupid to close things down," Navarro said. "Unless you shut everything down, absolutely tight, and no one goes anywhere, it's not going to have any impact on a pandemic."[6]

The historians' 2006 report did not refute that belief. It didn't find evidence in the seven communities that general NPIs had done any good—including isolation, quarantine, social distancing, mask wearing, handwashing, and public information campaigns. "Despite these measures, most communities sustained significant illness and death; whether these NPIs lessened what might have been even higher rates had these measures not been in place is impossible to say," the report concluded. As to protective sequestration of troops, the scholars said it might work, if tried early and maintained strictly, but the report didn't give the idea a ringing endorsement.[7]

Fortunately, the research didn't stop there. A doctor in a central role challenged the contention that it was "impossible to say" whether NPIs had reduced death rates in 1918. He was Marty Cetron, director of global migration and quarantine for the Centers for Disease Control, who had been given the task by the Bush administration of writing a pandemic plan. In the 1990s, Cetron had worked to build sentinel networks to catch rising flu outbreaks as they approached, and he also worked with the scientists sampling the frozen bodies in Brevig Mission. Cetron had read about plagues through history and respected the written testimony of people who lived through them. He knew isolation and quarantine had been used for millennia—the Book of Leviticus provides detailed instructions for precautionary quarantine of potential lepers.[8] "Five thousand years of human experience played a huge role in these tools, which sometimes is all we had," Cetron said. "That's a lot of smart minds of history to be blatantly ignored."[9]

Cetron blames intellectual fashion for discounting isolation and lockdowns. Presumed truths can be passed down through generations of doctors, from older professors to young medical students, without being carefully examined. The evidence never supported the confident assertion that NPIs do not work. Cetron said three factors drive epidemics: pathogens, hosts, and the milieu (social environment). The rise of germ theory in the nineteenth century and discovery of viruses in the early twentieth century put the focus on pathogens. New understanding of immunology based on experience with chemotherapy side effects and HIV highlighted the importance of hosts' susceptibility. "That sort of denied the role of milieu in shaping the course of an epidemic," Cetron said. "I was never really willing to give that up, especially with the nature of the work that I've been doing, which is around populations, immigrants, refugees, migrant workers, the social determinants, disparities, the role of conflict in accelerating epidemics, malnutrition. I mean, there's just so many things that actually speak against that. And so, to me, I didn't buy that part."

Cetron called on leaders in the then-developing field of network modeling to update the conceptual understanding of how pandemics spread. And he turned to the University of Michigan historians to find quantitative evidence about how non-pharmaceutical interventions could slow an outbreak. That work would require finding two strands of long-forgotten information from the 1918 pandemic: the timing of interventions American cities tried, and the rates of death before, during, and after those restrictions. To find out what cities tried—such as school closures, cancellations of public gatherings, isolation, and quarantine—researchers read newspapers from each of the largest forty-three cities over twenty-four weeks from September 1918 to February 1919. The lockdowns were widely covered in the papers, of course, but the team chose three newspapers from each city to capture a span of political perspectives, accounting for any bias in the coverage. They also gathered official death records from each city to track daily changes in excess mortality during the period, showing how lockdowns and other interventions correlated with the rate of deaths.[10]

The results were unmistakable and profound. In city after city, death rates dropped when interventions took effect. And among cities, those that acted most decisively suffered the fewest deaths. The modeling buttressed the validity of these correlations, as did the fine-grained historical research. Cities learned from the experience of those hit first and successfully adjusted their own measures. Officials in St. Louis saw devastation in Philadelphia, acted in time, and suffered far fewer deaths. In cities where public health authorities commanded resources and authority, such as New York, they acted effectively and saved lives. NPIs worked. Cities acting early with layered interventions delayed the peak of excess mortality, lowered the peak, and had lower total morality during the pandemic.

Cetron and the Michigan historians published the findings, ending the debate about the effectiveness of lockdowns, and the CDC released the pandemic plan before Bush left office in 2007. In the process, Cetron coined the phrase "flattening the curve" to explain how lockdowns and social distancing could help public health officials manage a pandemic, giving society and the health system time to prepare and reducing the total number who would die through the entire event. He also borrowed the Swiss cheese analogy we introduced in chapter 1 to explain how layers of interventions could work, even if each layer was imperfect—with Swiss cheese holes—to form a combined, coordinated strategy to save lives in a pandemic. The document predicted a flu pandemic would create shortages of ICU beds and ventilators, and it showed how early action to adopt non-pharmaceutical interventions before an exponential rise of infections could prevent the worst of the surge and buy time for vaccine development.[11]

That work would change the course of history.

We interviewed Cetron in the spring of 2021, after a full year of pandemic death and disruptions—a disaster that had devastated the country despite his successful research on how to respond. We asked him how he felt having answered such an important public health question so definitively.

"I'm proud of it in retrospect. At the time, I was just blown away. But right now, in the middle of all of this, I just feel sad as to how ineffective I and others were," Cetron said. "As a country, we came up with this. Our documents on how to handle these things were translated into multiple languages. We had big programs in which we educated across the globe these tools, and exercised them. And many, many countries did so much better, by following the US playbook. And we did so poorly as a country in comparison. And yet we kind of knew what needed to be done. We just didn't have the gumption to get out there and communicate it, and sell it, and overcome the countermanding forces. And it's so sad."

RECOGNIZING THE COMING WAVE

Esther Nash, David's wife, who is also a physician, began losing sleep thinking about the consequences of a potential pandemic after the novel H1N1 swine flu emerged in the spring of 2009. Esther had gone to work in management because of her frustration as a clinician in a broken system. The medical market rewarded volume, but not positive outcomes. She wanted to help align incentives for doctors, patients, and payers with good health. That led her, eventually, into a place many physicians consider the belly of the beast: working as a physician executive at Independence Blue Cross, the dominant health plan in the Philadelphia area, which controlled 65 percent of the regional market. As director of population health and wellness, she set up programs to make plan members healthier, keeping them out of the medical system and reducing costs for the plan. Her group addressed chronic conditions such as diabetes and heart disease as well as prevention. The job was something like a high-level position in public health, except that the company's incentive for backing Esther's ideas was not necessarily health for its own sake—every program she oversaw needed solid evidence of real savings to the plan, with a positive bottom line on a detailed spreadsheet.

The news that kept her awake told of a new H1N1 influenza virus that especially affected young people and for which available vaccines were ineffective. Esther had read about Philadelphia in 1918 when the flu was spreading and authorities refused to cancel a Liberty Parade for World War I—the virus exploded exponentially, killing 17,500 people in the city, with mass graves and other horrors.[12] A new flu epidemic could overwhelm Philadelphia again and cripple the health system. Independence Blue Cross functioned mostly from a single skyscraper in downtown Philadelphia, with workers who reached their offices by public transit. A severe flu epidemic could halt the company's operations and its critical work in the region's health care. But no one seemed to be grappling with these issues or the many other hazards of a potential plague. In the uncoordinated health system of a major American city, Esther began to understand she might be in a special situation, with the resources, span of responsibilities, and motivation to respond.

At home, David pooh-poohed the whole thing. While Esther urgently brought in a supply of the scarce antiviral drug Tamiflu for the family—the three Nash children were still at home—David said she was overreacting. He reasoned that the world was vastly different than in 1918 (and, at the time, he hadn't studied that pandemic closely). Today, Esther charitably notes that David was bound to be a skeptic. He grew up as an optimist, living in a gilded ghetto on Long Island where he rarely encountered prejudice, with parents who constantly encouraged his ambitions—and with some amazing good luck (as we will learn in chapter 8). Esther's parents, by contrast, inculcated a cautious outlook and a habit of anticipating the worst. Her mother, a pioneering psychologist and feminist, always encouraged her, but she had never escaped the influence of severe poverty and deprivation from the Great Depression. Esther, as first in her class in medical school at Brown University, also learned to look for the worst as a diagnostician, always ruling out the most dire possibilities first.

"I'm reading the science and beginning to think about if this happens, and I begin losing sleep at night," Esther recalled. Hospitals could be overwhelmed without enough ICU beds or ventilators, and with no system in place to share the load through the region. "My head was spinning, and who was preparing?"[13]

Philadelphia had a public health department, but surrounding counties did not, and none of the government health agencies was adequately funded. Esther used her position with the largest health plan in the region to pull together a task force that included regional representatives, the hospital systems serving the area, the other health plans, and even medical ethicist Art Caplan. They inventoried hospital capacity and critical equipment such as ventilators and modeled what might be needed in a severe outbreak. They developed a regional sharing agreement to move ventilators and staff in case a particular facility or area became overwhelmed (although they didn't plan for what happened at the Covid peak, when every facility reached capacity over long periods, because they didn't consider that possibility). "We were operating with limited knowledge. We were scared," Esther said.

At the height of national concern over the shortage of Tamiflu, Esther tried to convince her health plan to buy and stockpile enough doses for all its millions of members. The drug was available. But she couldn't prove the benefit on a spreadsheet. Her superiors, skeptical of the need, said no. When the pandemic passed with far less impact than expected—in the United States, fewer died from the novel virus than are lost in a typical year of flu—Esther felt her political capital at the company diminished by a perception she had been a Chicken Little, falsely warning the sky was falling. David's point of view seemed to be vindicated, even though it had been informed by nothing other than his innate optimism. This time, expecting everything to turn out fine worked out well, but a closer look demonstrated worrying weaknesses in readiness to address a pandemic. Of course, Esther was relieved at the outcome, but she hadn't been wrong—instead, the city had been lucky. Neither hospitals nor underfunded public health agencies had brought together a coordinated, city-wide group to prepare for a severe pandemic threat. Instead, it had taken a sleepless health plan executive to make that happen. And then, after the threat retreated, the group dissolved.

In 2014, a frightening virus again tested US health care, when a Liberian man visiting family in Texas came into a Dallas emergency room with Ebola. Bruce Meyer and other doctor executives helped lead the response in the twenty-four-hospital Texas Health System, which included Texas Presbyterian Dallas, where the Ebola patient had arrived. After two nurses came down with Ebola virus, caught from the original patient, the crisis exploded into political and public hysteria. (The original patient died, but the nurses survived.) The Obama administration dispatched a full-court press of agencies to Texas—even the FBI—but Republican politicians attacked, saying it wasn't enough. In Dallas, Meyer and his colleagues couldn't get support they needed from state and local elected officials and ended up working with a county judge for public health authority. Meanwhile, calls flooded in from people afraid they had Ebola, even if their only symptom was a low-grade fever.

Ebola is highly infectious through blood or bodily fluids, and deadly, killing half those who are infected.[14] Among the measures the team took, Meyer recalled setting up training and refreshers for donning protective suits in the hospital and for EMTs, who might not have used the gear in years. A member of the team invented a way to test a suit's seal around the body with food dye and pepper spray—if dye made it through, you could see it, and you could feel the pepper spray. He wanted the gear worn widely in the system's hospitals to protect employees who might encounter the virus and to prevent its spread. But management balked, limiting protective equipment to certain hospitals and units. That decision left staff without protective equipment feeling betrayed.

"There was full panic mode at the institutional level that no one would ever come back to the emergency room at Presby Dallas," Meyer recalled. "So, what that did was disrupt your relationship with the staff. People felt like the institution wasn't making decisions in their best interest. . . . I left four years afterward, and I would say that relationship had still not recovered at that hospital."[15]

In 2018, Meyer became the president of Jefferson Health, the fourteen-hospital system at Thomas Jefferson University in Philadelphia, where David has spent his career. He brought his Ebola experience. Many of the features of that crisis would be repeated during the Covid pandemic in the United States, including confusing, contradictory health messaging influenced by political opportunism, as well as disjointed responses among government and health care organizations. But Meyer planned to get his part right as the head of a large health system. He said he had learned three lessons: plan ahead for a worst-case scenario, be early and courageous with decisions, and, at the top of his list, protect the staff.

Jefferson did many things right. It's an example of using what we already knew. The health system had a pandemic plan. In addition, during a disaster exercise two years earlier, executives imagined what would happen if a deadly plague were released at a Philadelphia Eagles football game. They realized that with so many sick and contagious patients, every hospital would need personal protective equipment for every doctor, nurse, and support person—so the company bought and stockpiled a one-month supply of PPE for all 34,000 employees. In addition, Jefferson structured the executive team to allow bad news to get to the top quickly. In January 2020, the head of infection control, Kelly Zabriskie, brought concern about the new virus in China to Jonathan Gleason, then the chief quality and safety officer, who reported directly to the president, Meyer. In many organizations, the safety position sits layers lower in the organizational chart, and those messages can get lost. Gleason and Meyer are both physicians, so they understood the threat. In addition, John Zurlo, the physician chief of infectious disease, studied the outbreak and correctly predicted its course. Zurlo, who trained with Anthony Fauci, told Meyer that containing the novel coronavirus in China was unlikely and Jefferson should prepare.

Top health system leaders began weekly meetings, and, on January 23, Meyer sent a memo to everyone in the organization alerting them to the coming crisis. The first case had been identified in the United States only two days earlier, in a man in Washington who had returned from Wuhan, China, and the CDC was still expressing uncertainty about the ability of the virus to spread between people.[16] The WHO wouldn't give Covid-19 its name for three more weeks.[17] Meyer's message that day, and with every other email for the next year, asserted Jefferson's top priority in the crisis: staff safety.

The response was costly and speculative. The money might have been wasted. Meyer said it helped that Jefferson Health is a nonprofit organization. He could spend money on something that might not happen without answering to stockholders. "Our values are putting people first, doing the right thing and being bold and thinking differently," he said. "And what we talked about internally on the health system side was we're going to put our people first. Protect your staff. If you don't have care providers, you can't provide care. And if you can't provide care, people are going to suffer."

The system also prepared by cross-training six hundred nurses into ICU positions. Primary care nurses were teamed with acute care hospital nurses to support them and bolster their numbers in dealing with difficult Covid patients. Some hospitals in the system were designated for Covid and others to remain free of Covid. When patients with Covid showed up at emergency rooms, the system would adjust, transferring them to a hospital with capacity or transferring respiratory therapists or critical care physicians. All this action was transparent to everyone. Employees could access a dashboard from any computer in the system displaying all the current stats about beds, supplies of PPE, Covid volumes, and deaths.

Experts at Jefferson had authority to go beyond CDC guidelines in protecting against the virus. The leadership ordered every employee to wear a mask in early March 2020, well before that became a national recommendation, including having workers don masks on public transit on the way to work when no one else was wearing them. Everyone who could work from home did so before lockdowns were ordered. Consequently, Meyer said Jefferson maintained an infection rate among staff below 1 percent. The quality of care never slipped.

We learned in Philadelphia that using the knowledge we already had and prioritizing health in a systemic way could get us through, at least within an organization. Despite the best preparations, however, the tragedy and pain of the pandemic year remain—at Jefferson and all other health care organizations—as it always will, for caregivers who went through the most traumatic and difficult moments of their lives on the front lines.

THE WAVE HITS

One day in late March 2020, Rachel Nash texted to family, including her parents, David and Esther: "There's no way I'm not getting this." Rachel had arrived at work at Cooper University Hospital in Camden, New Jersey, amid the first spike of Covid cases and found no one wearing masks except where they were in direct contact with Covid-diagnosed patients. In a doctors' work room, she sat with ten physicians in close quarters, without barriers, none of them masked. After mask use increased, the early shortage of PPE hit, and for a few days Rachel had to reuse masks and don a reusable poncho instead of a gown. But soon masks and gowns were available, and she felt the hospital pulled together well. Management kept everyone informed. When David and Esther pushed hard for her to leave and avoid the disease, she said no.

"This is my job. I took an oath. This is what I signed up to do," Rachel said later. "Never in a million years would I say I didn't sign up for this or I'm not going to do this. That thought didn't cross my mind. To me, it's a duty. And I'm lucky enough that I was in a hospital that felt the need to protect me and us."[18]

Rachel followed in her parents' footsteps with her love of studying health and choice of internal medicine. As a hospitalist, she sees only adults sick enough to need acute care, and only during the time they are in the hospital. The job allows her to spend half her time teaching resident physicians. In the low-income communities that Cooper serves in Camden, Rachel often feels she cannot make a definitive change in her patients' lives, because factors outside the hospital—called social determinants of health—overwhelm what medicine can accomplish. In the hospital she can stabilize a patient with diabetes, for example, but that doesn't do much good if they go home and cannot afford insulin. Teaching, however, gives her more fulfillment, as she trains doctors as part of a large, collaborative team. She enjoys the bustle and energy of the work.

With Covid, an eerie quiet fell over the large, teaching hospital. As program director for internal medicine residency, Rachel was accustomed to having half a dozen medical students, residents, and interns accompany her on rounds. Family members or other advocates would be in the rooms, and she would rely on them for important information about her critically ill patients. Nurses would come in every hour at least. Now the hospital was mostly empty except for Covid patients. Safety protocols even kept nurses out of rooms unless necessary. Rachel would talk to specialists and other doctors, but she alone would examine the patients. Often, in these lonely rooms, she encountered stark terror, as victims of Covid lay in bed alone, contemplating death. Even as they gasped for breath, they frequently also feared that if they were sedated for intubation, they would never wake up. At that point in the pandemic, CDC data shows, 23 percent of hospitalized patients were dying.[19]

Rachel's first Covid patient was an adorable little old lady in her nineties who had fallen. Her Covid test was positive, but she had no symptoms. She was isolated, confused, and afraid. She couldn't receive a needed MRI because of concerns that she would contaminate the equipment with the virus. As Rachel examined her, the woman cried, because she didn't understand why she was all alone. Covid or no Covid, Rachel couldn't help giving her a hug. Another early patient she recalled was an African American staff member from a nursing home who was obese and had a serious case of Covid. Half of her nursing home patients were already in the hospital, and now she had followed them—and Rachel had to send her to the ICU (early in the pandemic, 60 percent of ICU patients died).[20] Rachel prepared another patient for discharge who had survived thirty-two days in the hospital. The wife of a doctor, the patient had been saved by an extraordinary and costly procedure to remove her blood and oxygenate it artificially, called extracorporeal membrane oxygenation—a technological miracle. But with many other patients at discharge, she had difficult conversations about sending them home to quarters that were too small to isolate from other family members they might infect.

The hospital provided daily podcasts on what was happening, and specialists outside the wards gave guidance on treating patients and new ideas on how to manage the disease. But Rachel often felt helpless as she watched Covid take its course with so little she could do to help.

"It was extremely hard," she said. "You're just throwing random stuff at them. Random. It felt like random treatments to use something one week and then to find out the next week that you actually might have caused harm—it is very disturbing, because we're taught evidence-based medicine. And this is sort of the opposite of that."

At first, Rachel was coming home to her boyfriend, Neil Makhija, at their townhouse in South Philadelphia, but it seemed impossible to keep him from getting infected if she caught the virus, so he left to live in his parents' basement on the north side of the state. The separation lasted a few months. Neil and Rachel's relationship flourished via FaceTime and Zoom, and, remarkably, she never got infected with Covid. She also got through the January 2021 surge of Covid, which was even worse than the peak in the spring, Rachel said, partly because the hospital was full of other patients as well. The couple planned their wedding for the fall of 2021, but a surge of infections from the delta variant of Covid forced a postponement. By the time you read this, we hope they will have been married.

We know Rachel's story best, because she is a family member. But more than thirty-six hundred health care workers in the United States died of Covid in the first year of the pandemic, according to an investigation by Kaiser Health News and the *Guardian* (the government did not track the number).[21] They contracted the disease at three times the rate of the general public, and in many cases their infections were directly traced to the shortage or denial of masks and other personal protective equipment.[22] For many of those who survived, scars remain. They carry the psychological trauma of having helplessly ushered innumerable Covid patients toward death.

So much of this tragedy could have been avoided. Better planning and leadership could have protected many of the health care workers who lost their lives by providing protective equipment and, more fundamentally, by preventing infections in the community that they had to treat. Deborah Birx, White House pandemic coordinator under

President Trump, later said most of America's deaths after the first one hundred thousand in the spring surge could have been avoided by a more robust response.[23] With over eight hundred thousand dead, that estimate suggests the administration was responsible for more than three hundred fifty thousand excess lives lost. The real number cannot be known, and it will long be debated. But we cannot proceed to our systemic investigation of America's Covid failure without looking at the malfeasance of the one man most directly responsible for so much suffering and death: President Donald Trump.

LEADERSHIP

The enormity of the pandemic year was only beginning to dawn, in mid-March 2020, when NYU sociologist Eric Klinenberg noted that America stood at a turning point.[24] Klinenberg had made his name studying another public health crisis, a 1995 heat wave in Chicago that killed more than seven hundred people, who were mostly older, poor, and Black—all avoidable deaths in a city with plenty of air conditioning and cold water. All that had been needed then was for neighbors to reach out. But that didn't happen, largely because Chicago's mayor denied the existence of the crisis for self-serving political reasons, weakening the response and dividing the community at a critical moment.[25]

As the pandemic spread, with its unequal effects on poor, urban people, NPR's Ailsa Chang asked Klinenberg whether Americans could pull together this time.

"In various cities we have been witnessing people hoarding food, hoarding medical supplies, toilet paper, basically acting for themselves and not for the greater good," Chang said. "Is there something that you, as a sociologist, can put your finger on that makes people flip a switch and act selfishly rather than come together and think of the greater good?"

Klinenberg responded, "When you don't believe that the government is telling you the truth, when you don't believe that there's a public and shared system that will provide you the care and support that you need, the message becomes, take care of yourself. Protect yourself and your family because that's the only way you're going to get through it. . . . And so this is a testing moment, because we are at a switching point in history, and we are going to figure out how many people live and die in this crisis, how much economic damage there is, what kind of world we rebuild when this ends. . . . If we can muster up that better part of ourselves, we have a chance to turn it around and to build something incredible when this is over. But if we can't, I fear that this event will be much more deadly than it needs to be."[26]

President Trump was already leading toward denial, division, and self-interest, as he looked to the fall election and sought to maintain the allegiance of his base of voters. As Bob Woodward substantiated with Trump's own words, he knew the severity of the crisis by January 28, 2020, but lied to minimize it and shunt off responsibility. He made no effort to prepare the country or develop a strategy to protect the public.[27] Unlike leaders at Jefferson Health, the president did not warn stakeholders, develop a stockpile of protective equipment, or mobilize and cross-train workers—on the contrary, he discouraged awareness and preparation and silenced those in the federal government who tried to raise the alarm. When governors and public health authorities called for lockdowns and mask wearing, Trump made them into adversaries, ginning up hostility to the mandates and issuing calls to "liberate" states under pandemic orders.

The shortage of personal protective equipment early in the pandemic is among the most vivid of Trump's failures. As the virus approached, the administration ignored calls to increase production of masks or to halt their export. The national stockpile of PPE was inadequate and out of date, never having been replenished after the H1N1 flu pandemic, and it quickly ran out. Facing a catastrophic shortage, Trump told governors they were on their own, unleashing a mad free-for-all among states and hospitals, who desperately bid up prices of PPE and, with lives in the balance, grabbed for supplies any way they could. Governors deployed state troopers and National Guard units to defend truckloads of masks. A VA hospital near Washington, DC, salvaged old masks from a dumpster and had security officers protect them. After Trump assigned his son-in-law, Jared Kushner, to address the problem, his chaotic new effort sent PPE around the country without tracking, allowing private companies to control the flow to favor their own clients. Officials could not determine where equipment was located or how to get it to facilities with the greatest needs. The situation persisted for months, into the early summer.[28] And this was only one set of examples from the Trump administration's senseless waste of lives.

By October, even the steadfastly apolitical *New England Journal of Medicine* could not remain silent about the historic, tragic incompetence, and it published the first political editorial in its 208-year history, signed by each member of the editorial staff. Editors said they had a moral imperative to speak up in the face of the Trump administration's attacks on science and promotion of misinformation.[29]

> This crisis has produced a test of leadership. With no good options to combat a novel pathogen, countries were forced to make hard choices about how to respond. Here in the United States, our leaders have failed that test. They have taken a crisis and turned it into a tragedy. The magnitude of this failure is astonishing.[30]

The editorial went on to provide a concise inventory of the failures and their consequences—without mentioning Trump, which was unnecessary—including the terrible toll on communities of color, which surely contributed to a national convulsion of protests and violence during the summer of 2020. Early in the pandemic, America performed uniquely badly in responding to Covid, while waiting for vaccines, with unparalleled health care capacity and a woeful harvest of death. And after the United States produced vaccine surpluses, its death rates remained high, largely due to infections among people who refused to get the shot, who often were Trump followers influenced by his hostility to public health and science messages.[31] By April 2021, per capita deaths in the United States were 4.5 times higher than the global average.[32] Trump was the one person most to blame.

These are painful memories and it is tempting to put them away, but Trump remains a force in the Republican Party and his Covid denialism remains deeply entrenched among his many followers. He campaigned for reelection at mask-less rallies and falsely claimed he had won the vote. By late November 2020, many of his followers had split into an alternate reality, committed to counterfactual beliefs generated by Trump and his media engine. Nurses in "red" states told of patients who denied the existence of Covid with their dying breaths. In that upside-down world, Trump followers saw mask wearing and public health interventions as part of a malign plot and health care heroes as villains.[33] This mass delusion remains a serious threat. Scientists, doctors, and journalists must vigilantly fight for truth, not throw up our hands.

But in our investigation, we also need to separate the aberration of Trump's leadership from the systemic failures that he did not create. The editors of the *New England Journal* pointed only to leadership. We find many deeper, structural causes of America's Covid failure. We should not allow Trump's wrongdoing to eclipse our view of these problems or to protect from accountability others who caused harm.

Evidence suggests, for example, that the initial surge of Covid in the United States, in the spring of 2020, could have been blunted by earlier testing for the virus, but the country lagged far behind the world in deploying tests. This shocking failure cannot be blamed directly on the president. (We will discuss in chapter 3 how a major investment in testing could also have reshaped the pandemic experience through 2020.) One can easily imagine a scenario in which the United States would have fielded a test as early as countries such as Thailand and South Korea, gained awareness of a virus that we now know was circulating in American cities as early as December 2019,[34] and enacted public health measures to limit the spread before wide-scale community transmission produced exponential growth of infections.

The World Health Organization published instructions for producing a working Covid test on January 13, 2020. Countries that were successful in preventing outbreaks immediately adopted that test and developed their own to supplement it, finding cases right away, tracing their contacts, and isolating exposed people. Thailand, with CDC-trained scientists, was a stand-out success with this strategy and stamped out Covid completely for much of 2020.[35]

But in the United States, the CDC decided to design its own, more complex test that would also check for antibodies to coronaviruses from animals and from past outbreaks that had passed, reasoning it might be better at detecting variants. The story was well documented by the *Washington Post*'s investigative reporting.[36] The new test was difficult to create and to manufacture, and the CDC produced contaminated test kits that did not work when they were distributed to state labs. A state lab in New York reported that the test found copious amounts of virus in distilled water (a federal inspector later found that substandard lab practices at the CDC had likely contaminated the kits).

Meanwhile, labs around the country prepared their own tests but were not allowed to use them by the Food and Drug Administration, which put up various bureaucratic barriers to emergency approval. A University of Washington lab spent one hundred hours filling out FDA paperwork for approval only to have its emailed forms rejected by the agency with instructions to instead send them through the US Postal Service. Scores of scientists wrote to Congress on February 28, saying no lab had succeeded in getting through the FDA process.[37] In New York, the huge Northwell Health system and a state lab were ready with a test and the capacity to use it widely for weeks before they could get approval, Northwell president Mike Dowling told us. He said those missed weeks could have allowed New Yorkers to see the problem developing and begin protective measures earlier. Dowling asked Governor Andrew Cuomo to intervene with the White House. Only after the political explosion did the CDC and FDA relent and allow testing to proceed. By then, in early March, forty-six days after the WHO test became available, the virus was already widespread in parts of the United States, the possibility of containment was long gone, and the death of many thousands of people was all but assured.

How could the CDC, the world's preeminent public health agency, have made such a deadly and historic blunder? The *Post* established that the blame did not belong to Trump (at least directly). CDC director Robert Redfield consistently downplayed testing problems to White House officials and repeatedly told them the test was almost ready. Likewise, awareness of the barriers at the FDA did not make it to the top until political pressure came from the outside, and then the administration immediately broke the logjam. (Certainly, however, better leaders would have inquired on their own and forced a solution sooner.) The *Post* blamed the problem, instead, on hubris. We agree. The CDC was too famous, too important, too far above other laboratories—it prioritized a technically better test with its own imprint over adequate tests made by others that could have been deployed quickly and easily. Other nations didn't make that mistake, and they suffered far fewer infections and deaths in the early pandemic.

In the previous chapter, we discussed the concept of the authority gradient. Power, expertise, and elite status can become a trap. Recall the example of the surgeon who is about to operate on the wrong body part. A nurse sees the mistake but says nothing, because the institution in which they work has put the doctor so far above the nurse that speaking up is too daunting. The doctor contributes to the problem, too, with haughtiness and a sense of superiority that blinds him or her to other perspectives. That's a trap, because no matter how excellent an individual is at a task, a qualified team of collaborators is always better at catching mistakes. The situation concerning the CDC test is analogous. Even if the CDC had succeeded in producing its superior test in a timely way, the country would still have been better off if every reasonably accurate test had been put to use as quickly as possible.

The result was terrible, but for systemic improvement, this finding actually is good news, because it suggests an avenue to make positive change. We can't prevent bad leaders from being elected. That will happen again. But we can address a systemic problem to improve health care. The authority gradient between the CDC and other public health agencies and state laboratories exists as a part of our culture, and culture can be changed. We will look at public health in coming chapters. Strengthening public health agencies and broadening their activities would be among the most important steps to improving Americans' health in general. In addition, for responding to the next disease outbreak, we should connect public health into a collaborative national system capable of responding to an emergency with all material and intellectual resources mobilized, listened to, and empowered by the national agency.

This change is already happening. The Covid pandemic washed over the landscape of health care and moved around familiar landmarks. The testing fiasco, and other mistakes, knocked the CDC off a pedestal. No one involved will soon forget these lessons.

TOWARD A JUST CULTURE

We began this chapter looking at the knowledge American institutions acquired through research that would have allowed us to prepare for the pandemic and respond to it effectively (and that did help some other nations). We also profiled those who saw what was coming and who did everything they should have done. Unfortunately, their successes were notable in contrast to the disastrous broader response—nationally, but also within regions that failed to work effectively together. Americans lacked the tools for a strong, coordinated Covid fight because of our health inequities, weak public health organizations, and fragmented providers—all topics for the chapters ahead. Failures of leadership made those problems worse. Political divisions and false beliefs ripped apart Americans' common resolve and, when vaccines became available, undercut our most powerful weapon, as many people refused to take the shots that would protect them and end the pandemic.

In chapter 1, we introduced the concept of just culture as the basis for a high-quality health care system. Within a group of doctors and nurses working with a patient, a just culture means treating team members with the respect that will allow each to voice concerns and contribute their best. We've suggested that the nation's health care system—in all its diverse parts—also must develop a just culture in order to better care for its citizens. For example, the CDC's disastrous decisions on testing look like an example of the authority gradient, something David might see in an investigation of an error by a doctor. Of course, the CDC is an institution, not an individual, and its failure involves many people whose exact actions and motivations we cannot know, but we think the comparison works and uncovers a valuable systemic truth.

We have tried to make the complex Covid story manageable with such metaphors and stories. Our central idea is to take the broken pieces of this crashed airliner and find out what went wrong. We are looking for the systemic flaws that brought down the plane—not only its improperly designed machinery but also the practices of the designers and the economic incentives that influenced those design practices. Using that framework for the pandemic, we intend to take apart the health system (which includes health care, the social structures that determine our health, and the culture that establishes our social structures) as an investigation into the fatal flaws that the crisis exposed.

As a starting point in that analysis, we know that the one nation with the most expensive and technically advanced health system on earth—the United States—fared among the worst in protecting citizens from the disease. Enough was previously known to greatly reduce that impact. The United States developed the technical skills and public health playbook for early testing and non-pharmaceutical interventions, but it did not effectively use those strategies. Some institutions responded effectively and saved lives, including Jefferson Health, with planning and preparation, early reaction, and priority on staff safety—actions that many more institutions and governments in the United States failed to take.

If we had the tools and knew how to use them, what aspect of our culture prevented that? In the next chapter, we will explore America's unique cultural fabric, with its weave of unhealthy practices and attitudes. We will ask what cultural flaws make Americans' health outcomes mediocre while our spending on health care is astronomical. This kind of examination is a central part of population health, which recognizes that what happens outside hospital doors is most important to staying well and that intervening in health upstream of the doctor's office reduces suffering, cost, and death.

Covid is a vivid example. By the time ambulances queued at hospital entrances, many Covid patients were already doomed. We must travel backward to the points where different actions could have changed those outcomes, finding the deeper causes that contributed to these deaths and that could be addressed to make Americans healthier and more fulfilled in the future.

Chapter 3

American Culture Makes
Us Vulnerable

Everyone has a Covid lockdown story, but we're not telling them much anymore. As weird and upsetting as many of these tales are, they won't regain the sense of novelty needed for good storytelling until another generation grows up whose members don't remember those difficult months as their own experience. We are no different. The many months of disruption and disconnection passed with a peculiar timeless quality, a claustrophobic purgatory of strange experiences—empty city streets and airports, two-dimensional online relationships and rituals—and with loss. We personally were lucky, but there was suffering for everyone. And then, when things began opening up again, and we once again dined in restaurants and returned to offices, that more intense Covid period took on a dreamlike quality. Did that really happen?

One of the oddest aspects of living near the sequestered urban centers of the eastern United States was hearing what was happening elsewhere. In areas of the US South and West, some governors and many individuals refused to wear masks or take the same precautions as in our region, and later had more vaccine refusal, and elevated infection rates and deaths followed in those areas.[1] In a few other countries, the populace followed the rules during strict, short initial lockdowns, and they then emerged to live normal lives, having defeated a disease that still raged in the United States. In November 2020, a commentator in the *New York Times* related how idyllic life remained in the Covid-free Atlantic provinces of Canada while so close at hand, on our side of the border, nothing was normal and the dying continued.[2] Why did these enormous differences develop, and what could we learn from them to fingerprint the systemic flaws that led to so many Americans being lost to Covid?

China mounted an extraordinary fight against the virus after initial attempts to cover up the outbreak in Wuhan. The all-powerful government mobilized enormous resources and controlled the private behavior of its citizens, an ability that both impressed and disturbed us as we followed it in the media. By January 2021, when the United States was in the depths of its worst Covid wave, China had already turned a hastily built hospital in Wuhan into a museum about a disease that was now in the past. In one gallery, visitors could leave virtual flowers for Li Wenliang, the ophthalmologist who first exposed the state's cover-up of the infection on social media, was punished by police, and then died of Covid, only to have his name rehabilitated by the government and be declared a martyr. The exhibit did not mention that he had been punished.[3] Surely there is a way to block an infection—solving this age-old collective action problem—without creating an Orwellian society that manipulates and subjugates its people.

New Zealand succeeded as a democracy, with an early, tight lockdown and an effective travel policy, which essentially walled out the virus, and only forty-seven total Covid deaths in two years (still a higher per capita death rate than in huge China).[4] But New Zealand is an island nation of less than five million, around the size of Wisconsin. Not only small nations did well, however. Australia, also a democracy, succeeded early with unified political messaging, strict public health and travel measures, and respect for the rights and special health needs of its indigenous people.[5] It is also an island nation, but its population would put it near the second largest US state, Texas, which had about seventy-five thousand Covid deaths compared to Australia's twenty-one hundred. And to eliminate the distinction about islands, we can look at Finland and Norway, which have about eleven million citizens between them (equivalent to a top-ten US state), are continental and western, and had about twenty-five hundred total Covid deaths, a rate about a tenth of the United States, per capita—and yet Finland and Norway were able to reopen their economies after an initial, strict lockdown.[6]

American exceptionalism helps us reject these comparisons. We're like an out-of-shape athlete or a back-row student, coming up with any number of reasons for exceptionally poor performance, when the scale of the failure is so profound as to put the lie to any of these excuses.

We cannot blame our size, geography, or form of government, although these may have contributed to the larger systemic failure. We suffered the many losses of the pandemic—worst of all, the deaths—through successive preventable waves. Before the wave in spring 2020, we lacked testing surveillance and pandemic preparation; before the wave that summer, we came out of public health measures prematurely; and before the mountainous winter wave, we traveled to holiday gatherings and persisted, Covid-weary, with indoor activities. As we saw in the previous chapter, research on the 1918 influenza pandemic had given Americans the tools needed to prevent many of our deaths even before the advent of vaccinations or therapies—masking, closure of bars and restaurants and similar unmasked places, testing, contact tracing, and isolation. Other countries, using the knowledge developed in our country, fared much better by anticipating and preparing, imposing strict public health measures to control the spread, and then maintaining control through testing, contract tracing, and travel policies. Within larger countries, travel limitations between subnational units also helped, as among the provinces of Australia and China.

Only in the spring of 2021, with vaccinations, did Covid markedly improve in the United States. The American capitalist system had excelled at what it does best: with a strong profit motive, and with financial risk mitigated by the federal government's Operation Warp Speed, pharmaceutical companies created several astonishingly effective vaccines with unprecedented rapidity. Despite the slow and chaotic distribution of the vaccines—again, a failure of government—immunity increased to break the pandemic in areas of the United States with high vaccine uptake by the early summer of 2021, allowing normal life to return. But then, as we will explore later in this chapter, the pandemic returned with a vengeance as the more transmissible delta variant spread in the politically "red" states, widely infecting people who declined to take the vaccine.[7] Again, infections overwhelmed hospitals. Vaccination also lagged in poorer nations without adequate vaccine doses or in those countries with less effective vaccine strategies. For example, Europe had invested in a single vaccine candidate, from AstraZeneca, which ran into problems, while the United States bet on many horses and had several successes along with failures. That difference neatly reflected the difference between European-style, government-managed health care, characterized by a unitary approach, slow innovation, and controlled cost, compared to free-market American health care, with many competitors, rapid innovation, and high cost.

With our advantage in innovation, we won the vaccine race, but by then too many Americans had died unnecessarily. The outcome fit a familiar pattern. So often, Americans neglect relatively inexpensive preventive and lifestyle interventions, instead requiring heroic hospital measures and, at last, the high-tech miracle of cutting-edge science that finally saves the day. Our Covid experience was analogous. We were weak on testing and prevention. We filled our hospitals, requiring heroism from our health care providers. At the end, incredible breakthroughs in vaccines promised to save us, and they did allow those who took the shot to return mostly to normal life with reasonable risk. But the crisis continued, as increasingly infectious variants swept through the unvaccinated population.

The systemic analysis of this unhealthy pattern takes up the first half of the book. There are several contributing factors. In chapter 5, we will discuss how our country neglects public health in favor of medicine, to the detriment of our wellness and our finances. As we will see, economics goes a long way to explain that flaw in the system, as huge profits flow to organizations providing care and drugs, but public health and prevention are seen only as costs. But our investigation in this chapter will look at another level, below economics, to the roots of our behavior—the "why" behind our choice of this kind of system in the first place.

More factors than economics are at play. Consider the economic incentives of a typical patient seeing a health care provider with warning signs for future heart problems. Most doctors have counseled such patients about the necessity for diet and exercise, which are proven to help avoid cardiac issues with little cost. The prototypical American patient, we know, ignores that advice and ultimately needs expensive surgeries or dies prematurely. For the patient, every economic incentive is on the side of prevention. But away from the doctor's scolding advice, cultural norms for overconsumption and inactivity hold more sway, profit-making companies push temptations, and economic disparities can make healthy foods and gyms unavailable to marginalized groups.

President Trump played his part in this repetitive drama of denial and rescue with his own course of Covid, in October 2020. His age, obesity, and sedentary lifestyle put him at high risk. He refused to take precautions to avoid infection, became severely ill, and received world-class, experimental hospital treatment. Afterward, he emerged as if a victorious hero, unrepentant and still disrespectful of basic prevention. Collectively, we Americans have behaved similarly. We are, on average, obese and sedentary. Our society received the necessary advice to avoid infection, but we followed it inconsistently. By late 2021, approximately half of the US population had been infected.[8] Our scientists intervened with expensive, innovative medicine to save us— but only after we paid a terrible price in lives, as well as economically.

Now let's look in the mirror and ask why we continue to behave this way. To build a better health system, we first must understand the cultural footing under its foundations.

UNDERSTANDING AMERICAN CULTURE

In the United States, your chances of dying from Covid depended in part on the political party of the governor of your state. Public health researchers at the Medical University of South Carolina and Johns Hopkins University looked at the correlation of Covid statistics, including deaths, with the party affiliation of the governor of each state (each party had half the governorships at the time). At first, Democratic states had more cases and deaths, likely reflecting the initial arrival of Covid in Democratic New York, New Jersey, Washington, and California. But on June 4, 2020, Republican-led states overtook Democratic states in rates of infection, and on July 4, 2020, death rates grew worse in Republican states, and the numbers stayed worse into December 2020, when the study ended. To clarify that this difference in death rates related to the party of the governor and not some other factor, researchers made statistical adjustments to account for population density, rural versus urban life, demographics, socioeconomics, number of physicians, obesity, cardiovascular disease, asthma, smoking, and presidential voting in 2020.[9]

Apparently, Republican governors were more lethal because their public health policies were weaker. A group at Binghamton University made this link by compiling a Public Health Protective Policy Index that captured fifteen policy categories—such as travel limitations, bans on public gatherings, and restaurant shutdowns—and scored each policy based on how restrictive it was (for example, scores would reflect whether restaurants were fully closed, could offer take-out, outdoor dining, limited indoor dining, and so on). The work captured in real time the kind of information Marty Cetron's team had used to study the 1918 pandemic, and the result was similar. The index showed Republican governors' policies were 10 percent less restrictive, as a whole, and modeling suggested that would account for 7 percent higher Covid case rates in their states.[10]

The social scientist who led that work, Olga Shvetsova, director of Binghamton's Covid-19 Policy Response Lab, used a political lens to understand the relative failure of Republican governors to protect their people. "They want everybody to be healthy, but they prefer somebody else makes unpopular policies," she said.[11] In part, the Republican governors had already rejected responsibility for health as part of their role in governance. Many of these Republican states had previously blocked provisions of the Affordable Care Act within their borders, refusing to expand Medicaid or create state insurance marketplaces. Shvetsova believes President Trump affected the response, too. After initially downplaying the severity of the virus, he tried to save face by discouraging testing, denigrating public health officials, and attacking protective measures. That messaging gave cover to Republican governors who wanted to avoid actions that would impose economic hardship.

The federalism of the American system allowed Trump to pass responsibility to the states and, to some extent, allowed governors to pass it down to local governments or to say public health measures were strictly matters of individual choice. We have already noted, in the previous chapter, how Trump's direction to states to obtain their own equipment and supplies created a chaotic and self-destructive scramble that could have been avoided by having a central, national process. The same lack of national planning and coordination undermined vaccine distribution, which could have been managed with a single, transparent set of rules, priorities, and processes (Google had built a national appointment system, but it could not be used because nearly every state created a different vaccine priority hierarchy).[12] A crazy quilt of local systems arose that favored those with technology skills or personal connections and allowed state and federal officials to shift blame back and forth for failures.[13] The fifty state travel policies and public health rules also probably created confusion and mistrust.

However, the layered governmental structure of federalism did allow states and local governments with competent leaders to protect their own citizens in ways that the failed national leadership did not. Trump would not impose mask mandates, but many governors and mayors did. Similar patterns can be seen in the health care system before the pandemic, both good and bad. Fractured authority has made it difficult to bring change nationally, but states that want to innovate independently have been able to move ahead (Massachusetts and Maryland, for example).

Rather than get too wrapped up in politics and governmental arrangements, however, let's look to a deeper difference among the states that may have mattered more than politics. Note that the South Carolina–Johns Hopkins study of Covid death rates adjusted for Trump's support and still found worse results in those states led by Republican governors. And Republicanism itself wasn't always a predictor, as some states with Republican governors invoked strong public health rules, including Maryland, Massachusetts, and Vermont. Each of those three states had something else in common—an eastern US cultural outlook. Vaccination rates followed the same pattern. By September 2021, only 60 percent of White Evangelicals or rural Americans had received vaccinations, compared to 82 percent of college graduates and 77 percent of urban residents (Democrats were 90 percent vaccinated and Republicans 58 percent).[14] Those numbers overlaid geographically with where the virus continued to spread. Could cultural differences among the regions of our huge, diverse nation, rather than politics, have affected the ability of states to respond to Covid?

Cultural differences within a state did seem to make a difference. Charles spent time in Alaska in 2020 and 2021, a state with a Republican governor and a strong Trump vote, but also a historical memory of the 1918 pandemic (which was particularly deadly there), as well as distinct cultural groups with their own values. Covid restrictions varied in different parts of the state, which is immense in area but has a small population, and the overall death rate remained low through 2020. Some deeply communitarian Alaska Native villages, governed by tribal elders, kept Covid cases to zero and had almost everyone vaccinated early. Meanwhile, in extremely libertarian White communities, with proud frontier attitudes of self-reliance, masks were rare and vaccine rates stalled at low levels, with Covid outbreaks continuing.[15]

These cultural differences were evident even within a single Alaska town, from an auto parts store (where no one wore a mask) to an art gallery (where everyone did). Then, in the fall of 2021, when the delta variant arrived, the cost of these difference became clear, when the health care system collapsed under the weight of Covid infections. Alaska's largest hospital set up portable toilets in the parking lot for those who couldn't get into the emergency room, and doctors reported letting patients die for lack of equipment.[16] At the height of the crisis, confrontations between the opposing groups devolved into violence and an anti-Semitic demonstration.[17]

All this suggests that Americans' values and outlook—their cultures—might be as good a predictor of protective public health policies as the party of their governors. Leaving Trump aside, perhaps Republican governors who eschewed the advice of public health experts were accurately representing their constituents' wishes. Ron DeSantis, the Republican governor of Florida, remained popular as an outspoken opponent of Covid public health measures.[18] Covid had killed sixty-two thousand Floridians through 2021. Nationally, Republican individuals were less likely to observe social distancing in their daily activity, according to a study based on cell phone location data.[19] Conservative intellectuals reflected this preference as well, with learned as well as popular writers downplaying the importance of Covid, saying it was overhyped by the media and that hysteria and intrusive public health measures arose from some ulterior motive on the left. Polling showed that this denialism drove the largest group of vaccine refusers over time—not, as happened early on, anxiety about vaccine safety. These unvaccinated people were often young, evangelical Christians who would not normally refuse vaccines but turned this one down because they were skeptical about the severity of Covid.[20]

A strand of thought in American conservatism puts ideology above science, going back to the debate between evolution and creationism. The desire to avoid communitarian solutions to problems seems to influence belief in the existence of the problems themselves. Conservatives doubted the science of climate change long after it became irrefutable, although, for many, their real concern seemed to be the specter of international government and the loss of liberty implied by climate solutions. Conservatives in Congress opposed the mandates of the Affordable Care Act, but they did not address the issue of health care access. This perspective on Covid was presented vividly in a book review published in the conservative *Wall Street Journal* in December 2020, at one of the darkest hours of the pandemic, when Covid was the nation's leading cause of death, every day taking as many lives as the September 11 attacks. Writer Barton Swaim characterized the pandemic as a "moderately serious problem" that had been blown out of proportion by overwrought journalists and manipulated by egomaniacal politicians who, for some reason, wanted to impose draconian economic shutdowns.[21]

"Public-health experts, particularly the highly accomplished ones who are employed by elite universities, don't seem to understand American culture," Swaim wrote. "Contact tracing and isolation . . . require the kind of coercive governmental measures that East Asian countries mostly permit and the U.S. Constitution mostly does not. An immense, decentralized nation like the United States, whose citizens jealously guard their personal liberties and often feel no obligation to comply with the dictates of bureaucrats, was always going to do a lousy job of breaking the chains of transmission."[22]

Leaving aside the incoherence of these arguments—that Covid was exaggerated to impose public health measures but, at the same time, that Covid overwhelmed public health measures—we should engage with the contention that Americans are culturally incapable of complying with non-pharmaceutical interventions. It is a sobering thought. What if Covid had been much more lethal? Would our country lack the capacity to avert complete destruction from a pathogen, while Asian countries could stop one in its tracks? And does that also suggest our health care system cannot be mended—for better results, lower cost, and access to all—because we are culturally incapable of preventing disease or working together to protect public health?

We don't think so. In fact, preliminary research that retrospectively modeled the counterfactual (what if we had not used NPIs at all?) suggests many times more people would have died but for the wearing of masks, closure of restaurants, and the like.[23] Americans did respond to Covid, but we did so less effectively than other nations, and that is why the cultural issues must be addressed. Conservatives invoke American exceptionalism in a perverse, negative way when they say our country is so different from others that we have nothing to learn from their successes. Rather than throwing up our hands, our goal should be to understand our culture, and those of other nations, so we can prescribe changes to improve our health care system in this milieu.

In our investigation, we are searching for systemic flaws, as in an aviation disaster, and here is one: a reluctance to use simple and effective preventive measures. The Asian countries that stopped Covid much more effectively—including China, Taiwan, South Korea, Vietnam, Thailand, and Singapore—are like aircraft that barely deviated from their schedules while ours fell from the sky (we cannot consider more than eight hundred thousand dead over two years a "moderately serious problem"). Those Asian countries are truly different. Their region had more experience with pandemic response, having dealt with the previous epidemic of SARS (which they halted before it reached the United States). Their populations are more culturally homogeneous than the diverse United States. Their political systems vary, from dictatorship to modern democracy (not all East Asians lack civil rights, as Swaim suggested), but they share social attributes that contrast to our country, with stronger group bonds and habits of respect, cooperation, and obedience.

A researcher looking for patterns among nations' response to Covid stumbled on statistical evidence of this difference. Leah Windsor, an associate professor in the Institute for Intelligent Systems at the University of Memphis, wanted to examine the claim that women leaders had been more successful in bringing their countries through the early months of the pandemic (New Zealand, Norway, and Germany all came to mind). She analyzed death rates in the ninety days after the first case in each of 175 countries along with a long list of national characteristics. Besides the sex of the leaders, she included in her analysis the land area of each country, the length of its borders, its wealth, political freedom, life expectancy, and the age of the population, as well as each of six cultural traits. She found no statistically significant evidence for female leadership decreasing Covid numbers and scant evidence for the influence of any of the characteristics, including some cited as important by many commentators (including us), such as borders or freedom under the governmental system. With only 175 countries in the world and so many possible factors, and a great deal of chance thrown in, finding any statistically powerful association is difficult. But one trait stood out with high statistical confidence.[24]

"The one that was the most strongly predictive of how a country did during the pandemic was whether your culture is individualistic or collectivist," Windsor said. "More individualistic countries tended to do worse and collectivist countries tended to do better."[25]

The Dutch social psychologist Geert Hofstede defined the dimensions of culture used by Windsor and many other researchers beginning in the 1970s, when he analyzed 100,000 attitude surveys of IBM employees around the world. Over the decades that followed, many other researchers and millions of survey respondents added to the system of six unique cultural dimensions that broadly characterize the norms and outlook of societies at the national level. (Hofstede emphasized that the patterns show up only at the broad, societal level and cannot tell us about the psychology or motivation of any individual.) In addition to individualism, the dimensions include power distance, uncertainty avoidance, masculinity versus femininity, long-term or short-term orientation, and indulgence versus restraint.[26] Countries are scored on each dimension using the surveys. The United States scores the highest of all countries on individualism, 91 out of 100, while the six Asian countries we mentioned all scored an 18 or 20.[27]

"The issue addressed by this dimension is an extremely fundamental one, regarding all societies in the world," Hofstede wrote in 2011. "On the individualist side we find cultures in which the ties between individuals are loose: everyone is expected to look after him/herself and his/her immediate family. On the collectivist side we find cultures in which people from birth onwards are integrated into strong, cohesive in-groups, often extended families (with uncles, aunts, and grandparents) that continue protecting them in exchange for unquestioning loyalty, and oppose other ingroups."[28]

Neither type of culture is good or bad—no objective viewpoint exists to judge the value of such a fundamental aspect of humanity—but societies could be relatively good or bad at certain endeavors, such as compliance with mask wearing or innovating new vaccines. An individualistic culture, emphasizing personal achievement and prioritizing tasks over relationships, is well suited for an economic system—or a health care system—based on competition. Not all societies are competitive. Many collective societies that share resources have existed on Earth, as Charles has written elsewhere.[29] Today, capitalism has spread internationally, but the market economy began as an invention of the West, first described during the Enlightenment by Adam Smith, and was equated with liberty in the founding of America.

This cultural dimension of individualism could help explain why US health care spends lavishly on elderly patients who are dying, a key driver of the high total cost of our system. Medicare patients in their last year of life consume 21 percent of its funds (a pre-pandemic figure based on the traditional program).[30] A more collectivist, rationalized system would invest care in younger patients, who would receive greater benefit, and would deny expensive procedures to people nearing death in their old age. In the United States, that kind of rationing is unthinkable: the decision to spend even millions of dollars on futile end-of-life care is left to the individual. For those under sixty-five, however, we do ration care, based on socioeconomic status, with access and often quality of care determined by the ability to pay. As a society, we have accepted this arrangement, which is unique in the developed world, partly because our cultural frame associates wealth and status with individual effort and merit. In the response to Covid, it became a fatal flaw, delivering inferior health services to those who needed it most during the pandemic and contributing to America's awful count of deaths (as we will discuss more in the next chapter).

Here we have arrived at one of the conclusions of our systemic investigation. Our culture weakened our response. Many Americans resisted public health measures as an expression of their individualism. And the health care system itself, built on our competitive, individualistic culture, failed to deliver equitable, high-quality health care at a reasonable price.

But those conclusions are far from the end of this discussion. Cultural norms are not destinies. Consider that the second-most-individualist country on Earth, according to the Hofstede model, is Australia, and it did particularly well in managing the virus. Culture does not determine our fate. Instead, we think of these dimensions of cultural difference as being like the topography of land on which our institutions are built. The United States is steep ground for constructing a just health care system, but that only means we need a better design.

UC Berkeley sociologist Claude S. Fischer has explained the contradictions in the American cultural identity in a more hopeful light. International surveys, he agrees, do show that Americans tend to see the individual as uniquely responsible. But in other questions on the same surveys, Americans are also more strongly affiliated with groups compared to citizens of other Western nations. Americans are more likely to put group and family interests above personal interests, including obedience to law and employers and respect for morality defined by religion, and are more patriotic, believing in service to the country whether it is right or wrong. Compared to other Westerners, they tend to see themselves as free to change churches and other affiliations, but they are more committed to the teaching of the church and more loyal to the mission of the group once they join.

"We have mis-specified the nature of American distinctiveness. It is the principle not of individualism—egoism or social withdrawal—but of voluntarism," Fischer writes. "Unlike individualism, voluntarism incorporates, even celebrates, group affiliation. Indeed, in this worldview, individuals pursue their personal goals through the voluntary association."[31]

This insight fits our intuition about the country we love. Americans have accomplished great things together. The nonprofit Jefferson Health system and Jefferson University, where David has spent his career, stands as an example: it was created long ago for its public mission, which it still fulfills, growing progressively stronger with the commitment of thousands of people. It is one of thousands of such mission-driven organizations that are an essential feature of our society. As we investigate the failure of the US health care system—and later prescribe for its improvement—we should also remember the strength in our culture for people to join together and solve problems when we are inspired to do so.

GOING UPSTREAM

When Leana Wen took the job as Baltimore's top public health official in 2014, she had her own ideas of what to work on, but meeting with a group of the city's children, aged eight to thirteen, changed her mind.

"I was new to the city, and I said to them, 'Look, I'm now running the health department, what do you think I should focus on?' And I thought that they would immediately go to the things that you associate with public education and young people," Wen recalled. "Instead, all of them mentioned something related to addiction, mental health, and trauma. Some of them told me about what it was like for them to be living in a home where everybody around them used drugs."[32]

Baltimore, like other American cities then—and now—was in the grip of a crisis of opioid addiction. The number of overdose deaths from synthetic opioids had doubled from the year before.[33] (It continued to rise, with seventy-five thousand Americans dying of opioid addiction in the twelve months that ended in April 2021.)[34] Wen met children who knew what it looked like when a family member overdosed. They described it in shocking terms, more graphic than the clinical language Wen was used to.

She decided to focus on drug addiction as a top priority. She knew the city had a severe need for addiction treatment and rehabilitation services. Only one in ten people who needed treatment were getting it. "There just wasn't treatment where people needed it and they would have to wait for days, weeks, in order to access treatment, which is something that we would find unacceptable for any other illness," Wen said.

A parable about public health helps explain why treatments for addictive behavior—and addressing its root causes in society—are such a good investment. Imagine encountering people drowning in a river, streaming by one after another. Your first instinct might be to stay at the bank and wait as they come down, so you could save each one. But a better move would be to go upstream and find the spot where they are falling in, fixing the problem before anyone suffers a fall. Treating addiction goes upstream, preventing many more interventions in the emergency room and court room, and it often returns sufferers to productive life. To go farther upstream, we would prevent people from getting hooked on drugs, attacking the conditions that contribute to diseases of despair, such as homelessness, poverty, and childhood trauma. Instead, our health system invests in responding to overdoses and drug-related crime.

Wen knew that neighborhood resistance to drug treatment centers would make it difficult to increase beds. She chose instead to make a big push saving lives, pulling people out of the river. In 2015, after getting legislation passed, she issued a standing order that served as a prescription for the overdose antidote naloxone for all six hundred twenty thousand residents of Baltimore. She and her staff went into the streets to train residents to use the shot, in homeless shelters, restaurants, and anywhere else people congregate, offering thirty thousand training sessions in total. Ultimately, everyday residents used naloxone to save lives more than three thousand times, Wen said.

Wen would have preferred to prevent overdoses by treating addiction. But the naloxone program allowed her to do that, too. With media exposure and awareness created by all the lives being saved, she gained the political capital for investments in drug treatment. Next came around-the-clock stabilization centers and drug treatment facilities based in hospitals and community health centers. She said that upstream work happened because the naloxone project had changed the community's understanding. Later, some other states and cities around the country started to follow Wen's example, in the same order, with naloxone programs followed by treatment investments.

"I didn't come to Baltimore to work on naloxone. That was a means to an end," Wen explained. "Of course, it is an end to itself, because there are people who are overdosing right now. If we can't save their lives right now, today, there's no chance for a better future for them tomorrow. . . . But it was chosen as a strategy very, very intentionally."

Americans are good at saving people when they are drowning but don't like to go upstream to keep them from falling in—staying out of the river is, presumably, an individual responsibility. Wen figured out how to go upstream, and win investments in drug abuse treatment, by taking advantage of that preference for last-minute heroics. After citizens got on board with being life savers with naloxone, they needed less convincing to support the more effective, longer-term intervention of treatment.

But something else was going on upstream as well. Bad actors were pushing people into the river. Evidence now shows that the drive for corporate profits helped create the opioid crisis. Purdue Pharma, the maker of Oxycontin, pled guilty to three felonies in 2020 for sending the drug to doctors who were diverting it, giving them kickbacks, and lying about it to regulators. The plea made Purdue a convicted drug pusher.[35] But while Purdue got most of the headlines, and paid the biggest fines, other companies and thousands of doctors also participated in getting Americans hooked on these drugs. Most of the time, doctors acted unintentionally, following bad advice from self-serving drug companies to overprescribe the drugs. But many providers and pharma executives simply didn't care enough about patients' health when they could make money from the drugs. In the history of the injunction "first, do no harm," there rarely has been more egregious damage done by members of the health care industry.

Consider, however, that from the point of view of their stock price, these companies' biggest mistake was not harming millions of patients, but rather getting caught breaking the law. In our system, health care firms can produce these horrendous results and still have a positive bottom line. The opioid crisis may even have added to America's gross domestic product. Not only did the drug companies produce economic activity selling their pain killers, but hospitals were also able to bill insurance companies and the government for care of patients after they became addicted. When these companies are paid for providing goods and services, they profit regardless of their patients' outcomes. Our market-based health care system accepts this contradiction: we make money from people being sick, not from being well. Going upstream and keeping patients away from the hospital door can hurt the bottom line for hospitals and clinics. No wonder Americans don't take care of themselves and assume the doctor will be responsible for their health. Companies that control more than a sixth of our economy sell that product.

We do not believe most individual workers in the health care system care more about money than their patients' health. Our investigation is systemic, not about individuals. We find that the system itself incentivizes the production of health care services as a product, not as an outcome. Practitioners respond to that system. The worst of them profit in the role of drug pushers. But all of us are caught, to some degree, in a culture that discounts healthy living in favor of medicine.

"I actually think that this is exemplified in coronavirus," Wen said. "We knew about distancing, about testing, and all the measures that are hard. About avoiding indoor gatherings, et cetera. They are things that are difficult to do. We as a society, basically, chose not to do it. Individuals did it, but as a society, we did not do these hard things. We relied on the silver bullet, a vaccine to come in the future."

Wen delivered her second child in a hospital gripped by the first wave of the Covid pandemic. Through the pandemic year, she served as a key public health voice on CNN and in the *Washington Post*. As she observed federal health officials being silenced by the Trump administration, she helped fill that vacuum as a calm, straight-shooting doctor giving truthful advice and criticizing bad policy. She continued when President Biden's CDC told vaccinated adults they could not reduce their precautions, such as masking and social distancing—a policy she said did not make sense and discouraged people from getting vaccinated.[36] That point reflected her savvy thinking, similar to her strategies in Baltimore. To motivate Americans to get vaccinated, one should appeal to their self-interest, not only the wider social benefit of pushing back the disease. With the promise of returning somewhat to normal life, people would get the shot.

That kind of thinking should also guide us as we search for solutions to cure the US health care system. Our prescriptions must take into account the culture in which we live and the motivations of the players in the system. How can we manage, within a market economy and an individualistic culture, to improve quality, equity, access, and the cost of care?

WHAT WOULD HAVE WORKED, AND STILL COULD

The United States spent $6 trillion responding to Covid, more than its entire budget pre-pandemic, and more even than it spent, in inflation-adjusted dollars, fighting World War II.[37] It is an unfathomable amount of money that could have bought almost anything. It did buy Operation Warp Speed, the unfortunately named program for fast vaccine development that yielded a modern scientific miracle: three vaccines that nearly eliminated the risk of severe Covid infection. As we have seen, that policy followed the American cultural tendency to bet everything on the silver bullet of technology while neglecting the upstream behaviors that would yield better health quicker and cheaper. It worked for those willing to take the vaccine, but it didn't stop the pandemic, because those reluctant to wear masks and avoid infection also resisted vaccination.

What if, in addition to spending on vaccines, a good portion of Covid funding had been invested in rapid testing? Operation Warp Speed consumed "only" $18 billion of the trillions the United States spent as of spring 2021 (the global program by the Coalition for Epidemic Preparedness Innovations spent less than a tenth as much).[38] A similar fraction of Covid funding spent on testing could have changed the shape of our pandemic years, as David has written elsewhere.[39] Short of vaccines, testing was the most effective intervention against Covid, and enough testing could have controlled its spread. Imagine, for example, if inexpensive rapid tests had been manufactured and distributed to homes all over the United States, allowing each family member to test every morning, with an answer within thirty minutes, before making a decision about whether to leave for work or school. In fact, only 50 percent of residents testing just once every four days would have been enough to reduce the reproduction rate of the original coronavirus below 1 (the level at which the spread eventually dies out).[40]

This strategy worked where it was tried: some colleges, the National Basketball Association, and the country of Slovakia all used wide-scale, non-symptomatic testing to find Covid cases before they could spread, and all controlled the virus enough to go back to work. With the scientific and industrial might of the United States, and its unlimited spending, the same strategy could have worked all over the country. And it would have dovetailed with Americans' cultural tendencies, as we would each take responsibility for our own testing.

Technology, thoughtfully applied, can help us go upstream with health care, too. We can use that lesson after the pandemic. As we will discuss in chapter 9, the computers that almost everyone now carries— our smartphones—can monitor our health and report to doctors or artificial intelligence when we need attention. They can also help positively modify behavior to support better health.

We can also adopt business models that work within our economic system but reward outcomes rather than procedures. As we will learn in chapter 7, these models already exist and are working in the United States, and in some of those examples we also saw superior responses to the pandemic. At the same time, however, various attempts have failed to control the cost of health care through outcome-based compensation, especially in the many experimental programs spun out by the Centers for Medicare and Medicaid Services based on the Affordable Care Act. Most of those experiments shared a key fault: they were voluntary, allowing providers to game the system by choosing outcome-based payment only if it would bring in more money than the traditional model.[41] The lesson here is the necessity of a program designed with the market and culture in mind.

One idea that clearly doesn't take those forces into account is Senator Bernie Sanders's Medicare for All. Patients under traditional Medicare often report they are happy with their coverage. That reputation provides Sanders with a good selling point to advocate giving the same coverage to all Americans. But the program has shown itself incapable of limiting cost, as it incentivizes doctors to provide more services and post more billings. Adding hundreds of millions of people to Medicare would expand a broken system with perverse, costly incentives.

Within Medicare, another option offers much more promise. Medicare Advantage is a managed care concept that has shown success in addressing seniors' overall health and removing incentives for excessive services. Could it be a model for a single-payer system in the United States? We think not. America's individualistic culture prohibits moving the entire, enormous health care sector into the control of a single federal program. In the real world, resistance would play out with the interests of voters holding insurance company stock in their retirement accounts, along with the legions of lobbyists and political consultants those firms employ. Pragmatically, no one familiar with American politics can seriously expect the government to nationalize the insurance companies, including the fifth-largest company on the Fortune 500, UnitedHealth (and many others on that list).[42]

But Medicaid Advantage could expand to cover more of the uninsured. That change, along with other incremental improvements, can start the transformation we need, which will have to come step-by-step within the American context, and with the cooperation of the people, institutions, and investors who already make up this vast system.

We will have much more so say about how that will look and how we will get there. But first we will continue our investigation into the flaws in the current system that contributed to the Covid catastrophe. Our goal is to find a better way. As we will see in the next chapter, our failure to equitably serve everyone in society caused many Covid deaths. We fell short of fundamental values. Even as individualistic Americans, we must commit ourselves to equity and universal access to health care. Without reorienting the system in that way, we cannot make the changes we need.

Chapter 4

Covid and Racism

When Covid first hit, patients rapidly filled safety-net hospitals, the public and not-for-profit hospitals that take uninsured and Medicaid patients, and where almost no one with commercial insurance goes. It happened in Philadelphia, Chicago, California's agricultural valleys, and many other places. The first to be overwhelmed was Elmhurst Hospital, a public hospital serving a million residents in Queens, New York—where 75 percent of the population is people of color and more than half speak languages other than English.[1] As internal medicine resident Eric Bressman recalled, "The latter half of March was a complete blur. Regular wards turned into ICUs overnight. Multiple codes an hour. An incomprehensible daily death count. Overflowing morgues and freezer trucks outside the building. Patients came in, got intubated, and died so quickly that often there was no time to obtain a family contact. They died alone, while their loved ones waited by the phone."[2]

Hospitals such as Elmhurst are called safety-net hospitals, but some just call them Black and Brown hospitals, because those are the colors of their patients. They have fewer resources, there are fewer of them, and they serve larger populations than hospitals for White communities, while the patients they see are sicker, needier, and, as Bressman pointed out, more grateful than typical patients at university or for-profit hospitals.

Covid crushed Black and Brown hospitals because of the way the disease hit communities of African and Latin American descent. And that shocked Americans who hadn't understood how race defines who lives and dies in our country.

"Coming into office, I of course knew that health-care disparities existed," wrote Chicago Mayor Lori Lightfoot, in the foreword to a

67

2021 book, "but the disparities became especially real for me in April 2020, when I first learned that Black Chicagoans were dying from Covid-19 at seven times the rate of every other demographic. That number literally took my breath away. The first raw emotion I felt in that moment was hopelessness."[3]

The pattern repeated that same month in Philadelphia, America's poorest large city. But despite the high rates of infection and death in low-income communities such as North Philadelphia, Covid testing went to residents of the affluent Center City area, where residents were being tested at a six-times higher rate.[4] Health care goes where the money is. Poor neighborhoods had far fewer clinics where testing could be done. City officials saw the problem, but they waited for funding to bring emergency testing to those neighborhoods, and funding wouldn't come for months.[5] The situation so disturbed Ala Stanford, an African American pediatric surgeon who grew up in North Philadelphia, that she decided to act on her own. She gathered test kits, volunteers, and a van, and she went to Black churches and into the streets of poor neighborhoods to give tests. Hundreds of people lined up. She told a TV news reporter, "I just couldn't be part of another town hall meeting or watch another webinar or talk about how pervasive the social determinants of health are, and not do anything."[6]

Stanford became a hero of the pandemic, heading a new organization called Black Doctors Covid-19 Consortium. Media attention followed, helping motivate other organizations to get involved and ramp up tests for Philadelphia's low-income neighborhoods, many using her example of going mobile and becoming agile to reach those in need.

"She absolutely made a difference and has continued to make a difference, and I think it also shed an important light—a persistent, glaring light—on where the other entities needed to deliver more focus subsequent to her work," said Sandra Brooks, who is executive vice president, chief community equity health officer, at Jefferson University Hospitals and an African American physician leader for health equity in Philadelphia. "I think Dr. Stanford has been fearless and she's a true heroine for what she has done."[7]

Stanford's life-saving work gave Philadelphia a feel-good news story during dark days. The media couldn't get enough. A year after her first mobile testing clinic, ABC's *Good Morning America* surprised Stanford with a live on-air segment at her vaccination site at a North Philadelphia church, congratulating her with singer Patti LaBelle and presenting her with a $10,000 check to support her work. Stanford cried when TV presenter T. J. Holmes held up a street sign with her name, saying, "This neighborhood that you have helped so much, you are getting your own street here in this community, dear lady. This is real. This is an actual street sign. And it is actually going up in this neighborhood."

In fact, that was false. The sign had been printed by the city as part of a publicity stunt initiated by ABC. There was no plan to rename a street for Stanford. The long, arduous political process for renaming hadn't even been attempted.[8]

We bring up this absurd incident, even though it is so minor in the scale of the terrible issues we have to discuss, because it is ripely symbolic of our society's response to the brutal health disparities between the races. We had a hero, we gave her an award, and even that was false. The inequity that Stanford tried to address had been well documented for more than 120 years without real progress. She stepped up when she was most needed, and every life she saved is worth celebrating. But Philadelphia is a city with four medical schools, not a place where volunteers should be expected to redress systemic racism. After a century of dismal failure to address these deep inequities, we find it fitting that the city's recognition of Stanford's work was also fake.

HOW RACE DETERMINES HEALTH

Before Ala Stanford came W. E. B. Du Bois. He worked in the streets of Philadelphia in 1896 and 1897, commissioned by the University of Pennsylvania for a sociological study of African Americans in the city (he had recently received his PhD at Harvard, the first African American to do so). The book he wrote, *The Philadelphia Negro*, became a landmark in sociology as well as racial justice. Detailed field work and statistics supported Du Bois's contention that the inferior health and welfare of African Americans—including their shorter lives—were due not to innate inferiority but to the places they lived, the food they could obtain, and their education. The book can shock a reader today because these same causes still shorten and impoverish the lives of African Americans in Philadelphia's poor neighborhoods. It also stands as a remarkable version—a century before its time—of the kind of systemic investigation we are engaging in to understand the failure of our country to cope with Covid.

Du Bois surveyed ten thousand Black residents, mostly by going door to door, in what was then called the seventh ward, a long, four-block-wide strip on either side of Pine Street across the Schuylkill River from Penn. Even in Du Bois's time the ward contained pockets of affluence, and today it is fully gentrified, but it also had streets and alleys of narrow, brick row houses for poor, Black families. Poverty often forced them to double up and take in boarders. Landlords who packed in people offered privies out back for toilets, which often stood in the alley and were also used by the public. The tenants paid abnormally high rents for these dark, damp, crowded spaces and could not demand repairs, because they had no options: they were practically barred from living in better areas. Working as domestic servants and laborers, they managed the high rents by stinting on food, clothing, and other necessities.[9]

Du Bois's survey of health conditions and causes of death disclosed extraordinarily high rates of a respiratory infection passed through the air—not Covid, but tuberculosis, which at that time was called consumption. African Americans were believed to be innately susceptible, and society at large assumed the deaths were unavoidable. But Du Bois's careful statistics and study of their homes showed the spread of the disease was driven by crowded, unhealthy living conditions, which were in turn driven by racism. "Particularly with regard to consumption it must be remembered that Negroes are not the first people who have been claimed as its peculiar victims; the Irish were once thought doomed by that disease—but that was when Irishmen were unpopular," Du Bois wrote. "Nevertheless, so long as any considerable part of the population of an organized community is, in its mode of life and physical efficiency distinctly below the average, the community must suffer."[10]

No one could seriously doubt Du Bois's case for how structural racism damaged the health and shortened the lives of African Americans in Philadelphia. But that was 121 years before Covid hit. Now some doctors said structural racism no longer existed in medicine and that health disparities were caused by poverty, with race merely as a proxy for that underlying cause.[11] We believe otherwise. Du Bois proved the relationship of race to premature death in his time, and our investigation indicates too little has changed since then to alter that conclusion. Racial bias in housing and economic opportunity continues today, and Philadelphia's neighborhood health statistics remain eerily similar to those found by Du Bois.

Through most of the twentieth century, housing segregation continued with government management. A federal agency distributed official maps and reports that explicitly entrenched racial housing discrimination by guiding banks as to where they should loan money for mortgages. The maps redlined the exact area Du Bois had studied in the 1890s. A 1937 report by the federal Home Owners' Loan Corporation noted, in those seventh ward neighborhoods, poor-quality housing and a high number of Negro families doubling up, and it said that home buyers there were of "low calibre."[12] The map designated the area as hazardous for home loans and said banks should avoid investing there.

Maps and reports like these eventually covered every urban area in country (you can see them online thanks to researchers at four universities who digitized them).[13] By blocking loans, the system kept slums in poor condition, without a tax base and without homeowner voices for schools, parks, or public improvements. The system also denied Blacks and other minorities home ownership, which was society's most important vehicle for upward mobility, wealth accumulation, and inheritance. It helped cement the health disparities Du Bois had documented at the end of the previous century.

The Fair Housing Act outlawed segregation in 1968, but the redlined areas often continued to be racial ghettos and slums. Once-a-decade federal investigations have shown housing discrimination continuing nationally, with, for example, minorities forced to pay higher prices than Whites to rent or buy the same quality of homes, much as they did in Du Bois's day. In some aspects, discrimination worsened from 1972 to 2012, as real estate professionals were found increasingly likely to steer families to areas segregated into residents of their own race.[14] In the most rigorous investigations, identically situated Black and White families posed as home buyers to record any disparate treatment. Using that technique in 2019, *Newsday* found that on Long Island, New York, Black homebuyers were discriminated against 49 percent of the time, facing higher financial requirements, receiving fewer choices, and being steered into less desirable, minority-dominated areas.[15]

Of course, racist real estate agents alone didn't keep Black and Brown people in poor neighborhoods. Government policy and a changing economy in the last forty years cemented the poor in place, even as the country produced an unprecedented crop of new super-rich families. As the US economy automated and globalized, jobs disappeared in well-paid, hands-on industries such as manufacturing, while new knowledge-based industries arose in which only the educated could compete. Philadelphia made this transition and eventually thrived, like other US cities that once made things and now do things. In 1970, the city produced ships and locomotives, carpets and clothing, hand tools and lighting fixtures.[16] Now those jobs are gone, but even greater numbers of people are employed in health care and pharma, higher education, and insurance. Companies abandoned factories, but office skyscrapers rose higher than William Penn's hat on the statue at the top of City Hall—once a taboo—and young urban professionals took over the formerly gritty neighborhoods nearby, including Du Bois's seventh ward, where yoga studios and wine bars replaced shuttered machine shops and repair garages.

But the wealth was not shared. Access to the new economy required good schooling, which was denied to most Black and Brown children in Philadelphia. Children of color make up 86 percent of the student body in the School District of Philadelphia. In 2019, the district reported only 22 percent of students were at least proficient in math, and fewer than half of younger children could read at grade level. A quarter of students were dropping out before graduation. Of those who did graduate, only a fifth met testing benchmarks for college readiness.[17] Dropping out of high school traps Americans in poverty—a third of former dropouts are poor, a number that has more than doubled in forty years. During the same period, Black men who finished high school but went no further suffered a one-third reduction in employment rates.[18]

In the 1980s and 1990s, both political parties also supported punitive policies against the poor. So-called welfare-to-work denied public assistance to adults. Racially biased drug laws imposed extraordinary sentences, filled prisons, and fractured Black communities, wasting vast human potential. Tax cuts for the wealthy and a stagnant, poverty-level minimum wage increased income inequality. Wages for those at the median income or below fell relative to inflation and the growing economy.

As income and opportunity declined for low-income Americans, so did their health. Gains in US life expectancy stalled around 1980, lagging behind other developed countries, even as our spending on health care ballooned. And the gap in life expectancy between rich and poor grew wider. Then, in 2014, Americans' average life expectancy began to fall, cut short by people, mostly poor, dying of drug overdose and suicide.[19]

As the Covid crisis taught us, however, health disparities eventually affect all of us, even those lucky enough to live in the suburbs and work from home, who were free to avoid the virus if we tried. More wealth yields longer life in America (a difference of fourteen years between the poorest and richest groups),[20] but even the most privileged White Americans have health outcomes inferior to the average in other developed countries.[21] Perhaps this fact supports Dr. Martin Luther King Jr.'s statement, in his *Letter from Birmingham Jail*: "Injustice anywhere is a threat to justice everywhere. We are caught in an inescapable network of mutuality, tied in a single garment of destiny. Whatever affects one directly, affects all indirectly."[22] Indeed, research from the World Bank shows that nations with greater income inequality tend to have lower overall life expectancy, and the United States is on the wrong end of that trend line.

We should have known this. Du Bois had already documented the higher death rates of Black Philadelphians suffering with crowded housing, inferior education, lack of nutritious food, and an unhealthy physical environment. Racist policies and traditions kept those disparities alive. They are visible today in the shadow of the old redlining maps, which still outline the persistent disadvantages of racially segregated US neighborhoods. These areas even get hotter in the summer. Mapping by Philadelphia's Office of Sustainability shows the city's low-income neighborhoods average as much as twenty-two degrees hotter in the summer than nearby affluent areas. They lack trees and greenspace and their dense streetscape traps heat in pavement and black rooftops.[23] Summer heat kills approximately twelve thousand Americans annually.[24] Those low-income areas, mostly in North and South Philadelphia, also share the highest rates of hypertension, high cholesterol, diabetes, smoking, and obesity, and the least access to medical care, factors that, even before Covid, led to a one-third higher likelihood of death from cardiovascular disease among Blacks as compared to the total population.[25] (The link of heart problems is so strong that clinicians can predict cardiac events by counting the number of social determinants of health facing a patient.[26])

Du Bois found higher heart disease death rates among Black Philadelphians in 1899, as well as pneumonia, stillbirths, and several other causes.[27] In 2019, these trends continued. Everyone, on average, lives longer than in Du Bois's time, but the racial death disparity he found remains. Residents of the poorest neighborhoods in Philadelphia, compared to the wealthiest, had around three times the rate of low-weight births, cancer, COPD, and stroke; they were ten times more likely to be victims of violent crimes or die by homicide or accident; and they were thirty-four times more likely to die of a drug overdose. Men in Philadelphia's Black Nicetown-Tioga neighborhood had a life expectancy of 63.9 years in 2019, compared to 82 years in White Center City, just a few miles to the south, where the median household income was more than three times higher.[28]

Tuberculosis is no longer a major killer in Philadelphia's poor neighborhoods, but Covid was, and for much the same reasons. Poor Black and Latino families tend to live in close quarters in multigenerational households, in dense neighborhoods with crowded indoor facilities (and neighborhoods such as Nicetown-Tioga are almost all Black and Latino). That's what people can afford. Family earners couldn't stay home during the pandemic, and when they caught Covid, they couldn't isolate away from other family members, and when they were released from the hospital with Covid, as we learned from Rachel Nash in chapter 2, they frequently had to return to the same crowded apartments.

And yet, in a city economically powered by health care and served by many great hospitals, these residents couldn't get tested, they often lacked access to treatment, and, when they got treatment, they tended to receive inferior care. We will investigate those shocking disparities, which cost many lives, later in this chapter.

In *The Philadelphia Negro*, near the end of the chapter on health, Du Bois offers this point: "The most difficult social problem in the matter of Negro health is the peculiar attitude of the nation toward the well-being of the race. There have, for instance, been few other cases in the history of civilized people where human suffering has been viewed with such peculiar indifference."[29]

We hope, and honestly believe, that this indifference is finally giving way to real concern and a will to change our society and make it more just, with the reward of longer life for all Americans. That would be a fitting answer to the tragedy of America's Covid failure, which, as we shall see in the next section, was deeply entwined with the injustice and inequality we had accepted for so long.

WHY PEOPLE OF COLOR DIED MORE FROM COVID

We have come to the point in our investigation to count the casualties and ask why some people were chosen by death and not others. The patterns will point to systemic problems, and identifying those problems will suggest solutions.

Covid washed over the United States in a series of waves. The first wave hit amid confusion and surprise in the spring of 2020, affecting New York and other urban areas hardest. The second wave, in the late summer, spread the crisis to areas that had prematurely relaxed public health measures, largely in Republican states, as we discussed in the previous chapter. The third wave, and the deadliest to that date, came in the winter, after holiday travel, and killed everywhere, but still with the highest death rates in places where elected officials resisted mask mandates or other non-pharmaceutical interventions.[30] When 2020 ended, 375,000 people had died of Covid, and the rate of deaths was still rising.[31]

Before vaccination, Covid killed rapidly in group housing quarters, including nursing homes, prisons, and mental hospitals.[32] People with intellectual disabilities got sick at the highest rates and were more likely to die than any group other than the elderly. Besides living in concentrated settings, many struggled with mask wearing because of cognitive impairments and sensory issues.[33]

The first person to be vaccinated was a Black nurse at Northwell Health in Queens, Sandra Lindsay, on December 14, 2020 (the event was televised nationally).[34] States varied in their vaccination priorities, but generally the first shots went to front-line medical personnel and those most susceptible to dying from Covid, including the elderly and those with certain health conditions. As vaccination ramped up, new infections ebbed. Deaths fell rapidly in mid-February 2021. By early summer, the pandemic seemed to be subsiding in the United States, with six hundred thousand dead in total. Then came the spread of the delta variant and increasing cases and more deaths, almost exclusively among those who had not been vaccinated. The unvaccinated tended to be in states with conservative cultural and political traditions and to be younger people. Vaccination rates also lagged for African Americans and Hispanics, although for different reasons.[35] By late July 2021, Massachusetts had 63 percent of its population vaccinated and hospitalizations were down 95 percent, while Missouri, with roughly the same population, but a 40 percent vaccination rate, had about thirteen times more seriously sick Covid patients, and hospitals were running out of ventilators and ICU beds.[36]

As 2021 drew to a close, America seemed to have broken in two. In areas with high vaccination rates, especially coastal cities and suburbs, Covid remained a concern, but infections were within the capacity of hospitals. Break-through cases in vaccinated patients tended to be mild. But in other regions, especially in the west and south, the pandemic raged on, taking more than one thousand lives a day, week after week, from late August to the end of the year.[37]

We repeat this familiar narrative to explain Covid's demographic profile. It changed over the course of the pandemic. At the start, the typical victim was older, more urban, and Black or Hispanic. Race made more difference than income: Covid increased deaths for the most affluent Blacks more than for the poorest Whites during the early period.[38] Later, patients became somewhat younger, more rural, and Whiter, as hot spots spread to areas with larger White majorities and as older people became vaccinated. The quality of care for those who caught Covid also made a difference, with people of color generally receiving inferior medical care and being more likely to die as a result.[39] We will explore each of these issues later in this chapter.

The tragic bottom line was that life expectancy in the United States dropped by 1.5 years in 2020. For African Americans the drop was 2.9 years, for Hispanics 3 years, and for non-Hispanic Whites 1.2 years. Nothing like this had happened since World War II. Covid contributed the most to the decline in life expectancy, but secondary impacts of the pandemic shortened lives, too, especially a huge increase in drug overdose deaths. However, the statistics showed little evidence of the anticipated burden of neglected health care due to the pandemic—mortality from cancer and heart disease declined, partly offsetting the loss of life expectancy due to Covid.[40]

People of color have no special susceptibility to Covid. They died more because their life circumstances caused higher rates of infection, they received inferior care, and, for reasons that were often related, they were slower to get vaccinated (although the vaccination disparity had been resolved by late 2021).[41] We discussed in the previous section how crowded housing made it difficult for families to avoid spreading Covid among their members. That was true in the old cities of the east, in barrios in the southwest, and in housing for migrant farm workers in California.

People in low-wage jobs couldn't work from home. Often their jobs were designated essential, while the people themselves were treated as expendable, packed closely together in kitchens or on food processing lines, or in frequent contact with the public, delivering packages or driving cabs. A study looking at essential workers who died in California in the first nine months of the pandemic found the five jobs with greatest increased chance of mortality were sewing machine operators, cooks, agricultural workers, meat and fish processing workers, and couriers.[42]

Journalists told of brutal and uncaring conditions confronting workers in low-wage jobs who could not stop working during the pandemic. Amy Maxman, reporting for *Nature*, documented conditions in California's San Juaquin Valley, where Covid spread in food processing plants and an Amazon distribution center, and among migrant workers picking fruit in farmers' fields. Pickers avoided Covid testing because their earnings depended on how much they harvested each day—evidence of infection might leave their families destitute. Undocumented workers avoided medical care even after they got sick with Covid for fear of deportation and separation from family.

At a huge chicken company, Foster Farms, Maxman met a worker who knew Covid was an issue in the plant but couldn't read notices that were printed only in English, a language most employees did not understand. When she asked a coworker to take a picture of a notice so her son could read it to her, the coworker refused for fear of getting in trouble, and she never did learn what it said. She tested positive for Covid. The plant assigned her additional shifts, but her son convinced her to stay home. As the outbreak raged on through the plant, the company for weeks successfully resisted local health officials who tried to shut it down, until eight workers had died. Then it finally did shut down—for six days.[43]

Researchers at Columbia University and the University of Chicago showed how livestock processing plants became nodes to super-spread the virus, causing high rates of disease in the counties where they were located. Bigger plants and faster speeds on the processing line correlated to higher death rates in surrounding communities (faster lines had workers closer together). Just a few huge companies control this industry. During the pandemic, they were designated essential and few plants ever closed. Their pay policies generally encouraged sick workers to stay on the job, and they employed many undocumented workers with no safety net or access to health care if sick. The Columbia and Chicago researchers found that by the summer of 2020, these plants alone had contributed 3–4 percent of all US Covid deaths among their workers and communities. Eighty percent of their employees were people of color.[44]

Researchers demonstrated through mobile phone data that low-income, racially disadvantaged groups were less able to reduce their movements during pandemic outbreaks and more frequently visited crowded indoor spaces where the virus was likely to spread—often places they had to go for work. Full-service restaurants topped the list of dangerous places (which helps explain the high death rate of cooks). Also, common destinations tended to be smaller and more crowded in low-income or minority neighborhoods—think of an urban bodega compared to a suburban supermarket, for example—and so more people caught the virus while shopping and doing other unavoidable tasks.[45]

If people of color picked up the virus at work, shopping, or elsewhere in the community, they also were more likely to have family at home with high vulnerability to a severe case of Covid. We've mentioned the generally worse health of people who live in poor, racially segregated neighborhoods, with high rates of obesity, type 2 diabetes, and heart disease, all problems associated with the conditions where people live, the availability of healthy food, and the lack of opportunities for exercise. People of color also tend to live with their family elders, who were the most vulnerable of all. Almost two-thirds of African American senior citizens cannot afford to live on their own.[46] The tradition of caring for aging parents and grandparents also reflects their lack of trust of the quality of care in institutions where they might go.[47]

Unfortunately, that mistrust is not misplaced. Nursing homes in the United States remain highly racially segregated, and their quality scores, as a group, line up consistently with the proportion of Black and White residents—more Blacks, lower quality. Until vaccines arrived, nursing homes were the pandemic's most dangerous places, with astronomical death rates. And those death rates also lined up with the race of the people in the beds—more Blacks, many more deaths. The reasons for that disparity extended beyond quality of care. Black nursing home residents tended to be sicker, and facilities serving them tended to be located in racially disadvantaged communities that had high rates of Covid infection.[48] But those factors also reflect racial disparities and the alienation of these communities from the health care system. The unavoidable question remains: How can those of us offering health care earn the trust of these communities who need us most?

RACISM IN MEDICAL CARE

The physician leader at Jefferson whom we introduced at the beginning of this chapter, Sandra Brooks, told us the story of her decision to work on racial inequity, coming to population health from her field as a gynecologic oncologist. It happened at the University of Maryland Medical Center, where Brooks saw patients from the most powerful to the least—patients from the governor's office and from the poorest neighborhoods. One day while she was practicing there, a medical technician working in the operating room approached her as a Black woman approaching a Black female physician.

"She said, 'Dr. Brooks, I'm having this problem, can you help me?'" Brooks recalled. "She felt comfortable to talk to me about it, because prior to that, she didn't feel like she could talk to anybody."

It turned out the tech had stage III cervical cancer, a preventable cancer that is curable in its early stage. (With Brooks's help, the tech did eventually have a positive outcome.)

"It just struck me as being so wrong that this patient worked in the health system but did not feel comfortable accessing the health system, and presented with a disease that really should have been detected five to eight years before," Brooks said. "That has stuck with me. And really, I then started to dedicate my life's work to trying to unpack those health disparities that relate to how people access care, how they experience care, and how we can narrow those gaps in outcomes."

W. E. B. Du Bois noted the reluctance of African Americans to seek medical care in 1899. Doctors treated them with brusqueness and a lack of sympathy, he wrote, and most would rather risk death than go to a hospital.[49] The Civil War was barely thirty years in the past, and many Philadelphians had come from southern states where they had been held as slaves. But it took another sixty-nine years—until 1968—before Black doctors could join the American Medical Association or the staffs of many hospitals.[50] Decades later, a tech in a Baltimore OR still felt shut out, even as a hospital employee. Brooks could easily imagine her bad experiences as a patient or a worker in health care.

"Research that shows that African Americans are more likely to say they've been mistreated in the health care system," Brooks said. "So not only the remote past but people's current experience did not lend to people having a high level of trust."

Many studies document harmful bias against African Americans in health care. For example, research published in 2020 (covering 1992–2015) showed that Black newborns were substantially less likely to survive childbirth if cared for by White rather than Black doctors. In our country, Black babies die in childbirth at almost twice the rate of White babies, but that difference is reduced by 39 percent through the single factor of having a Black doctor.[51] Another series of studies has shown bias in how doctors typically treat pain, allowing more suffering in their Black patients. In a survey, substantial numbers of White medical students betrayed their belief that Blacks have thicker skin and higher pain thresholds.[52] Health care bias became vivid during the pandemic when a Black doctor, Susan Moore, began recording social media videos of herself as a patient in an Indiana Covid ward, where, she said, White doctors doubted her symptoms, denied her pain medication, and discharged her early. "I put forward and I maintain if I was White, I wouldn't have to go through that," she said in one of the videos. Days after her release, she was readmitted and shortly afterward died of Covid. She was fifty-two.[53]

The ugly image we see in the mirror is of doctors without empathy for their Black patients. As Brooks said, we readily feel empathy for people like ourselves or with whom we are personally familiar, but too many White doctors have never spent time with diverse peers at work or during their training. Like most Americans, they grow up in segregated schools and neighborhoods. Medical training emphasizes technical ability, not empathy (as we will explore more in chapter 8). In hospitals, Brooks believes empathy should be measured along with other aspects of care to make staff accountable for how they treat everyone. "We celebrate technical expertise, but we don't always celebrate empathy, which is really what's important and critical to making sure the people get the best care," she said.

We agree. Empathy is a cornerstone quality of good doctors. A well-designed system would support empathy and include layers of protection to prevent biased doctors from giving inferior care based on race. Instead, the opposite is true: structural bias in health care imposes racial disparities despite the best efforts of some caregivers. In our systemic investigation of the Covid disaster, this glaring flaw is grossly evident, and it was responsible for some of the most terrible consequences of the pandemic.

David Ansell dramatically exposed the racial inequity in the quality of hospitals after a long career as a doctor in Chicago at public, not-for-profit, and university medical centers. Ansell's landmark 2017 book, *The Death Gap*, chronicled the journey along Ogden Avenue, where a short ride traversed neighborhoods with a twenty-year difference in life expectancy. Several hospitals stand near the street. Cook County's Joseph H. Stroger Jr. Hospital is diagonally across from the Rush University Medical Center, where Ansell now serves as senior vice president for health equity. In his book, he describes the stark differences for patients at the two facilities, one of which serves poor Black and Brown patients and the other the middle class.

At Rush, the right insurance card provides access to world-class health care and just about any service imaginable. . . . But if you have the wrong insurance card at Rush (or no insurance card), access to some doctors and services is blocked. At Stroger, a patient receives the best care the hospital has to offer without regard to ability to pay, but often after a mind-numbing wait. Some critical specialty services and even some basic care, such as screening mammograms and colonoscopies, are often unavailable in the county system. . . . Mostly poor minority patients dying there donate many of the organs used in transplantation at the wealthier transplant centers across the city. Yet in my twenty-seven years at those institutions, not one of my patients—or those of my colleagues—ever *received* a lifesaving organ transplant.[54]

Think of that ghoulish image, organs trafficked from trauma victims in Black and Brown hospitals to be implanted in White patients in the well-heeled university hospitals—one-way traffic only. Now update that image to the pandemic, when Chicago's Black and Brown hospitals were overwhelmed with Covid patients, facing shortages of personal protective equipment and running out of cash to buy more. Now the rich academic medical centers refused them as patient transfers to avoid financial risk.[55]

"These people were worthless, meaning they didn't have the good financial means, they weren't worth it," Ansell told us. "We have a capitalist health care system."[56]

The situation repeated all over the United States, but in Chicago, Rush had adopted an equity strategy and became the safety valve for exploding safety-net hospitals. Ansell called the CEOs of each and offered help. In 2014, he had stepped down as chief medical officer at Rush to focus on equity because, as he said, "I did it for ten years and I could be still doing it today, but not preventing one death." Covid was a chance to prevent many. Rush took the hardest cases from the Black and Brown hospitals in Chicago, regardless of ability to pay, and gave those patients state-of-the-art care, including setting up twelve extracorporeal membrane oxygenation circuits—a challenging and high-tech process of oxygenating the blood outside the body (this was the treatment Rachel Nash saw a doctor's wife receive in Camden, as we described in chapter 2). Rush accepted one thousand transfers, about five hundred of them very sick Black and Latino Covid patients, and in the process rapidly lost some $250 million, as the reimbursement for the patients was far below what handling these complex cases cost, Ansell said. Later, Rush received the same emergency federal funds as the other hospitals that had turned down patients from the safety-net hospitals. But Ansell doesn't regret the decision. He believes it saved many lives, as Rush posted a better death rate than the sending hospitals and may have played a part in Chicago having a lower overall Covid death rate than comparable big cities.

Black patients nationally were 11 percent more likely to die of Covid purely because of the hospital that cared for them, according to researchers at the University of Pennsylvania.[57] Gatekeepers maintained these brutal inequities. In 2020, the *Wall Street Journal* obtained emails among Southern California government officials, hospitals, and emergency responders showing that four major hospital systems with ample capacity refused or delayed transfers from overrun community hospitals in the Imperial Valley because patients were uninsured or on Medicaid. These "wallet biopsies," as one administrator called them, left poor Latino agricultural workers to die while nurses frantically called hospitals around California seeking room for them.[58]

In Philadelphia, we lost a major hospital serving low-income patients shortly before the pandemic, when a real estate investor bought the Hahnemann University Hospital, which had been operating since 1885, and closed it. The Center City property would be worth more as condos or offices. The owner even tried to "sell" the hospital's resident physicians to other hospitals for $55 million (the trainees would come with federal funding).[59] When Covid hit and the city government asked to reopen Hahnemann to provide urgently needed beds, the owner demanded a rent of $1 million a month. The city instead used a Temple University sports venue for patients.[60]

David Ansell said the system produces exactly the results it is designed for: refusing care to poor people, usually Black and Brown, who cannot pay. And he said it was designed as part of a system of White supremacy that was created with intent but now often goes unrecognized. At least until the impact of Covid hit.

"It was the best case-study for the uninitiated, White person in this country," Ansell said. "The realization that we're all swimming in this river together. This has nothing to do with personal racism or anti-anything, it just has to do with the foundations of everything so deeply embedded with this system that has never been fully dismantled—that becomes the challenge for health. And Covid just planted its roots right in those preexisting crevices, those chasms, in all sorts of ways."

Poor people are probably wise not to trust a system in which greed plays such a large role. But their mistrust also costs lives. For example, people of color were more likely to refuse vaccinations when they were first available and to postpone medical care. As we examine the Covid failure and seek solutions, mistrust appears as both a serious problem and a symptom of something deeper—the injustice that is the system's fundamental malady.

TOWARD JUSTICE AND TRUST

As early vaccination rates lagged, programs in many cities encouraged African Americans and others from neglected neighborhoods to get the shot as their best chance to beat the disease and return to normal life, and to help their communities and the vulnerable people within them. Jefferson worked with the city's public health department on one of these efforts. They ultimately proved successful nationally, as racial disparities in vaccination rates slowly disappeared.

But urging vaccination wasn't enough. The Jefferson team also focused on listening. The program converted census takers into door-to-door vaccine ambassadors, learning about people's concerns and the rumors they were hearing and addressing those issues directly and personally. Sometimes workers would talk to one person several times. They offered rides to vaccination sites. Brooks herself led a program called the Real Talk, starting with the health care staff at Jefferson. She offered more than information to the skeptical—she also offered empathy, respect, and concern.

Black health care workers would become important nodes in networks of trust. Some had their own doubts and histories of bad experiences as patients—like that Baltimore OR tech Brooks cared for years ago. Even Philadelphia's hero doctor of Covid, Ala Stanford, at first declined to be vaccinated. Her concern for the people she was helping changed her mind. During the Covid year, testing sites her coalition set up had become pop-up neighborhood health clinics for African American residents wary of the official medical system. As she worked there, patients frequently told her they would take the vaccine when she did. In December 2020, Stanford did get the shot, inviting the local media to cover the event.[61]

"It comes back to trust, right? Trust and caring for one another," Brooks said. "If we've neglected those things for extended periods of time, it's hard to build that up in a month. But I think that by working through these trusted messengers, we've been able to make some strides."

The vaccine effort encapsulated the challenges of eliminating racial disparities in health care. Trust was one part. Barriers to care may be a deeper reason (and they also add to mistrust). A national coalition of researchers and philanthropists called CommuniVax documented these issues while conducting hundreds of interviews to learn the true reasons for low vaccination rates in communities of color. "Our participant testimony shows that many unvaccinated people are not 'vaccine hesitant' but rather 'vaccine impeded,'" the researchers wrote. People of color reported difficulties with transportation, lack of internet access or computer skills to schedule vaccine appointments, and suspicion of the quality of the single-shot Johnson and Johnson vaccine that was targeted to their communities. They also talked about vaccine reactions and, if one happened, the repercussions of missing even a single day of work, or of being unable to care for children or elders, or of having to pay a doctor. Some feared deportation if something went wrong. Others simply didn't know enough about the vaccine. People excluded from the health information marketplace worked in the casual economy, lacked media or social media contact, and had limited English skills.[62]

Evidence was gathered in the summer of 2021 that being "vaccine impeded" was the real problem behind low vaccination rates. Surveys showed, by then, that minorities were not as distrustful of vaccines as some other groups, but their rates of vaccination still lagged behind the population as a whole. (As we mentioned in the previous chapter, the largest cadre of vaccine skeptics were conservative men, especially in Republican-dominated states, who tended to rely on information sources throwing doubt on the safety or need for vaccines.[63]) As social inequities impeded vulnerable people from getting vaccinated, community infections rose anew. King's statement again seemed relevant: "Injustice anywhere is a threat to justice everywhere."

We are all responsible to solve these problems. And solutions begin by identifying racism in the system and taking it on. David Ansell, at Rush University Hospital in Chicago, has advanced this process as far as anyone.

"Our comfort in naming racism and poverty as root causes of poor health arose from our long-standing approach to quality and safety rooted in, among other things, performing effective root cause analyses when harm occurred in the hospital or clinics," Ansell and his colleagues wrote in an explanation of their equity program. "If structural racism, economic deprivation, and neighborhood conditions were afflictions at the root cause of health inequities, we had an obligation as an academic health system to name these as the first step in identifying ways to address these inequities."[64]

In work begun in 2016, Ansell's team studied the needs of communities in West Chicago, where life expectancy was as low as sixty, listening and working side-by-side with people who lived there. Rush abandoned a mission statement focused on medical care and adopted a new one: "to improve the health of the individuals and diverse communities we serve through the integration of outstanding patient care, education, research, and community partnerships." With many partners in the neighborhoods, and others bringing resources from outside, Rush helped build a West Side United coalition governed by the area's residents, with the goal of reducing the disparity in life expectancy by 50 percent by 2030. The plan would address the economic and health disadvantages reinforced by structural racism.

A decades-long economic transition from industry to health care in Chicago's West Side, as in Philadelphia, had entrenched poverty in those neighborhoods. Rush and its partners—including six hospital systems in the area—decided to reorient their economic might to be part of these communities, directing employment opportunities and supply purchases to their residents. With a combined forty-three thousand employees and $4 billion in annual procurement, the hospitals' economic heft was as great as their state's largest corporation. In addition to economics, the effort focused on the physical environment, education, and, of course, health care. When Covid hit, West Side United jumped into providing an equitable response, providing food and masks, testing, vaccination, and thousands of wellness checks. During the racial justice protests of the summer of 2020, members of the group ran full-page newspaper ads, signed by thirty-six Chicago health care providers, calling racism a public health crisis.

Other medical systems—including our own at Jefferson—are taking similar steps, although none are further advanced than the program Rush instigated. We recognize that health depends on jobs, food, housing, education, and the other social issues W. E. B. Du Bois originally identified in 1899. That recognition, and the responsibility it entails, should force health care out of the model of providing elective surgeries for profit and into a role of promoting wellness and longevity equitably for the entire community.

That change will take us partway from medicine to another field that has always been more effective in adding years to our lives—public health. As we shall see in the next chapter of this systemic investigation, gaps in public health may have been the deadliest of all during the pandemic.

Chapter 5

Public Health

Public health saved your life today; you just don't know it. So goes a saying we've heard repeated by doctors who *do* know, and we agree. When Edwin Chadwick published the first public health report in London in 1838, members of the upper classes were dying, on average, at thirty-six years of age, tradesmen at twenty-two, and laborers at sixteen. In Massachusetts, in 1850, one-fifth of babies died at birth. Scientists didn't fully understand the causes of disease, but they could deduce that the filthy conditions of new industrial cities were killing people, with dirty water to drink, stinking air to breathe, and deep piles of rotting garbage and human waste on the curb.[1] By 1880, the average American's longevity and physical height had been declining for a century. A new movement to clean the cities and build sewers and water systems reversed that decline, and the public health work that followed transformed what it means to be human, with each generation living longer and more robustly than the one before.[2]

Public health applies science to devise social changes addressing disease and premature death. Public health practitioners gather information on causes of ill health and prescribe solutions through the political process, public persuasion, and work with individuals. Public health can be accomplished by public works, as in the construction of sewer systems; by direct interventions, such as vaccinations or well-baby visits; by lawmaking, such as seat belt or helmet requirements; or by communication, with information campaigns on the hazards of smoking, for example, or the need for social distancing during a pandemic.

Today, health care is responsible for, at most, 15 percent of variation in premature death. The social determinants of health are far more important, dwarfing the impact of hospitals and clinics.[3] But public health policies often are politically controversial and opposed by powerful interests—such as the tobacco industry, in the case of smoking—and their potential supporters belong to an invisible throng who may not even know they are beneficiaries. Public health victories are crises that never happened. When public health works, you don't notice it. That's a difficult basis for building a political constituency. This problem helps explain a long-term decline in funding for public health despite a return on investment for every dollar invested of $14 to $88, by different calculations (it is also difficult to determine the exact value of health problems that don't occur).[4]

During the twentieth century, life expectancy increased thirty years in the United States, with twenty-five of them attributed to public health.[5] From 1990 to 2015, life expectancy increased 3.3 years, a comparatively paltry improvement, but still additional years worth living (since then, it has declined). Researchers at Harvard and the University of Michigan found that 45 percent of the most recent longevity increase was due to public health and 13 percent due to medical care.[6] Yet medical care now consumes more than thirty times more money than public health—of the $11,582 per person Americans spent on health in 2019, a mere 3 percent went to public health activities.[7] State public health spending varied from a high of $140 per capita in New Mexico to a low of $7 in Missouri.[8]

Public health agencies lost capabilities as funding declined. Over the last decade alone, the state and local public health workforce shrank by sixty-six thousand full-time employees.[9] During various crises, Americans briefly recalled the importance of public health. Effort ramped up for the H1N1 flu virus and for Ebola. During the Zika outbreak in 2017, federal support went to mosquito control, laboratories, and staff support in hot spots. But that funding lapsed the next year and much of the work was abandoned. Funding for the Public Health and Emergency Preparedness Program—the node for the nation's network to respond to disasters—declined significantly through the many emergencies from 2002 to 2020. And funding reductions have consequences. For example, as money for addressing sexually transmitted diseases declined—by 40 percent over fifteen years—the problem increased to highs not seen in decades.[10]

The loss of spending power for public health came at the same time that society's income inequality increased (as we discussed in chapter

4). Public health depends on a willingness to contribute to the common good. But as wealth disparities grew, more money went into medical services for individuals—even as those individuals arguably could have received greater benefit from investments dedicated to the good of all. One economist has called this the "wrong pocket" problem. The cost of public health comes largely from the pocket of the taxpayer, often at the state and local level, but the benefit goes to health insurance plans and the individuals who avoid harm, and they receive those benefits whether they contribute or not. Meanwhile, most health care providers receive no financial benefit at all—they make more money from sick people than well ones, and the savings achieved by public health may reduce their bottom line.[11] In a society pulling apart as if by centrifugal force, our dedication to the common good may have weakened too much. Even with huge potential gain, we were too divided to invest in one another.

Then Covid hit, and we learned the cost of this neglect. Our public health system was unready and collapsed. Errors and incapacity crippled agencies on the local, state, national, and international levels, with failures in science, surveillance, communication, contact tracing and isolation, and vaccination. Amid the failure, people who had previously starved the system turned against it. Public health leaders were threatened and vilified. The most visible officials needed police protection. During 2020 alone, almost two hundred public health leaders around the country resigned or were fired.[12] Public health should have been society's immune system. Instead, the body politic treated it as an allergen.

This situation calls for systemic investigation. Using the terminology of an aviation accident probe, we see public health's failure as a central component in the chain of causation. But the failure was symbolic, too, representing many aspects of the health care system's sorry response to the pandemic. In this chapter, we will examine public health and Covid, and consider how to fix the system. As always, we will avoid blaming individuals. Public health workers strove courageously to protect the public. The system and larger society let them down.

Anne Schuchat, a doctor and the highest career employee at the CDC—the world's most respected public health organization—recognized these difficult truths in a widely quoted retirement address in June 2021. She had worked at the agency for thirty-three years. Schuchat said,

> With prior responses—including the hantavirus outbreak and bioterrorist anthrax, pandemic H1N1 influenza and the Ebola and Zika epidemics— the public health front line has been the little engine that could. For each of those responses, state and local public health departments absorbed the initial shock until emergency funding came through—and then repeatedly watched resources ebb as the crisis abated. Over the past few decades, public health experienced a progressive weakening of our core capacities while biomedical research and development accelerated into the future. With Covid-19, we were the little engine that couldn't.[13]

WHAT WENT WRONG

In April 2021, a year after Covid turned the United States upside down, the National Academy of Medicine published an analysis of what went wrong in the public health response, written by a team of experts in the field. The paper had plenty to say about the lack of funding, which contributed to many other problems, but funding was far from the only cause of the system failure. "While health departments had faced numerous challenges during Covid-19, the roots of these problems— institutional silos, rigid funding streams, ambiguities over authority, and neglected infrastructure and workforce development—long pre-date the pandemic," the paper said.[14]

Early in the emergency, the federal government discarded its pandemic playbook—the strategy devised by the CDC's Marty Cetron, as we described in chapter 2—and pushed responsibility down to the states. But in the United States, many states lack strong centralized authority for public health. In addition to fifty-seven state and territorial health departments, health powers also reside in many tribal systems and in an estimated twenty-five hundred local health departments (apparently, the exact number is not known). Some states share authority with local departments, some hold power centrally, some cede most control, and in some states there is no fixed pattern, the academy report said. These arrangements rendered a coordinated response impossible and made it difficult to know even who was in charge.

In addition, the capabilities of these many departments varied widely. Some had advanced laboratories and highly qualified medical staff, but more than a third were unaccredited because they lacked the resources or employee qualifications to meet standards. Many departments relied on outdated technology, using fax machines rather than computers for communication. Some departments needed help from private-sector partners just to publish online their Covid statistics on cases, hospitalizations, and deaths. Reporting sometimes failed in astonishing ways, including instances of loss of enormous numbers of Covid test results. Many agencies were unable to produce basic data at all on factors such as the race of victims.

Karen DeSalvo, a doctor, led the team that documented these issues in the National Academy paper. She had become a leading public health expert without ever planning to work in the field. In 2005, when Hurricane Katrina hit New Orleans, she was a professor at the Tulane University School of Medicine and its vice dean for community affairs and health policy. Hospitals flooded and could not function, power and potable water supplies went out, the 911 emergency system and other communications went down, and troops patrolled flooded neighborhoods in a state of martial law. DeSalvo had no official role, but, with students, hospital residents, and other doctors, she drove back into the city and began offering urgent care in the streets. To get away from the hot September sun, and for a place to store gear overnight, her team broke into empty buildings—usually with the help of the police—first setting up an emergency clinic in an empty Covenant House Shelter, and then more in churches and grocery stores around the city.

The experience taught her what can be accomplished with the freedom to ignore how things are usually done. There were no rules. DeSalvo quickly set up clinics and innovated new systems. Her team created electronic medical records to track trends and patient needs and to share information with a higher-level emergency clinic set up by doctors from Louisiana State University in a Lord and Taylor department store. Old paper records had held back the adoption of electronic systems in medicine, but now, in New Orleans, the paper was soggy and useless, and it was possible to start from scratch. DeSalvo built a simple spreadsheet to track what the pop-up clinics needed—a necessity, as donations of useless items were pouring in (huge numbers of unneeded crutches, for example)—and to help deploy mental health volunteers and other personnel where they could do the most good.

The spreadsheet showed that front-line doctors needed tetanus shots and diabetes medications. Where were those drugs, as well as the flu vaccines that had supposedly been sent into the area?

"The hospitals were closed so the feds couldn't figure out how to get vaccines to the population," DeSalvo said. "So they sent it to the health department, who, instead of sharing it with the partners and trying to get everybody vaccinated, put it in a warehouse. And they were doing this with all kinds of supplies that they were getting, like tetanus shots, diabetes medications—this is like a recurring theme, because they didn't have a culture of partnering and they didn't have a culture of trust."[15]

DeSalvo and her medical colleagues learned during the crisis what could be accomplished when doctors went into communities and responded to health needs firsthand, solving the problems as they found them rather than offering the predefined services provided by institutions. Amazing things happened when people from different kinds of organizations rallied to address needs without worrying about established systems and hierarchies. As they emerged from the crisis, they also wanted to fix New Orleans's public health system to bring it into that same collaborative approach, she said.

The long drought of funding—dating to the 1980s—had shaped many public health departments into insular systems without community connections, DeSalvo said. Forced to pursue grants, including federal categorical funding and philanthropic giving, their work became oriented to the goals of donors, not their communities. Carrying out public health programs to comply with grant requirements, they lost touch with the constituents they were supposed to serve. Collaborative relationships atrophied. Other organizations that should have been partners instead became competitors for grants, kept at arm's length to defend potential funding opportunities. Successful agency heads were managers rather than leaders, skilled at fulfilling grant agreements and keeping clean books, not innovating, building partnerships, or investigating and responding to community needs. Agencies narrowed and lost the energy and capacity to respond to a crisis like Katrina or Covid.

When New Orleans's new mayor asked DeSalvo to take over as public health commissioner—and to make the transformation she had been calling for—she learned a more hopeful lesson about public health. It turned out the health department was full of talented people dedicated to their mission of keeping people well and doing their work with skill despite low pay (which is endemic in the field and makes it difficult to keep energetic young people who come into public health with idealism). DeSalvo's surprise at the quality of the public health staff forced her to reevaluate her attitude as a doctor, and it suggests why even people who should know better look down on public health workers. Indeed, DeSalvo initially turned down the job. Her colleagues and mentors told her it would be a step lower and would damage her career, which was rising in the more prestigious field of academic medicine.

"I didn't listen to them, obviously, but I also thought that when I went to the health department, I was going to go help them because clearly they were incapable of doing anything. And I was so wrong," DeSalvo said. "I realized there was this entire universe of knowledge and skill and experience and relationship with community that I never saw because I just didn't have the respect."

Where does our culture's disrespect for public health come from? DeSalvo suggested it developed with seemingly miraculous advances in medicine, such as antibiotics, dialysis, and cardiac catheterization. These death-defying innovations, and the incredible technology of modern hospitals, glorified doctors and gave them unique stature. Think of all the television programs focusing on hospital heroics. Meanwhile, public health workers used simple and unexciting tools and frequently served unpopular constituents—the poor and homeless, sex workers and drug users, for example—and produced incremental or invisible results. And there was a key economic difference, too. Medicine can make a lot of money, and doing more procedures on more sick people makes more money. Traditionally, doctors were among the best-compensated and most respected people in their communities. Public health doesn't make any money, no matter how many people it keeps well, and its workers are poorly compensated and anonymous.

But that could change. Public health has natural allies in business and government. The companies and organizations paying for medical care through health insurance premiums should support public health. It can save them money. And DeSalvo believes those collaborations can strengthen the public health system in many ways—with technology, political support, and new levels of professionalism. The incentives already align for these partnerships to happen, but it would take strong, innovative leadership to make the connections. We will explore those ideas more later in this book, because these are critical linkages to fix the health care system.

THE INFODEMIC

Karen DeSalvo stayed in public health, taking a high-level position in the Obama administration, where she coordinated the adoption of information technology in health care and oversaw the US Public Health Service as assistant secretary of health. She went back to academia after Obama left office, but in 2019, not long before the Covid crisis, she became Google's chief health officer. Within months, in January 2020, she was at Google's London office when she read a news article saying the US government would be screening passengers arriving at airports for the new coronavirus. She had been involved in similar decisions during the Ebola epidemic and knew it would be a huge effort. The article got her attention.

That night at her hotel, when she Googled the coronavirus, she got an old webpage from the previous SARS pandemic. But a group at the company, based in Israel, was already working on the problem, figuring out what information should be presented to users when they asked questions about the new virus. DeSalvo helped shape the plan and became a member of Google's crisis response team, as a doctor and public health expert, and as a person with experience in handling crises. Google adopted the role of a public health information source for the hundreds of billions of inquiries it received. Users looking for Covid information would be given local, official sources with authoritative guidance, not the latest trending rumor. The company also gave free ads to health agencies to amplify their messages. Curating the flow of Covid information and pushing out health messages became a company-wide project involving health workers, technology experts, advertising designers, and content reviewers. DeSalvo also talked to top public health officials to help them understand the potential power of these tools.

"I am your megaphone," she told them. "Tell us what you want the world to know. We want to help. It's not like in public health where you're trying to get on the local TV station or local radio and get the word out. People are coming to us, and so I've got to have the right thing to say, and we're not going to invent that. I want to amplify the message of public health."

The company removed hundreds of thousands of videos containing Covid misinformation from its YouTube platform, using the same techniques it used to shed videos depicting child pornography or beheadings, DeSalvo said. False information was spreading rapidly. Researchers have found that most false Covid posts and videos were created for profit, to sell advertising or products, or for political ends, and they were spread by people whose cultural or ideological worldview was reinforced by those messages.[16] For example, President Trump gave dangerous advice, with his disparagement of non-pharmaceutical interventions and his suggestion that people inject disinfectant, and was heeded by his followers.[17] Each of the social media companies tried to cleanse Covid nonsense from the world's information flow, but they did not succeed. The viral information pandemic eased the way for the deadly biological virus to spread.

Social media had already contributed to the nation's unprecedented partisanship and division in the years leading up to the pandemic. Tech companies designed algorithms to maximize usage and ad revenue, serving users with the most provocative and extreme voices that reinforced beliefs and prejudices they already held. That mechanism segregated Americans into narrow information diets without many contrary views or challenging perspectives. With the pandemic, those divergent channels produced mutually exclusive realities. One reality connected with science and public health and another presented an *Alice in Wonderland* world of Covid denial, quack cures, and conspiracy theories.

Information is a key tool of public health. Effective media has saved millions of lives. In 1964, the US surgeon general gathered existing research on smoking and released a report that linked it to cancer and heart disease. The blanket media coverage of the report immediately transformed Americans' understanding of the hazards of smoking, a change revealed only decades later with the release of private polling by the tobacco companies.[18] The companies fought back, trying to obscure the truth with junk science, and they invested heavily in lobbying and public relations campaigns to defeat anti-smoking legislation. But consistent messaging by public health, based on real science, helped develop social norms against smoking, which influenced local and state laws. By the fiftieth anniversary of the surgeon general's report, the culture had changed. The report and publicity that followed it had saved eight million lives, adding an average of twenty years to each, and was responsible for 30 percent of the substantial increase in life expectancy of forty-year-olds during those decades.[19]

Perhaps the tobacco companies could have foiled that change in the age of social media. Without journalistic gatekeepers to moderate the flow of information to the public, it has become far easier for self-interested liars to poison the public's understanding of science and health. We might still be smoking but for the unquestioned authority of Walter Cronkite, the *New York Times*, and similar trusted news sources, who reached everyone with messages that were assumed to be true. During the pandemic, social media informed a large segment of the populace that public health officials were part of a conspiracy to harm them—and they believed it. Consequently, many refused to wear masks, avoid crowded places, or take vaccinations, and those decisions increased infections and deaths.

Possibly, public health had no chance to communicate effectively in this degraded information environment, especially after lines of authority became confused and fractured among thousands of agencies. But repeated errors made the situation much worse. In our systemic investigation, we locate a key, cascading failure in the lack of transparency in communications about the virus at all levels. Public health and elected officials squandered trust and invited the proliferation of malign alternative voices. They should have known better.

We'll explain that accusation below with examples ranging from the WHO downward. But first, what is transparency, and how does it fit into the idea of establishing a just culture to avoid medical error?

Transparent communication shares emergency health information without holding anything back, in a two-way exchange that considers the needs and competencies of all audiences, and with disclosure of the scientific or evidentiary basis behind statements and decisions. In the first SARS outbreak, a lack of transparency contributed to rapid spread, and full transparency later helped stop the virus. After using that epidemic as a case study, scientists came to understand that trusted communication can mobilize a population to join authorities in fighting a disease—which may be the only effective tool in countering a novel pathogen. Transparency builds trust in public health officials by showing they will convey information regardless of whether it serves their purposes and by taking control of the communication marketplace. That second benefit is a lesson from corporate disaster communications. When a company makes a big mistake, consultants advise rapid release of the bad news to drown out alternative voices that would extend and worsen the process and, in the process, damage the credibility of the company itself.[20]

Transparency helps establish a just culture because it promotes equality. Recall our repeated example of a nurse in an operating room whose status under the surgeon is so inferior as to prohibit the nurse from speaking up when observing a serious error. That is an example of an excessive authority gradient. Leaders who withhold information increase the authority gradient between themselves and their teams. Knowledge really is power, and without it we can become distrustful and disconnected. In the grip of a pandemic, every citizen is a team member with the ability to help slow the spread. Without transparency, citizens are disempowered like the nurse who allows the surgeon's error.

After the public health emergencies of the 2000s, the WHO studied transparency and produced guidance on the subject for public health leaders. An international group of scientists who watched this process found three main reasons public health agencies fail to be transparent. Error one: They wait for scientific certainty before giving cautionary guidance to the public. Error two: They allow consideration of collateral damage of information release to affect the honesty or directness of their statements, such as backing off due to economic consequences. Error three: They keep strict communication control within the organization, allowing bureaucracy to create barriers to the free flow of information.[21] In the Covid crisis, we saw each of these errors. The WHO itself committed all three.

On January 14, 2020, the WHO announced "no clear evidence of human-to-human transmission" when the transparent truth would have been that, while scientific proof was lacking, transmission between humans appeared likely.[22] Details were lacking due to China's refusal to allow access to Wuhan. That was an error of the first type the scholars identified. On January 30, 2020, the WHO announced an official "Public Health Emergency of International Concern," essentially saying a pandemic was underway, but avoided using the word *pandemic* and otherwise downplayed the message to avoid panic, specifically warning against shutting down international air travel. Most nations ignored the announcement entirely.[23] Error of the second variety. Through the first year of the pandemic and into the second, the WHO (and the CDC) resisted accepting overwhelming evidence that the primary transmission pathway for the virus was in tiny airborne droplets called aerosols. Later investigation by journalists showed that scientific conservatism and an unwieldy bureaucratic process within the WHO had prevented the agency from updating its advice. That was a huge mistake. With the right information, more attention could have been focused on indoor ventilation, saving many people from getting sick, and less attention could have been given the futile cleaning of surfaces and the shutting down of parks, playgrounds, and other places for outdoor gatherings, lessening the disruption of the pandemic.[24] The WHO finally changed its guidance, without fanfare, in May 2021, after 3.3 million people had already died globally.[25] Error type three.

Public health officials argue that communicating science is difficult because science changes. That's true. But the best way to address that challenge is to transparently disclose uncertainties in the evidence underlying decisions. Being honest about uncertainty prepares the public for when the evidence changes. Anthony Fauci, whom we admire, erred by not disclosing his uncertainty early in the pandemic when he advised Americans against wearing masks, along with the CDC and WHO. Neither he nor the agencies provided any scientific backing for this policy, which they later had to reverse, with a loss of public trust.[26] Fauci offered a two-part explanation after the fact. He said evidence hadn't been solid about the benefit of masks and that masks were needed for health care workers—and so he fell into errors one and two. Common sense and experience suggested masks would be a reasonable precaution, even if scientific proof was lacking, and the desire to keep masks for health care workers, although an important goal, should have been kept separate, not influencing comments about their efficacy.[27] The price of transparency sometimes includes motivating conduct you don't want—such as people rushing to get masks that are needed by health care workers—but Fauci's statement lost trust that ultimately cost much more in the long run. Transparency forces leaders to share power with the public, and sharing power is always risky, but without being empowered, the public cannot help.

In fact, Fauci's blunder was far less egregious than many other errors in public health communication during the pandemic. Local, state, and federal officials repeatedly issued changing and contradictory rules for social distancing and other non-pharmaceutical interventions without providing evidence to back them up. The public understandably became cynical about rules that closed schools but kept bars and restaurants open; or that allowed indoor dining and gym use, but with a 10:00 p.m. curfew; or that called for entrance door temperature checks, long after experts had found them largely useless.[28] In Rhode Island, at one point, outdoor gatherings of even two people were prohibited, but twenty-five could gather in a restaurant, and seventy-five if the food came from a caterer.[29] That these dictates lacked a scientific rationale was obvious to all. They were clear examples of error two—public health messaging manipulated for economic or political purposes. After nine months of this confusion, the winter holidays arrived in 2020 with public health advice to avoid family gatherings, but with restaurants remaining open. Millions of Americans ignored the advice, went home for the holidays, and set off the biggest wave of the pandemic to that point.

Making decisions during a public health crisis is difficult. Definitive information is rarely available, and it is always necessary to balance interests. Sometimes concerns other than disease prevention *do* need to take precedence, when the harm of an intervention is greater than the benefit, or the harm and benefit are distributed unfairly. But when those trade-offs are necessary, they can be communicated transparently, too. If the trade-off is valid, the public is more likely to comply. If it is invalid—such as the decision to close schools but open bars—transparency will help reveal those flaws and force leaders to be less self-serving in their choices.

Social media amplified the sense that public health officials were dishonest and their rules were arbitrary. People were angry when they were forced to make sacrifices—sometimes life-changing sacrifices—but believed the rules that affected them were opaque and unfair. Opportunistic politicians added fuel to the backlash.

This poisoned atmosphere helped cripple contact tracing and isolation in the United States. Distrust of government officials in traditionally neglected minority communities also played a part. Many people wouldn't answer the phone or, if they did, wouldn't cooperate with contact tracers to report their activities. The weakness of public health agencies contributed to the failure. Agencies lacked funds to staff up quickly, and when they did, training was often inadequate, or they used call centers that had no connection to the communities they were contacting. Besides, for much of the pandemic Covid test results came back so slowly that contact tracing was rendered useless.[30]

Then came the miraculous vaccines, and the same errors repeated themselves. The CDC issued national standards based on scientific considerations for the priority of vaccine delivery, which, if followed, would have allowed for a national vaccine scheduling system and simplified distribution of shots. Google built such a system, DeSalvo said. But few states adopted the CDC standards. Instead, their often complex and contradictory priority systems, promulgated without scientific bases for the differences, created a crazy quilt of vaccination plans and added to the chaos. Some Republican leaders bizarrely attacked vaccines and demonized public health leaders for advocating them. In Tennessee, the state public health director was fired after Republican legislators objected to a program to inform teens about their eligibility to get vaccines without their parents' permission.[31]

Public health ultimately demands a social commitment to a common cause of good health for all. That unity of purpose gives us the ability to invest in the public health infrastructure we need and to follow its guidance when an emergency arises. We failed to support public health agencies, allowed them to atrophy in an outdated structure of tiny fiefdoms, funded them with top-down grants that separated them from their communities and made them compete rather than cooperate with sister agencies, and evolved our habits of communication in ways that made it especially difficult to hear their warnings. The collapse of public health during the pandemic happened for all these reasons. Systemic investigations of failures in the health care system rarely reveal simple solutions, but the picture is becoming clearer about the problems in our society at the base of this chain of causation.

Next, we will look at how these broad societal problems can be solved. There's hope, because the kind of change that is needed has happened before.

SOCIAL DETERMINANTS AND PUBLIC HEALTH

Covid created an immense social experiment demonstrating how public health works—and why. When public health supports were crippled, we saw the results. In good times, the public health system holds a defensive circle around our system of medical care, addressing the social determinants of health that are the most important factors in extending our lives, along with staunching the flow of sick people arriving at hospital doors. As we have pointed out, during the pandemic, when Americans avoided routine medical care due to the fear of Covid, little evidence emerged of a population-level reduction in their well-being, despite concerns to the contrary. The same cannot be said of public health, as the loss of its work during Covid correlated with increases in drug overdoses and gun homicides, accounting for tens of thousands of deaths. Therein lies an important lesson for the future: this is an opportunity to understand the diverse and largely invisible ways that public health strategies can address the social determinants of health.

Many examples demonstrate how these linkages work. Americans' leading cause of death is heart disease, but the numbers have gotten better. The risk of heart attack for middle-aged American men is half of what it was in the 1950s, mostly thanks to public health advances that addressed the social determinants. Advances included reduction in smoking, elimination of trans fats from our diets, less air pollution, public awareness of how to respond during a heart emergency, and increased access to health care through government programs. Medicine contributed as well, but less, with amazing imaging, diagnosis, and surgical capabilities, drugs to reduce hypertension, cardiac rehab regimens, and improvements in quality and safety in the hospital.[32]

We have a long way to go to finish that partial success story, however, and we're headed in the wrong direction. Obesity is a major risk factor for heart disease, stroke, type 2 diabetes, and severe Covid. Obesity is increasing rapidly among Americans across the board, but with big gender, racial, and ethnic differences.[33] In the first half of the twentieth century, weight gains from better nutrition contributed to greater health in the population, but since the 1980s Americans overshot ideal weights, and our collective fat has rapidly accumulated in ways that are bad for us. Forty percent of Americans are now categorized as obese. Why this happened is a subject of debate, but an interesting argument by a group of Harvard economists put the blame on processed foods, especially snacks, which are a particular part of contemporary US culture (and we are the world's fattest nation), and which became ubiquitous around the same time weights started to rise rapidly. In countries with lower use of snacks and premade, microwave food, the problem is less severe.[34]

Public health has failed to reverse this negative trend, but at least most people know that real food is better for you than processed meals and fatty snacks. Then came Covid. Obese people who got Covid were more than twice as likely to be hospitalized as people at normal weight, and they were also more likely to die. Obesity reduces lung capacity, increases blood clotting, and reduces the effectiveness of the immune system, and obese people are more likely to have other health problems that contribute to bad Covid outcomes, in their hearts, lungs, and pancreases.[35] The pandemic again highlighted a failure in our health system—in this case, the public health system's inability to address a key social determinant of health: our diet.

Is it unfair to blame public health for Americans' sedentary lifestyles and tendency to reach for a bag of chips or a frozen dinner rather than healthy food from the farmers' market? Yes, it is unfair, especially considering how the public health system has been weakened. But this can work. Public health has proven through experience that its communication of science can change social norms that transform our health. We have mentioned the smoking example. The temperance movement similarly was an astounding success. Prohibition didn't work because of the social side effects, but the movement did change Americans' norms for drinking alcohol, and our per capita consumption remains only a third of what it was before campaigners began their messaging in the nineteenth century.[36] More recently, we learned to wear seat belts and put children in car seats. Laws backed up the changes, but not many people had to be cited to obtain near universal use of seat belts. Today drivers commonly feel uncomfortable without buckling up. Our norm has changed. As for child car seats, any parent without one today would be pilloried in the grocery store parking lot. When we were children, we didn't even know what a child car seat was. Since 1966, vehicle deaths per mile traveled have gone down by 79 percent.[37]

Not every public health success comes about because of public health agencies. Not every success is even recognized at the time as a success. Until Covid, we failed to see the impact of public health, social services, and education in reducing gun homicides. Murder in American cities hit a horrific peak in 1993, and then it dropped by almost half over the next decade and continued to stay near historic lows (mass shootings account for a tiny percentage of gun homicides and didn't affect the overall statistics). Other violent crime dropped 75 percent. A similar trend happened in major cities all over the United States, including Philadelphia, but patterns were not the same: policing tactics, economics, and racial segregation all seemed to affect the numbers. Homicide death rates for young Black men are many times higher than for any other demographic group. Academics debated all the causes for the decline in gun violence, but they could not reach a consensus.[38]

Then, in 2020, amid the pandemic, homicides increased 25 percent nationally, taking the death rate back to what it was in the late 1990s. In Philadelphia, the situation was even worse, with numbers back to near all-time highs and constant fear of shootings returning to African American neighborhoods that had been relatively peaceful for a generation. The nonprofit journalism group ProPublica probed the human cost and the causes of this collateral disaster from Covid. As reporter Alec MacGillis wrote,

This soaring toll, which is heavily concentrated in Black neighborhoods, has brought new urgency to understanding the problem. But the terrible experience of the past year and a half has also offered an opportunity to make sense of what drives gun violence, and how to deter it. The coronavirus pandemic, and the decisions that officials made in response to it, had the effect of undoing or freezing countless public and social services that are believed to have a preventative effect on violence. Removing them, almost simultaneously, created a sort of unintended stress test, revealing how essential they are to preserving social order.[39]

The decline in violence surely had many causes, and that was one of the lessons during Covid. In Philadelphia, strategies included organized citizen mediation of disputes in neighborhoods, grassroots programs for dialogue between teens and with police in rec centers, and work in libraries and schools. Some youth even received trauma counseling and cognitive behavioral therapy to address the cycle of violence. Research had shown that community anti-violence programs work. With the pandemic, the programs stopped (or went virtual) when indoor spaces closed, along with the closure—now clearly misguided—of the outdoor public places where teens could congregate in positive ways, such as public pools and athletic courts. Virtual interventions did not work with kids who usually met on the street. Schooling didn't work either, and class attendance in low-income areas fell drastically. Then came the murder of George Floyd, widespread protests and looting, and violent responses by police that shattered positive police-community relationships that had taken years to nurture.

The ProPublica project documented how these events spiraled by talking to community members in Philadelphia's neglected neighborhoods.[40] With more murders and a lack of help to deescalate conflict, and with police regarded as the enemy, young people began carrying guns to protect themselves. Federal stimulus checks for Covid fed the gun buying.[41] The ubiquity of guns then produced more shootings. Social media played a big part, too, with young people relating there instead of in person, and with the tendency of online communication to escalate conflict and spur expressions of disrespect—which became sparks for real-world violence.

The qualities of a murder outbreak are notably similar to those of an outbreak of disease. Community programs and positive engagement with young people had functioned like an immune system against the flashpoints of anger that led to shootings. It didn't always work, but it worked often enough to keep the problem from spiraling out of control. When the pandemic deactivated those antibodies—the neighborhood peacemakers—acts of violence began replicating like a virus, with more guns, more fear, and negatively altered norms for how to respond to provocations.

The outbreak of violence was a health disaster, and recovering from it will take time, but at least now the prescription is clear. The city needs mental health and community programs, one-on-one support for young people, functioning schools and rec centers, and all the other small, thoughtful investments we can make in one another.

As we have learned from public health, however, prescribing for the current ailment is not enough. To continue the metaphor, a public health solution should address the underlying conditions in the community to make it less vulnerable to violence—a step similar to getting in shape and eating right rather than only taking medication for your heart. That larger solution would reach far beyond rec centers and youth meetups. It would change the quality of where the young people live, their opportunities in life, and their hope for the future. Real public health for urban violence calls for effective public education; good skilled jobs; safe, comfortable housing; and an end to the racial segregation and institutional deprivation that have trapped generations in violence and fear.

As we see in the next section, those bigger, longer-term, and more basic changes become possible as we widen the view of what public health means.

SOLUTIONS

Leana Wen, the doctor we met in chapter 3 who led public health in Baltimore, said collaboration with the food industry could help address Covid and other diseases.

"African Americans and Latinos are disproportionately affected by severe outcomes when it comes to Covid. Why?" she asked. "It's not the virus that's doing the discriminating. It is our health care. It is our existing systems. Who is most likely to have severe outcomes? It's people who have underlying conditions, diabetes, high blood pressure, heart disease, obesity. Who has those? Well, it turns out the same populations, Latino Americans, African Americans, are disproportionately affected by these illnesses, too. And why? You go one step further and you see that, for example, in Baltimore, one in three African Americans live in a food desert compared to one in twelve whites."

Wen's team set out to fix that in her time in Baltimore, before Covid. They worked with corner stores in low-income neighborhoods to stock fresh fruits and vegetables. They gave the stores subsidies, helped them buy refrigerators, and connected them with farmer's markets. In another program, the agency partnered with ShopRite, a grocery store chain, to deliver food directly to urban people and through hubs at libraries and senior centers.

DeSalvo cited these kinds of collaborations as key to future successful public health in her National Academy paper on Covid. Collaborating with other elements of society, in business, government, and communities, public health could lead toward social changes that address ever larger segments of the social determinants of health. To do so, and to marshal resources for a surge of big collaborations, we would need strong, focused leadership empowered to tackle big ideas.

The public health system as currently configured cannot do that, with its inadequate funding, lack of autonomy, and tiny, fractured areas of authority. What we have in mind is much bigger and would require a new commitment to building a just society in America.

Imagine the health benefits of addressing problems in housing, health care access, and healthy food. We would find ways to equalize incomes, eliminating deep poverty and ensuring that everyone can get an education that will support a good career in the knowledge economy. We would provide universal access to mental health care and substance abuse therapy, especially for people without homes. We would house everyone. The resources exist for these changes. We already spend more on health care than we spend on housing, and a quarter of that health spending is wasted.[42] And if such a costly effort seems improbable, we counter that it would cost much less than current ideas of nationalizing the health care system and would create a far greater return on the investment in terms of improving the health of the population.

In coming chapters, especially the final chapter, we will discuss these issues, and how to make them the responsibility of health care, with its prodigious wealth. Here, we hope we have established that public health and the social determinants of health are fundamental to the health care system. Covid churned the dark waters of our long-standing national failure to address these problems. We have learned a hard lesson about not taking care of our own. We have learned that we are all connected, and keeping our communities healthy is a common responsibility. We've also seen the result when we don't do that and a virus is able to attack our sickly society and turn it upside down.

That's the downside we can avoid. The upside is equally large. In a 2020 report, the consulting firm McKinsey & Company documented the enormous economic benefits of public health, with its ability to increase the size of the workforce and its productivity and to improve the quality of life for everyone. McKinsey economists estimated a third of economic growth in the past century could be attributed to health improvements, almost as great a contribution as was made by education. Simply applying globally what we already know now—mostly in public health—would contribute $12 trillion to the world economy in twenty years, or about 8 percent of global GDP. As the consultants say, "Over 70 percent of the health gains could be achieved from prevention by creating cleaner and safer environments, encouraging healthier behaviors and addressing the social factors that lie behind these, as well as broadening access to vaccines and preventive medicine."[43]

None of this would cost more money. The report assumes merely shifting current health spending from treatment to prevention.

The numbers are startlingly large. They demonstrate how foolish we are to continue to ignore inequities and the social determinants of health, a senseless choice with this much wealth at stake. But, of course, health is worth more than money. McKinsey also estimates that we could add ten more years of robust, middle-aged life by adopting these changes in the next two decades. The real reason to address the social conditions that make us unwell is to allow all of us, collectively and individually, to live long, fulfilling lives—and to make us resilient the next time nature challenges us with a novel virus.

Chapter 6

Crisis in the Hospital

Northwell Health, in New York, began planning for the coming pandemic in January 2020, without knowing exactly what it was planning for. President and CEO Mike Dowling told us he expected Covid to hit early in the global hub of New York City. As the largest health care provider in the state, Northwell opened its incident command center, mobilized its huge lab capacity to develop a Covid test, and managed warehouses of stockpiled PPE to protect its seventy-five thousand employees. The system controlled enormous resources within its twenty-three hospitals and 830 outpatient facilities.[1]

"The problem at the time was, we didn't know what it was," Dowling recalled. "It's one thing to plan for something that you can anticipate. If you have a hurricane or a bad storm, you pretty much can outline the problems that you're going to be seeing. But this one, we knew it was going to be bad, but we didn't know what it was and how to deal with it. And we didn't have treatments."[2]

In March, with the number of cases still manageable, sickness hit the command center itself, where fifty to sixty Northwell leaders had been meeting since January. The head of the children's hospital, a clinical leader, and an administrator all came down with Covid, which we now know had probably been circulating for many weeks, Dowling said.

"We were all sitting close together. We were sharing stuff. And of course, the question was, when that happened, 'Oh, my God, maybe all of us are infected,'" he recalled. "And then, right at that moment, we disbanded the Central Command Center and we went remote. And that was a bit of a scary moment, because we had never done this before. We had always managed crises in person, when you're sitting across the table, you're looking at the dashboard and looking at the metrics."

By early April, Dowling said, "All hell broke loose," with more than 3,500 Covid patients in Northwell hospitals. Dowling kept walking the halls, meeting nurses and other employees. Doctors advised him not to do that, but Dowling believed he needed to be on hand as a leader, as the situation daily developed into something like wartime. He also felt safe in his protective equipment, which had been issued early on to all employees.

"The only way I knew how bad it was, was to walk the floor," Dowling said. "You had to see it to understand it."

Staff had converted waiting rooms and conference rooms into Covid wards. Orthopedic surgeons and dermatologists worked in ICUs and acute care units. And ever greater numbers of patients arrived at the emergency room or through the system's many outpatient clinics. But despite the urgency and crowding, an eerie quiet hung over the hospitals.

"The thing that I will never forget was the quiet," Dowling said. "I walk through the hospitals all the time and it's bustling. It's a little bit noisy. There's lots of activity going on. There's people moving around. This was a completely different circumstance. Everything was silent. There were no noises. Any noise was very muffled because everybody was masked. None of the patients were talking. They were all so sick, and back then a high proportion were intubated. There were no visitors. The first thing was the eerie quiet."

Dowling had spent much of his life in hospitals. He grew up in deep poverty in Ireland in a dirt-floor house, with a troubled family, and was expected to do no more in life than work for local farmers. Instead, he made his way upward through education and sports to get a college degree and emigrate to America, where he worked on docks and at construction sites before joining academia at Fordham University in New York. There, Governor Mario Cuomo recognized his talents and turned to him for advice about poverty (which he understood firsthand) and other social issues. Dowling eventually became head of health and human services for New York state and a top leader in Mario Cuomo's administration. When Covid hit, he had already known Andrew Cuomo, the current governor (and Mario's son), for forty-five years. That relationship, combined with his experience in government and health care, made him especially valuable during the terrifying early weeks of the pandemic in New York.[3]

Dowling recalled seeing patients too sick to speak lying behind a glass wall, where doctors made notes about their respiration and oxygen levels with markers on the outside of the glass, as if on a classroom board. The patients were silent and alone.

"Especially in the units where people were being intubated, back in the early days—and I would see patient after patient—you knew that, at the time, 60 percent of them, 70 percent of them, are not going to make it," Dowling said. "The staff, and their commitment, was absolutely extraordinary, especially the nurses. And then you realize how important some other staff are that you sometimes don't think about. The respiratory therapist. The environmental cleaning people. The people on the front desks. The security people in the hospital. We had twenty-four employees die from Covid. A number of them were security people. So, you would think, 'Why? They're not actually treating patients.' But they're the ones that meet them at the front door coming in, and they're potentially very exposed."

Northwell soon had dozens of patients dying daily of Covid. With nowhere to put so many bodies, the company hired sixteen refrigerated trucks to store the dead—some for an extended period—and Dowling ordered entrance shelters built so bodies could be moved from the hospital to the trucks without being seen or photographed. That was a minor expense compared to the unbudgeted $500 million Northwell poured into Covid response. Dowling had discarded the budget and told executives to spend whatever it took to get through the disaster.

Despite being stretched to the limits—and expanding them—Northwell never became truly overwhelmed. It persevered through the crisis as a large, coordinated system, with robust, centralized leadership and a nonprofit mission. It even became a key support to other hospitals, helping manage the crisis for the region. Tragedy washed through its halls. When a flood of pandemic patients reaches hospital doors, it is already too late to avoid that outcome. But we can learn a lot from a system that functioned well amid the toughest circumstances, as well as those that did not.

In this chapter, we investigate America's different kinds of health care providers, their economics and leadership, and identify systemic errors that contributed to our national Covid failure. Here is rich evidence in our search for root causes. Over the first two years of coping with Covid, every hospital and health system was tested (although few faced the pandemic in the same way as Northwell, as the breaking wave of an invisible tsunami). Some did well, innovating and flexing to respond; some failed, with shallow resources and brittle networks to obtain help; and some turned their backs on the crisis, protecting themselves and their bottom lines, and betraying the very purpose of the medical profession. We see a pattern in the kind of systems that excelled, and that pattern points to hope for the future.

What worked? Big, integrated systems proved more resilient, as they could shift loads and deploy resources to manage the crisis. Virtually every hospital adopted the incident command structure, unifying oversight of the emergency, and that worked, but it worked better in larger systems that had more muscle to flex. Health systems excelled when they prioritized employee safety, issuing personal protective equipment early and emphasizing the needs of hard-pressed, front-line workers (as we discussed in chapter 2). Related to protecting and respecting workers, systems that had planned for an emergency and stockpiled supplies, without relying on government help, proved more robust—and, as we shall see, often those were organizations that prioritized mission over profit. And the best systems also prioritized equity, teaming with Black and Brown safety-net hospitals and going into low-income communities with testing, vaccination, and home care.

What didn't work? For the most part, economics collapsed for traditional American health providers. Hospitals and practices funded by the fee-for-service model—billing insurance or patients for each visit or procedure—lost huge chunks of revenue while incurring exceptional costs. The cost of clinical labor leaped upward for all hospitals due to huge overtime costs.[4] Meanwhile, insurance companies kept banking payments from policy holders and posted windfall profits. The government stepped in quickly with the CARES Act, giving relief payments that saved hospitals, the most vulnerable of which had helped needy patients at great cost, but the formula for those payments perversely benefited the hospitals the most that needed the money the least (as we will document later in this chapter). Hospitals that turned away the sickest, neediest patients did best of all. For small providers, especially the self-employed doctor or small clinic, the economic shock of the pandemic may have produced a final push toward oblivion. Medicine as a small business could end—and, as we shall see, that could be a good thing for the quality and cost of care.

What else didn't work? Cost cutting that left hospitals short of supplies (if they relied on just-in-time inventory) or short of staff (if they had not cultivated their human resources). Small, independent hospitals often didn't work, nor did systems without interoperable electronic medical records or plans for how to transfer patients—some patients probably died because hospitals could not communicate. Most outrageously, some rich hospitals refused Covid transfers from struggling safety-net hospitals or rural hospitals, putting their financial results above human lives that were not backed by good insurance plans. That approach may have worked for their year-end financial results, but it did not work to promote basic human decency.

As we explore each of these issues, a commonality will become increasingly clear. Health care failed when the *market* for health care services failed. In fact, as we will discuss, the health care market in America proved nonexistent and the laws of supply and demand did not apply. Most provider organizations had been built to sell medical services like widgets, with their profitability linked not to patient need but to the ability to build more facilities and do more procedures. This society-wide crisis instead demanded coordination, strategic thinking, and equity. But large, mission-driven systems did excel if their leadership had focused on community health. And best of all, organizations did well if they had been designed to promote health, rather than sell health care services, and especially if they owned their own health plans, receiving payment directly from policy holders.

We didn't expect that. (We didn't expect the pandemic at all.) But now it seems clear that the best models for meeting the Covid crisis are also best for fixing America's expensive, mediocre health care system. Our investigation continues as we seek to understand those connections and find the good that can come out of this vast tragedy.

THE HAZARDS OF HEROISM

At the height of the early pandemic crisis, a young man approached Mike Dowling in one of Northwell's hospitals and asked to take a selfie with him, as often happened when he walked the halls. Dowling was constantly in the news at the time as the face of Covid hospital care. He posed with the nurse, both wearing N95 masks, the nurse also wearing a shield, and shared the moment of comradery.

"You're fighting a war, so everybody bonded," Dowling recalled.

Before he parted from the nurse, however, a supervisor pulled Dowling aside and told him it had been a tough day for the young man. His father had died on the floor above just two hours earlier. Dowling expressed sympathies and asked the nurse why he was still at work.

"This is where I am needed," Dowling recalled the nurse saying. "There's nothing more I can do with my father now. That will take its own course. I'm staying with the team. I'm finishing my shift, and I would probably come in again tonight, a double shift."

Dowling came across similar stories of heroism in his hospitals many times. We all saw and read about extraordinary acts of selflessness, resilience, and commitment to others during the pandemic. Many health care workers gave their lives for others. Many others, nurses and doctors, rushed to New York City to lend a hand. Early on, signs sprouted that said, "Thank you health care heroes," showing up in windows and on front lawns across the region. Charles, in New Jersey, saw a butcher refuse payment for a purchase from a nurse in scrubs, and the other customers in the butcher shop applauded her. David, in Philadelphia, heard ordinary people banging pots and pans, clapping and cheering from windows and front steps, as they did in many cities at 7 p.m. nightly to pay tribute to the health care workers who were giving so much.

And then there were the television commercials, tearjerkers showing exhausted nurses and doctors, or depicting heroism in essential workers—all aired, not coincidentally, by companies seeking to burnish their own brands. Heroism became a commodity for advertisers, with images of nurses used just as video of puppies or babies had been used at other times. New York governor Andrew Cuomo became a hero, and briefly a national star, with his straight-talking, fact-filled daily briefings, which he parlayed into a $5 million book deal before being disgraced and forced to resign over sexual harassment allegations.[5] Some other attempts at heroic gestures immediately fell flat. The Trump administration sent the hospital ship *Comfort* to New York, amid great fanfare, but it proved unsuitable, unable at first to take any Covid patients, and had little impact (Dowling, his hospitals straining with patients, told reporters the ship was "a joke").[6]

The laurels of heroism don't last. After the pots and pans went silent, health care workers continued to work beyond any reasonable expectation of endurance, and in obscurity, all across the country, often without hope for reinforcements or even support from their communities. The pandemic divided public opinion in many places (as we discussed in chapters 3 and 5), and some misguided people became hostile to doctors and nurses as representatives of the idea that the disease should be taken seriously. After financial losses hit hospitals in 2020, many facilities laid off hero nurses who had just finished serving in the Covid wards. Some of the hospital administrators making those decisions were reportedly working remotely from summer homes.

Expressions of appreciation for health care heroes rang hollow when the society they served was unable to pay their salaries or provide them, in the heat of the crisis, with personal protective equipment. In fact, hero worship wasn't what anyone needed. A well-functioning public health system able to avoid millions of Covid infections would have been much more beneficial. A stable and economically rational medical system would have been better, too.

Questions about the ethic of medical heroism had already spread before the pandemic. Tradition instills the norms of service and endurance in health workers, most of whom sincerely dedicate themselves to a mission of caring for patients and accept personal sacrifices to avoid harm. But in health systems stressed by corporate cost cutting or other financial imperatives, workers' willingness to sacrifice can be exploited. In 2019, New York physician Danielle Ofri noted that demands on doctors and nurses had increased over recent years without more time or resources to do the work. New scarcity and complexity created artificial crises that demanded heroism from doctors to keep patients safe. That seemed to be about money. Ofri believed that health care companies were cynically taking advantage of employees' willingness to sacrifice as a way to boost profits. She wrote in the *New York Times*, "If doctors and nurses clocked out when their paid hours were finished, the effect on patients would be calamitous. Doctors and nurses know this, which is why they don't shirk. The system knows it, too, and takes advantage."[7]

The roots of the heroic ethic run deep in medical education. Doctor training seeks to instill individual skill, willingness to sacrifice, and endurance in the face of hardship. Even after reforms, eighty-hour work weeks are common for residents, and new doctors are subtly encouraged to exhibit stoicism in the face of tragedy and work as hard as possible (we'll have much more to say about these issues in chapter 8). Personal strength is a good quality. But these qualities of go-it-alone heroism burn out doctors, sap their energy and empathy for patients, and lead to medical errors. A pair of physicians at the UC San Francisco wrote in *JAMA* about the impossibility of continuous, unending heroic behavior (and elicited many online comments from doctors who agreed).

"Occupationally related emotional exhaustion and distress, and, in extreme cases, depression, anxiety, and suicide can result from striving to meet impossible expectations," wrote Urmimala Sarkar and Christine Cassel. "After this pandemic year, it is past time for society to support health care professionals' capacity to respond to emergencies and for medicine and health care systems to encourage and support clinicians to embody teamwork, embrace vulnerability and humanity in the health care workforce, and ask for personal sacrifice only in exceptional rare circumstances."[8]

When investigating medical errors, David has often asked about the style of the doctors involved. The culture of medicine—and the wider culture of society—elevates the status of the highly skilled, expert physician, like a celebrity athlete or performer with unique abilities. The hero. But doctors who think of themselves that way, or strive for that kind of individualistic excellence, often practice medicine as loners. As we saw in chapter 1, loners don't necessarily make more mistakes, but the mistakes they inevitably do make are less likely to be caught before they hurt patients.

Being a loner has never been a good way to practice medicine, but today teamwork has become essential and unavoidable. The increasing complexity and specialization of medicine require that health care providers cooperate effectively. Systems that emphasize teamwork have better results and make fewer errors. Improving medical teamwork has become a critical area of research and reform, as important as the development of new therapies and drugs.[9] The pandemic underlined this truth, as large, integrated systems performed well, informing front-line doctors rapidly with research and insights consolidated from the experience of large teams of physicians (as we will learn in the next section).

The pandemic also accelerated the approaching extinction of the heroic doctor practicing on his own. Financial upheaval and supply issues crushed small private practices. Their revenues fell, on average, by a third, while their expenses rose, especially for personal protective equipment. Many small practices couldn't obtain masks or tests for much of 2020. The smaller they were, the worse and longer-lasting their supply problems.[10] That meant that many small practices could not see Covid patients for months. As small businesses surviving on providing individual services, paid by insurance, they simply couldn't stay above water through a year with few patients coming in the door, even after government aid arrived. Doctors quit their practices in huge numbers.[11] During 2020 alone, more than forty-eight thousand of them went to work for hospitals and health systems, giving up independent practice, often by selling or merging their clinics into larger entities. By mid-2021, almost 70 percent of doctors were employed rather than practicing on their own, an increase of eight percentage points from just two years earlier.[12]

This can be a good thing. We feel sorry for family doctors giving up small businesses they built, but this transition has been needed by the larger system for a long time. As we have discussed, the fee-for-service model of payment for medical care is among the most important barriers to improving the health care system. But the alternative—a value-based system that charges for wellness and outcomes rather than à la carte services—cannot work well amid a galaxy of tiny, disconnected medical practices. To effectively promote wellness, a system must provide services through many connected parts, addressing most or all of clients' needs. Those connected systems have other positive built-in qualities, too, as we will explore, including the benefits of teamwork and coordination.

When Covid hit, the emergency tested every health care provider. Large, integrated systems were able to cope with the crisis, especially those offering value-based care, as they pivoted rapidly, allocated people and resources where needed, and continued to collect premiums, staying financially strong. Small, private practices failed. They lost money, laid off staff, and often couldn't participate in helping address the emergency—some merely referred patients suspected to have Covid to emergency rooms. The pandemic had become a Darwinian event, thinning out these weaker, smaller providers. As a result, the entire system may emerge stronger, with more doctors receiving paychecks rather than sending out bills, and working within teams of health care providers rather than as lonely heroes.

We cannot build a medical system on heroes. It's not good for the heroes—or for the rest of us. But issues remain in our investigation. Did large health systems really address the challenge of teamwork and coordination, or were they just big enough to weather the storm? We will look at that question next.

IS BIGGER REALLY BETTER?

As the enormity of the Covid crisis loomed, Governor Andrew Cuomo called Mike Dowling and asked him to coordinate hospitals—not only his own but also the public hospitals and the other nonprofits—while working with the head of their trade association, Kenneth Raske. Modeling projections indicated New York wouldn't have enough beds, ICU beds, or supplies. The heads of the hospitals met on Zoom as often as daily to deal with the issues. Dowling said creating beds was easy—you can always put more beds somewhere—but finding supplies and ventilators for ICU beds was much harder. Staffing the beds with qualified doctors and nurses could be harder still.

As the wave of sickness rose, safety-net hospitals staggered under overwhelming numbers of extremely ill patients in low-income, Black and Brown neighborhoods. Dowling likened the situation to panic. Hospitals were running out of oxygen for patients. He got another call from Cuomo. Northwell agreed to step in to support five safety-net hospitals.

"I told the governor they will not cause you a problem, either with the press or anybody else, because we will make sure that we take care of them," Dowling said. "So we temporarily adopted those hospitals, and I was in communication with the heads of those places. And I had my staff out there. And I would say, 'Any problem—any problem—you call me, don't go to the press, don't create hysteria.'"

In addition to making sure the under-resourced hospitals had oxygen, Northwell mobilized its transport system to begin moving patients from struggling hospitals to sites with capacity to care for them. It also sent a team of administrators to the Javits Center, the convention center in Manhattan where the army had installed four 250-bed medical stations designed to shelter victims in natural disasters. The facility wasn't initially equipped to handle Covid patients or, indeed, many other kinds of patients coming from urban hospitals. It needed supplies of oxygen, ventilators, and other ICU equipment. The Northwell administrators managed the facility at Javits, and it got up and running, eventually treating a total of over one thousand patients.[13]

Each of these examples buttresses the point that, at least in this pandemic, big was better than small at dealing with the crisis. But did patients get better Covid care in big health systems? Hard data is not yet available at this writing, but the answer could be yes. Ira Nash (who is David's physician brother), a senior vice president at Northwell, wrote that his system had the sophistication and resources to make important plans before the pandemic hit, including assembling the right teams of experts and developing standardized treatment protocols to protect patients and staff. After Covid hit, Northwell developed its own test for the virus and doctors initiated clinical trials to find effective treatments, communicating discoveries rapidly to front-line doctors in the system's many hospitals.[14] A clinical advisory team staffed by Northwell's top doctors met daily—or more often—to review issues and decide on clinical guidelines for every unit in the system, digesting experience across a vast number of cases and defining new best practices that could be implemented everywhere, all at once. It also decided which non-Covid cases could not be delayed and brought them into the mix in the crowded hospitals.

"It wasn't like every hospital administrator or every hospital chief medical officer was making clinical decisions independent of one another. That would have been chaos," Dowling explained. "Everything had to come through the central clinical group every single day. We issued thousands of communications, continuously. Which, by the way, the staff was so thankful for—that they got continuous communication about 'This is the new way you handle this,' or 'This is the learnings from yesterday, or two days ago, and what happened, and this is the new policy now.'"

Small hospital groups or single hospitals didn't have that advantage. They did receive new knowledge about the disease. It developed many places and spread through online servers and ad hoc communications channels among doctors. But surely having a formal system is better for sorting and analyzing new evidence and treatments about a novel disease. An expert from the University of Kentucky confirmed to us the challenges small hospitals and rural states had during the pandemic. Lawrence Prybil, the Norton Professor in Healthcare Leadership (retired), said expertise in handling advanced pediatric care existed in only a few places in his state as the delta wave of the virus began to hit children in the summer of 2021. Small Kentucky hospitals lacked expertise or places to transfer young patients.

"It's intuitive and obvious that organizations that were larger—had more capacity or the ability to bring supplemental capacity in—were able to handle the onslaught of the Covid surges," Prybil said. "What many of the smaller hospitals had to do was to desperately find places to send patients that were beyond the capacity of their organization to deal with."[15]

In some places, those transfers were hindered by receiving hospitals that resisted taking money-losing patients lacking commercial insurance, as we discussed in chapter 4. In others, the practical barriers of disjointed systems slowed transfers between hospitals without common computer or communication systems. In chapter 9, we will dig into the failure of the United States to develop information technology to coordinate medical care, but here we must note the impact on patients. In 2020, the *Wall Street Journal* documented a terrible crisis in California's Imperial Valley, where the city-owned El Centro Regional Medical Center, overrun with Covid patients, had to rely on phone calls and text messages to find beds for transfers. The state's hospital association said it took an average of forty phone calls to find each patient bed. Patients were sent as far away as Sacramento, six hundred miles north, although there must have been beds available in the southern half of the state. The process took so long—up to four days—that poorly managed patients would arrive at receiving hospitals with aggravated cases, almost certainly leading to unnecessary Covid deaths.[16]

In the highly complex, expensive, teamwork-based enterprise of modern medicine, large entities perform better in a global crisis. They even proved more innovative and agile than their smaller competitors, because they had the expertise and centralized research capabilities to make their own decisions. To revisit an example we mentioned in chapter 2, Jefferson Health defied the CDC's early guidance not to use masks outside of clinical settings. Northwell made the same decision at about the same time. In Philadelphia, Jefferson evaluated, on its own, the science about aerosolized virus particles and decided to mask up the entire thirty-four-thousand-employee company, onsite and while out in the community, before many Covid cases had shown up, as we were told by Jonathan Gleason, who was then the system's chief quality officer and a physician (and whom we introduced in chapter 2). Gleason made the call by applying recognized principles of health care quality, including reliance on expertise and total transparency. The choice generated controversy from other hospitals and some alarm from members of the public—it seemed radical, David recalls—but Gleason proved correct. Thanks to that decision, Jefferson won loyalty from staff, who saw the company prioritizing their safety and that of their families. And Jefferson's leadership avoided the loss of credibility suffered by the CDC and Anthony Fauci, when those authorities had to reverse their recommendation and call for wider use of masks (as we discussed in the last chapter). A smaller organization might have lacked the internal expertise to choose such a contrary direction.

Although our investigation has established the positive attributes of size and consolidation during a crisis, we do not believe increasing size alone is enough to heal the health care system. Patients in these large systems may have fared better during the pandemic, but the creation of huge organizations may be making our overall system worse in some ways.

Consolidation exploded after the passage of the Affordable Care Act in 2010. Growing systems rapidly bought up hospitals and clinics. The trend happened in nonprofit systems as well as investor-owned hospitals—and in many cases nonprofits have behaved as aggressively and with as strong a bottom-line motivation as those with Wall Street owners. As a financial solution, consolidation worked, because economies of scale allowed for cost cutting and because buying up the competition allowed large systems to raise prices. With their often-dominant economic power in many markets, they can name prices to insurance companies without the worry of being undercut. Insurers cannot afford to have these huge systems outside their networks, so they sign contracts and pass the increased costs on to premium payers.[17]

Cost cutting at large consolidated systems caused problems during the pandemic. Reduced staffing and just-in-time supply chains weakened the response to the surge of patients, as the *Wall Street Journal* documented in another excellent piece of journalism, which focused on the huge nonprofit Banner Health in Phoenix. Before the pandemic, Banner thinned staffing and expenses to bank enormous retained earnings (and paid its CEO $25 million one year). But during the Covid surge of summer 2020, Banner's cost cutting hampered its response. It recovered, using its vast hoard of past earnings, by hiring traveling nurses at very high wages to staff its hospitals. For the region's health system as a whole, however, that didn't solve the problem, because smaller hospitals could not afford to compete with the emergency wages and were left short-staffed.[18] Cost cutting by the corporate giant had created a deficit of capacity for society as a whole. When the disaster hit, no amount of money could produce new nurses to instantly fill the void.

Top-down cost cutting can diminish the quality of care in other ways, too. Administrators of health systems are contracting out ever more core services to save money, a practice that grew by 37 percent in 2017 alone, but recent research shows these outsourcing arrangements can lead to medical errors and inconsistent standards of care. By outsourcing emergency care, lab work, radiology, or even janitorial work, hospitals fracture their teams, with consequences for communication, oversight and accountability, and staff morale. A decision in the executive suite for short-term savings can become a long-term cost.[19]

During the pandemic, big health systems such as Banner, Jefferson, and Northwell served as ships in the storm, able to stay afloat, navigate, and, in some cases, take the smaller members of the fleet in tow as they helped overwhelmed hospitals. But big health systems alone are not a solution. They cost more and they have not been able to deliver a superior clinical product over time. In January 2020, an important study of hospital mergers showed that patient outcomes generally did not improve after consolidation and that the patient experience got worse, with a decline in satisfaction equivalent to reduction from the fiftieth to the forty-first percentile. The researchers could not say definitely why the patient experience deteriorated after mergers, but it makes sense if these business deals drove cost-cutting pressures or reduced local competition, allowing systems to lower their standards and make more money.[20]

What's going on here? If bigger is better during an emergency, why haven't bigger systems paid off with better care and savings? Consider the problem of unexplained clinical variation, the phenomenon of physicians making different treatment choices when faced with the same set of symptoms. Researchers have studied the problem for fifty years. It is a major concern for medicine as an evidence-based practice: In most cases, there should be a single best treatment option for a particular condition, but in fact physicians are often all over the map in how they address similarly situated patients, with differences depending on doctors' personalities, the habits of their hospital colleagues, and even their region of the country.[21] The problem links closely to the cost of care, because the differences in doctors' choices can yield unnecessary procedures and hospitals stays. Study shows that Medicare spends 50 percent more on patients in some regions than others, mostly for acute and post-acute care, without an apparent reason for the difference.[22] Even in a nationalized system—military health care—individual service members receive different amounts of care as their assignments move them around the country, with cost variation of up to 70 percent.[23]

Sometimes the problem starts with vague criteria for when procedures are warranted. That is a hard problem to address. Doctors need discretion in day-to-day decisions because so much of medicine remains art rather than science. Only 18 percent of what physicians do is backed by the gold standard of scientific evidence: the randomized clinical trial. Much of the rest is based on case or cohort studies, or, at the lowest level, simply expert opinion from clinical experience, which is little better than anecdote. Our biases and habits of behavior easily influence choices based on our opinions, which creates risk for patients.[24]

With their wide span of discretion, doctors can feel justified in decisions that are unconsciously bent in the direction of their own financial benefit. This phenomenon arises, for example, among surgeons who perceive that many more people need their own specialty procedure than disinterested doctors believe.[25] Likely, some of the one-third of heart stent insertions that don't benefit patients may fall in this category (as we mentioned in chapter 1).[26] Charles may have encountered a similar situation when he went to an ear, nose, and throat surgeon in Alaska with a sinus problem. The doctor, in private practice, recommended an aggressive and expensive operation, which he would perform himself. A second doctor, employed at a university hospital in New York, instead prescribed a gentle regime of saline solution and medication (which worked). To return to our metaphor of aviation crash investigations, imagine the cost to safety if airline pilots exhibited variation similar to doctors, flying in a personal, idiosyncratic style, with cultural differences about how to take off and land in various parts of the country, and compensation depending on how much risk they were willing to take. To paraphrase our aviation expert, John Nance (introduced in chapter 1), you should not trust a pilot who says, "Watch this!" or a hero doctor's opinions based on personal experience.

At Northwell, during Covid, a centralized clinical team made the calls. In the aviation metaphor, that was like the FAA setting the rules for how to take off and land based on investigation of past incidents. Doctors can use these feedback loops to bring more science into their decisions, applying shared lessons to standardize care (as we will discuss more in chapter 11). Northwell's Covid experience suggests that a large health system could use this mechanism to tackle unexplained variation. But outside the pandemic emergency, David hasn't seen that happen. Hero doctors trained for individualism rather than teamwork resist threats to their autonomy. Large health systems generally haven't reduced unexplained clinical variation, despite its cost and harm to patients.

Large systems also haven't made a dent in the biggest driver of excessive cost, despite their penny pinching, which is low-value care that doesn't help patients, including all those unneeded heart stents. Consolidated systems may have learned how to provide stents a little more cheaply (even while they charge more), but they didn't stop doing unnecessary procedures, which would have saved more money for the society and saved their patients from harm. The reason is not hard to find. Consolidation didn't help because it didn't change the incentives or culture of a medical system that profits from low-value care, a system that is essentially designed to do procedures, charge fees, and make money. Solving these problems would not increase profits—on the contrary, solutions would more likely save money for patients and insurers and cost revenue for health care providers.

This key finding will lead us into the second part of this book, as we consider the path to change. Our investigation tells us that large, coordinated systems can do a better job, marshalling resources and connecting doctors to address problems of disjointed care, to respond robustly in emergencies, and to rapidly apply new discoveries to patients' health. Coordinated systems are a prerequisite to creating the integrated health organizations that can take responsibility for all of a patients' needs, for health care and for wellness, because they can assemble the top-to-bottom services to "own" the entire patient. But size is not enough. Without transforming the economic environment in which health care is practiced, it turns out large and small systems perform pretty much the same.

In the next section, we will investigate how the economic system works—and how Covid is changing it.

THE FINANCIAL EMERGENCY

Health insurance companies and health care providers live in a state of constant war. The system relies on the dubious principle that a balance of power between these adversaries will control prices. Insurance companies collect premiums from employers and buy health care on behalf of their workers. The prospect for cost control in this arrangement assumes insurers will be smart shoppers, creating competition that drives providers to hold down prices and deliver better care. There are many reasons why that doesn't work well, some of which we have already alluded to. In many markets, too few providers exist to produce real competition. Hospital prices are secret and irrational, making it difficult for anyone to evaluate a good or bad deal (hospitals bitterly fought new regulations to make pricing transparent, information that now is showing they charge some clients many times more than others for the same services).[27] And, even without these problems, the system is too complex. Competition works best in our economy when a buyer judges the price and quality of a particular product and makes a decision on the spot, sending a signal directly to the market. In our system, employers pay monthly premiums to insurance companies as a form of employee compensation, making the individual employee the ultimate buyer of the service. But the employee's consideration of a health plan occurs only once, when accepting an offer of a job (if that factors into the decision at all). The employee's preference has no chance of arriving at the point where the price is set, in the annual negotiation between hospital and insurance company.

Let's see how this works when a patient seeks care. Policy makers and employers have tried to reduce cost by forcing each of us to pay more for care through large insurance co-pays and high deductibles, which commonly expose patients to thousands of dollars of out-of-pocket expenses before we can access insurance benefits. The idea behind these charges is to incentivize patients to avoid unnecessary care and to shop by price, creating competition among providers. Research shows it hasn't worked. High deductibles do keep some patients from going to the doctor or filling prescriptions, often denying them care they need but cannot afford (in that sense, this is a form of rationing according to wealth).[28] Once patients enter the health care system, however, deductibles have little impact on the cost of care. The system itself controls how much we pay and what services we receive.

A study by the National Bureau of Economic Research explains why. It looked at where patients chose to go for an MRI of a foot or leg—the most shoppable of medical procedures—and found that on average they drove past six lower-cost options of equivalent quality, paying 79 percent more out of pocket than if they had chosen the cheapest provider within an hour of home. Instead of shopping, patients relied on their doctors' referrals.[29] It's hardly necessary to explain to a reader in our society why a patient would make that choice. Who knows how to find alternate MRI providers, research their price and quality, and somehow make a choice contrary to a doctor's recommendation? Once we are under a doctor's care, taking control of costs or even the amount of care we receive requires unusual sophistication and assertiveness.

Doctors typically have no incentive to refer patients to lower-cost providers. The NBER study found doctors often referred patients for high-cost MRIs at facilities that were part of their own health systems. This is another way consolidation increases cost: large health systems combine with doctor groups, especially money-losing primary care practices, so the doctors will steer patients to their own profitable facilities. Frequently, patients don't care. Insurance insulates them from considering cost after deductibles are fulfilled, as they will be for expensive hospital visits. These factors help explain Roemer's law. Milton Roemer first observed in 1959 that when most people have insurance, new hospitals produce new patients. In a functioning market, hospital construction would generate competition and lower prices. Instead, it generates more care.[30]

Insurance companies do have an incentive to hold down prices, so they can make more money and sell more policies. But they have ways to profit without encouraging competition. When they refuse to pay claims, they keep more money, regardless of whether the claims are valid, and many valid claims are initially turned down. That encourages hospitals to inflate prices for the claims that are paid, covering unpaid work and the administrative cost of fighting with insurers. Theoretically, this is the part of the system that would address low-value care and unexplained clinical variation, because the insurance companies would refuse to pay for care that did not benefit patients. It should come as no surprise, however, that claim review by insurance company employees has not produced that result. The system is set up to pay for procedures, not outcomes, and connecting the two has proved complex and difficult in this economic model (as we shall learn more in the next chapter).

This rickety system has lumbered on for decades with these cracks and fault lines in full view. But when Covid hit, the cracks became chasms and the fault lines became points of failure.

At first, insurers classified the disease as pneumonia, providing much lower reimbursement than the true cost of a complicated case, as we learned from Bruce Meyer, the physician president of Jefferson Health (whom we introduced in chapter 2). And when patient numbers dropped for non-Covid care during the first pandemic surge, few claims were filed and hospitals lost money, but insurance companies continued collecting premiums and banked enormous surpluses.

In New York, Mike Dowling said Northwell lost 80 percent of its non-Covid business while pouring money into unexpected costs for Covid care. With revenue down $1.5 billion, the company faced the need to lay off the heroic nurses who had just pulled the city through the crisis. Some hospitals made that choice, but Northwell did not, instead asking for help from insurance companies that had held back payments.

"The insurance companies were a nightmare and a disaster," Dowling said. "They make it very difficult to get paid. We have reached out to all of the insurance companies that were holding hundreds and hundreds of millions of dollars of our money, asking if they would advance. And they basically almost universally said, 'No.' With minor exceptions, they were not players at all. So, this is where the insurance companies, in my view, demonstrated their true character . . . that they were not interested in any of this other than putting money in the bank."

With hospitals across the country facing financial calamity, Congress stepped in with relief packages that, in their final multi-trillion-dollar scale, exceeded any previous level of US government spending, in peace or wartime.[31] Northwell received over $1 billion and narrowed its loss for the year to about $100 million, Dowling said. For such a large system, that amount was hardly significant. Other, small hospitals faced financial difficulties even with the federal money, and they became targets for consolidation by the larger systems that ended up with healthier balance sheets.

As we learned in chapter 4, some hospitals serving middle-class patients with insurance reduced their losses during the pandemic by refusing transfers from safety-net hospitals that were overrun by poor Black and Brown patients. But they didn't miss out on the government support. Before the Department of Health and Social Services distributed CARES Act funding, it consulted with lobbying organizations representing large hospitals on how to write the formula to allocate the funds.[32] As it worked out, that formula directed twice as much money to the richest hospitals where most patients had private insurance, compared to the poorest, the safety-net hospitals that served the hard-hit Black and Brown communities, which needed money the most.[33] In many cases, those who did the least came out the best.

The insurance companies did extremely well. Remember, the system had received its usual revenue—employers still paid premiums—but insurers paid much less of that to providers. And then the federal government made up that money with huge payments to providers. Considering the health care system as a whole, including insurers and providers, the federal money created an enormous windfall of added funds. The net result: a huge transfer of funds from the federal treasury to shareholders of insurance companies.

That's the commercial part of the system, but more than a third of health care spending comes from Medicaid and Medicare, a larger amount than all private health insurance plans combined.[34] Contrary to the hopes of those who call for "Medicare for all," however, those programs have many of the same flaws as the commercial system. Most of the money flows to fee-for-service medicine that has the same incentives for low-value care (Medicare Advantage is an exception, as we shall see in the next chapter). Covid bared the flaws in the government-paid system, too.

Medicaid (the program for those without financial assets) pays the bills for about two-thirds of the daily care provided by nursing homes. Medicare (the program for the elderly) covers only one hundred days of nursing care, and it funds just 11 percent of nursing home days.[35]

Because Medicaid reimbursements rates are low, nursing homes can't make much money from daily care, but they can make much more by charging Medicare or private insurance for services such as rehabilitation and physical therapy on a fee-for-service basis. These incentives have pushed nursing homes to cut back on staff and cleanliness and to offer more medical services that pay better—even when those services were not needed.

These incentives proved deadly during the Covid crisis. According to an investigation by the *Washington Post*, when the pandemic hit, nursing homes full of vulnerable patients pivoted to offer more profitable Covid care. The *Post* focused on a Michigan nursing home chain with short staffing, filthy bathrooms, and a record of poor infection control, which responded to Covid by offering respiratory care and ventilators.[36] The virus predictably passed to the frail, elderly residents. Nationally, 186,000 residents and staff of nursing homes and long-term-care facilities died of Covid (by August 2021), accounting for 29 percent of all Covid deaths.[37]

The nursing home industry had been declining for some time, as more families chose home-based care and as the facilities struggled to make a profit on Medicaid payments. Covid's financial emergency accelerated that trend. Hospitals stopped referring patients to nursing homes for convalescence, and families began thinking of nursing homes as places where old people catch Covid and die. Although vaccinations rapidly reduced nursing home Covid deaths, beginning in December 2020,[38] the loss of business appeared likely to last much longer.[39]

How should we feel about these failures and the horrendous accumulation of deaths? We naturally feel disappointment when people we trust are overcome by greed during a catastrophe as severe as the Covid pandemic. We want people to be self-sacrificing caregivers regardless of the financial incentives they face (and many individuals do meet that description). But as James Madison wrote, in explaining why our American system of government needed to balance the opposing interests of selfish people, "If men were angels, no government would be necessary." We would offer a corollary: if doctors, hospital administrators, and insurance company executives were angels, medical care would not need a rational system of financial incentives.

Fortunately, we don't need angels or any supernatural help. We have an example of success during Covid. One set of health care providers made it through the pandemic in relatively good financial shape. Health care entities that collected premiums—whether combining insurance with a provider organization or as an HMO—did not suffer the financial crash that faced hospitals on the fee-for-service model. In the next chapter, we will learn more about Geisinger Health, in central Pennsylvania, which owns hospitals and an insurance company and weathered the pandemic. Other examples include the Kaiser Permanente managed care system, based in California but with more than three hundred thousand employees nationally, and Ochsner Health, in Louisiana. These vertically integrated organizations—firms paid to be responsible for their patients' whole health, not just individual visits or procedures—received the money they needed from the right people to take care of the patients who relied on them when the crisis came. In our investigation of this disaster, they were airplanes that made safe landings.

Covid showed that our health care system can work—if it is structured the right way. In the second half of this book, we will look at the hopeful lessons that came from the crisis, showing the path to deep, permanent improvements to the health care system that we know will work—because they already are working.

PART II

The Health System Healing Itself

Chapter 7

Rise of the Payvider

Aligning Incentives

In rural central and northeastern Pennsylvania, incomes tend to be low and the towns have seen better days, with long-closed iron furnaces and rail yards made into historic sites. Small businesses employ much of the workforce. The population is older and aging. More people die than are born.[1] The ingredients were present here for the Covid failures we depicted in the first half of this book—age, income and occupation, and distance from large, connected urban hospitals. Yet this unlikely place has produced an innovative health care system that successfully navigated the Covid crisis, emerging financially stable and with a record of caring for patients in ways that addressed many of the serious concerns of the pandemic.

The Geisinger system includes nine hospitals, many clinics, pharmacies, a medical school, research facilities, and a health insurance plan with more than half a million members. It is among the largest employers in the communities it serves and, as a nonprofit, accepts all patients, regardless of health care coverage. And it has taken on responsibility for much more than traditional health care, also reaching into areas usually thought of as public health and population health to address the well-being of the geographic area as a whole. With startling frankness, the company makes this statement about itself on its public website:

> The region we serve has struggled economically for decades; community health status proves that zip codes and income levels are as essential health predictors as cholesterol levels or BMI. Our communities have big problems with diabetes, heart disease, opioid addiction—all issues we

should be able to prevent. So, just as we tackle genomic factors, we must address social issues like poverty, and food deserts, environmental factors . . . everything that makes it hard to achieve and maintain wellness—for individuals, and for our communities.[2]

Doctors around the country have told us about their frustration with stabilizing low-income patients with diabetic emergencies in the hospital—at great expense—only to send them home to communities where the healthy food needed to manage the disease is unavailable or unaffordable. David's daughter Rachel Nash felt a sense of futility over this issue at her hospital practice in southern New Jersey, as she described in chapter 2. In chapter 5, we learned about the public health program Leana Wen created in Baltimore to bring fresh food to urban neighborhood bodegas. Geisinger's solution is more direct. Its doctors give "Fresh Food Farmacy" prescriptions to diabetic patients who lack food security. The prescriptions come with cooking equipment such as measuring cups, spoons and recipes, twenty hours of training, and ongoing provision of enough fresh groceries to serve ten meals a week to patients' entire families.[3] Feeding people healthy food works better and costs less than treating them in the hospital. Indeed, the value of all the food produced by every farm and fishing boat in America amounts to a fraction of what we spend as a nation on diabetes care, which by itself consumes a fourth of health care spending.[4]

No one should be surprised that hungry people tend to be unhealthy. Research shows that people who are food insecure are twice as likely to report poor physical or mental health and to heavily use the emergency room, and a map of food insecurity in the United States neatly overlays with rates of diabetes, obesity, and hypertension.[5] A history of malnutrition also is associated with severe Covid outcomes.[6] In any humanely designed health system, everyone would get the food they need. In our system, health insurance companies have begun to recognize immense cost savings could be available from providing food to some of their members.[7] A 2019 study in Massachusetts found that delivering just ten meals a week tailored to the medical needs of certain patients reduced their need for health care, saving an estimated $753 per recipient per month.[8]

Despite these obvious benefits, however, most hospitals would not establish a solution like Geisinger's Fresh Food Farmacy because they cannot capture the savings from prevention but would lose revenue from care. When patients with diabetes adopt healthy diets and come to the hospital less frequently, those savings go to the providers' natural adversaries: the health insurance companies.

But at Geisinger, the equation works differently. The company also owns the health insurance plan that covers many of its patients. The company does well when its members do.

"We've always been really big believers in population health and prevention," said Jaewon Ryu, Geisinger's president and CEO, himself a physician. "We've had our own health plan since 1985, and so with that comes the mindset of getting upstream, preventing, getting out into the communities, out into the nursing homes, out into the homes. These are all things that we've long believed, even from before anybody had even heard of Covid."[9]

Geisinger's reach into its communities allowed it to tackle aspects of the Covid crisis in a coordinated way that wasn't possible in places where hospitals, primary care providers, and public health officials all controlled different pieces of the problem. Early on, Ryu said, Geisinger teams went into nursing homes to help with PPE and infection control, because protecting residents there would keep them out of hospital beds later. Geisinger had built an at-home care program for the sickest 3 percent of its own patients. During Covid, this home care allowed patients to stay away from the hospital during times of high infection risk, without missing out on treatment during the lockdown, as so many patients did in other parts of the country. Geisinger also broadened the at-home program for other, less sick patients, as well as those with Covid. The program allowed doctors to discharge Covid patients earlier and still receive care, freeing up hospital capacity and reducing the risk of having them recuperate in nursing homes. The company even got its integrated pharmacy involved, ramping up delivery to patients during lockdowns so they could keep taking their medications without leaving home.

"A lot of the care that used to happen inside the hospital, we were able to do more and more of it out in the communities, out in the homes," Ryu said. "We were able to actually pivot our Geisinger at Home program to even take care of Covid patients that were probably a day or two shy of being able to go home. . . . We were able to expedite discharges and follow them up in the home with those care teams. For some folks, whether Covid or not, we were able to launch more services in the home and avoid an admission, which, of course, was critical not just from a capacity standpoint, but also just from a safety one. If there's anything we can do out in the home environment that avoids an admission, that's something that we're very interested in doing."

Across the country, public health departments traced contacts of Covid-positive patients to control the spread of the disease, but Geisinger took on that responsibility, too. As we learned in chapter 5, many communities struggled to ramp up contact tracing, fielding poorly trained teams or even using contracted phone banks that had no connection to the areas they were trying to serve—with high rates of refusal to participate. Ryu said Geisinger already employed preventive health teams that could move naturally into the role of finding contacts in their communities, where residents were familiar with those workers and the company.

"In our world at Geisinger, just culturally and how we are, we did very much view that as our role because it was a mere extension for our preventive care teams, filling care gaps, doing proactive outreach," Ryu said. "It wasn't that much of a departure for those teams to then also be reaching out to folks who had recently tested positive to do that contact tracing. And so we rolled out a program fairly early."

Ryu's own stellar career developed at the intersection of health care, the social determinants of health, and the economic policies that influence both. As the child of a physician family in the northern suburbs of Chicago, he launched early on the educational path to become a doctor himself, but his eyes opened to issues of equity and prevention as an AmeriCorps volunteer with the I Have A Dream Foundation, tutoring and offering emotional support to poor, inner-city children. That interest led to studies in health policy, public health, and leadership. On a break from medical training, he earned a degree in law and practiced as a corporate lawyer in health care; then he finished his MD and practiced as an emergency room doctor. He also worked at various organizations with unified systems of care, including at the VA, Kaiser Permanente (America's largest fully integrated health care system), and Humana (a large, publicly held health insurance company). With uniquely diverse skills—medical, financial, policy-related, and legal—he joined Geisinger in 2016, implementing its at-home program, and became the company's head in 2019.[10]

Geisinger is a vertically integrated health care system. It is a payer, with its insurance plan, as well as a provider, with clinics, doctors, and pharmacies. David likes the word *payvider* for this kind of organization, which unifies the incentives of traditional adversaries—on one side, the health plans avoiding paying claims and, on the other, the doctors and hospitals submitting them. Putting the two together does more than simplify the process of paying for health care; it also aligns providers with maintaining plan members' health rather than only healing them after they become sick. The alliance with the insurance plan is key. As much as Americans dislike health insurance companies—and polling indicates these are the most disliked and least trusted of organizations in health care—their role carries the strongest financial incentive to reduce unnecessary care and to keep patients well and out of the hospital.[11]

Consider, for example, the home care that helped carry Geisinger through the pandemic and that assists its sickest patients every day. Providers can't earn as much money from home care as they can by admitting patients to the hospital and serving them there. So why do it? Ryu said home care is better for patients. But the reason the company can afford to work in its patients' homes, despite lower payment, is because about half of them are also members of its own insurance plan. As a provider, Geisinger loses revenue for home care compared to hospital stays, but as a payer the revenue loss becomes savings.

Payviders do best by keeping members healthy, preventing illness, and providing the right amount of care for the lowest price. Attention to outcomes is built in, because high-quality care costs less in the long run, with fewer flare-ups of chronic conditions or failed procedures that call for follow-up care. Also, the market has a better chance to work— with customer choice influencing price and quality—because patients and employers buy from a single company that controls both the health plan and the provider system, rather than working with two companies at war over reimbursements.

Payviders did better during the pandemic. Their health plans brought in revenue to keep them financially stable, and their large, consolidated provider organizations helped them manage during the crisis. And the pandemic did well by the model, creating financial disruption that has unexpectedly encouraged the consolidation of payers and providers. In 2021, the McKinsey & Company consultancy advised health plans to buy providers or otherwise partner in integrated managed care systems, noting that payviders were more profitable and had happier customers, better outcomes, and lower costs.[12] Providers moved this direction, too: in November 2021, Jefferson Health acquired majority ownership of a nonprofit health plan covering elderly and low-income residents in Philadelphia, a way of better serving neglected communities and capturing overall savings.[13]

We will explore each of these issues and trends later in this chapter, in addition to looking at some of the other payment models designed to increase health care quality and lower cost. Even if that doesn't sound like beach reading, please stick with us. These are some of the biggest problems facing our country—regarding our well-being and our finances—and we will offer practical solutions to them. Yes, the topic can be complicated enough to trigger your amygdala's instinctive fear response, but please don't flee; we promise that the key concepts we have already explained will make it all clear.

And, finally, we will remember, before the chapter is over, that there is something more important than economics at the heart of these issues—good health itself, for one, and also the deeper community values that motivate us regardless of money. No prescription for reform should ignore the powerful pro-social energy inside all of us. Why, after all, do we care about the tragedy of strangers' Covid deaths and the outrageous inequities they exposed? Not because of money.

Economic incentives alone don't explain Geisinger's success, according to Jaewon Ryu. For one thing, the incentives aren't perfectly aligned. Geisinger is not the only game in town for health insurance or medical care. Half the patients it treats are not covered by its own health plan. It also serves patients with other kinds of health insurance, as well as those without coverage. And when Geisinger works on prevention, non-members benefit, too.

A sense of mission and community motivates many health care providers and organizations, including profit-making companies and not-for-profits such as Geisinger. When Covid hit, Geisinger began prevention work out of "muscle memory," as Ryu put it, with powerful awareness that in the small cities and countryside of central Pennsylvania, infected residents would come to the system's own hospitals. Going upstream would protect the system from being overwhelmed. Far from major cities, this connection between community and health provider is unavoidable, as sick people all end up in the same places.

Ryu said that connection has existed since 1915, when Geisinger was founded.

"Abigail Geisinger started this hospital so that people could get their care closer to home, and, oh, by the way, it happened to coincide with an outbreak of typhoid," Ryu said. "I really do believe there's something to that founder's story that's still amazingly part of our DNA, in that interconnectedness with our community. And lo and behold, a pandemic breaks out, and who does the community look to for health solutions to solve this on behalf of the community? They've looked to us, and it's a huge responsibility that our organization has, but it's a function of how closely knit we are with the communities in which we operate."

Is Geisinger's community connection unique? If so, perhaps its model cannot be replicated. Geisinger has attracted national attention for innovation over two decades, but some analysts view geography as the key to the system's success.[14] It is among the largest employers in the small cities it serves.[15] In larger metro areas, health care providers' community role is less obvious.

Cynicism comes easily in the big-money world of modern health care, but we think there is something real here that is worth considering for the creation of a better system. Every geographic area is unique, but communities exist in many kinds of places—recall, from chapter 4, that Rush University Medical Center has built community links to some of the most depressed urban neighborhoods in Chicago. Perhaps, rather than geography, the key to this kind of innovation is to create systems that value these human linkages. Most of us do put connections to people ahead of money. In communities, that can mean working together to build something good that we share. We will learn later in this chapter and later in the book about how connections and partnerships between businesses and organizations in communities can lead to better health. Just as we learned about Philadelphia's community-based violence prevention in chapter 5, these efforts are not flashy and won't make anyone rich or famous, but they can move the culture in better directions, with profound results.

One of the greatest benefits of fixing how we pay for health care may be to get money out of the way of these better angels of our nature. As we now begin consideration of the dismal science of health care

economics, this is a good impetus to get it right. We believe that perverse incentives have distorted health care into a system that rewards
mediocrity and divides people who should work together. If money
instead flows to a system built for prevention, equity, and quality care,
perhaps a virtuous cycle will ensue, as our instincts for caring and connection are allowed to reemerge.

THE PUZZLE OF PAYMENT

Why do Americans pay for health care through such a complex,
unplanned system that hardly anyone understands? The answer may go
back to our culture and form of government (as we discussed in chapter
3). When the modern practice of medicine arose early in the twentieth century, other industrialized Western countries adopted nationalized programs (Germany in 1883, France 1928, United Kingdom
1948). In the United States, with power distributed to the states and
a check-and-balance federal system that makes change difficult, doctors successfully resisted creating a national health care plan, and we
muddled through with regions and industries developing their own
solutions to the rising costs of an increasingly technical and professional medical system.[16]

Health care coverage became commonplace in the United States in
the 1940s. Hospitals had begun selling prepaid coverage during the
Great Depression as a way of obtaining steady revenue, plans that
coalesced into the nonprofit Blue Cross insurance company, owned by
the American Hospital Association. Doctors started Blue Shield as their
own version of that concept. These plans created the fee-for-service,
volume-based payment model. They set prices with a cost-plus method,
with doctors' fees based on "customary and reasonable charges" they
set themselves and hospital reimbursement based on their costs and
return on capital. The system encouraged price increases and facility investment, whether needed or not. When the federal government
started Medicaid and Medicare in 1965, it adopted the same model.
Fee-for-service coverage continued as the norm when Blue Cross and
Blue Shield severed connections with provider associations and became
indistinguishable from the other commercial insurance companies that
entered the market. Without a mechanism to control costs or effective

price competition, the payment system set off the race for unconstrained investment and fee increases into the 1970s.[17]

A parallel history also began in the 1940s, when California shipbuilding magnate Henry Kaiser and doctor and hospital founder Sydney Garfield began offering health care directly to Kaiser's workers during World War II. The system they rapidly developed included aid stations and hospitals, offering all the health care that workers might need. At the end of the war, they opened the system to other employers, evolving it into three parts, with an insurance company, hospitals, and a doctor group, all connected and coordinated under the same ownership, and providing the totality of health care for members whose employers bought in. To use the jargon of health care, the system was capitated (meaning a single price pays for all of a member's care) and closed (meaning members can obtain care only from the system's doctors and facilities). These two features allowed the company to capture savings from prevention and improvements in quality, and they took away incentives for increased volume and fees for services (there were no such fees).[18] Seventy-five years later, the Kaiser Permanente system now serves more than twelve million members in eight states and wins high quality rankings.[19] Its vertically integrated system, with salaried doctors who can spend more time with patients and address issues at home, with a strong emphasis on prevention, and with controlled costs, has become the model of successful managed care.

Unfortunately, the Kaiser model remains a niche, with only 8 percent of Americans enrolled in health plans offered by health care providers in 2015.[20] Kaiser Permanente was born at a unique moment in history, when World War II's economic disruption generated rapid change. Henry Kaiser faced a labor shortage and needed strong incentives to attract workers to shipbuilding. Free health care brought them in. Those circumstances have not recurred—until now. The economic disruption of the pandemic bears an eerie similarity to the 1940s. Once again, employers are competing for workers amid a shortage. Many are using Kaiser's strategy, offering more health care as an enticement, including huge employers such as Amazon, which added hundreds of thousands of workers during the pandemic, offering a health plan and bonuses for new hires with proof of vaccination against Covid.[21] (We will discuss more about employers' roles in chapter 10.)

Outside of times of national emergency, America struggled to manage health care as in the Kaiser model, with repeated advances and setbacks. In 1973, Congress passed the Health Maintenance Organization Act to encourage more Kaiser-like firms to form and enroll patients, with hopes for lower-cost care. Within twenty years, HMOs had thirty-five million patients.[22] But early models of HMOs made mistakes with a gatekeeper design that created incentives for primary care doctors to deny access to specialists. Also, Americans hated not being able to choose their own doctors. In 1996, a doctor testified to Congress that she had killed a patient by denying needed care when she worked as a cog in the machine of an HMO (although the situation she described could have happened under any insurance plan with exclusions for certain procedures).[23] Soon HMOs had become all-purpose villains in Hollywood movies, cursed by Helen Hunt in *As Good as It Gets* and even condemned in a children's movie about talking animals, *Dr. Dolittle*.[24]

Humana was the largest HMO provider, and the cultural backlash tarnished its image. Doctors boycotted some of its hospitals because of cost controls, and other insurers steered away from them because they believed Humana treated its own insurance plans better. The company was beset by lawsuits. In 1993, with a falling stock price, and anticipating passage of President Bill Clinton's health care bill, then pending in Congress, Humana unwound its vertical integration, selling all seventy-five hospitals.[25] (David was a Humana board member from 2009 to 2019.) The country seemed to be headed in a new direction, toward Clinton's concept of managed competition. But in 1994 the bill collapsed politically and Republicans swept into control of Congress for the first time in forty years.[26] The age of HMOs ended (today, few care even to use the acronym), and health care cost increases entered one of the fastest periods of growth.[27]

But managed care did make progress, with Medicare Advantage as the largest-scale success. Passed into law in 1997, Medicare's managed care option now covers 42 percent of beneficiaries, or 26 million older Americans, and it is growing at a rate of 2 million people a year.[28] Medicare Advantage pays private insurance companies a capitated fee—a set amount per person—to provide all care for seniors who sign up. Quality is assured by a star-rating system of forty measures, including points for medical outcomes and patient satisfaction, with insurers receiving bonuses of up to 10 percent for getting top scores (this is a form of so-called value-based payment). In 2021, plans earning four or five stars served 80 percent of those enrolled and received bonuses.[29] And Medicare Advantage plans also have more ability to decide where and how care is provided than traditional Medicare, using prior authorization, provider networks, cost sharing, and other ways of reducing use of medical care.[30]

Seniors like Medicare Advantage because they pay less and receive more services. Often the plans charge no premium; cover prescription drugs, vision, and dental care; and offer preventive services. Many even provide benefits such as free gym memberships or rides to appointments and senior centers. In 2021, 55 percent of Medicare Advantage plans offered home-delivered meals or groceries to their senior clients.[31] David's aged mother enrolled in a Humana home health subsidiary's plan. A Humana worker visited her Florida home and departed with the shag rug from her bathroom floor—a tripping hazard. For the plan, these extra expenses make sense because they can reduce medical claims. Active, safe, well-fed seniors need less medical care, and that saves money. If the plan succeeds in its prevention work and earns a bonus for high quality, it can make a profit, despite the flat payment from Medicare (but profits are limited, with excess going back to the government). It turns out that Medicare Advantage saves money for seniors and for the government.[32]

How did these plans fare during Covid? Unfortunately, the Centers for Medicare and Medicaid Services stopped collecting some data, and even froze some quality scores, due to Covid disruptions and to avoid unintentionally creating financial penalties for emergency innovations.[33] But the limited information we do have suggests that greater flexibility for at-home and nonmedical care may have helped keep Medicare Advantage users out of nursing homes and other in-patient facilities where they could have run greater risk of infection.[34] More fundamentally, healthier seniors were more likely to survive Covid, and the balance of evidence shows that people enrolled in Medicare Advantage are healthier, by self-report and outcome measures, and that they receive higher-quality care.[35]

Screenwriters may not have liked managed care in the 1990s, but Medicare Advantage seems to have proved the superiority of a well-designed managed care program over fee-for-service medicine.

The control in this vast experiment is the traditional Medicare program, which pays for care as bills come in from doctors and hospitals according to government-established standard rates. Medicare Advantage costs less, delivers better results, and is rapidly winning in competition with the traditional program during open enrollment periods, as seniors switch.[36]

Despite this evidence, however, the movement to value-based payment elsewhere in the health care system has stalled. The Affordable Care Act, which passed in 2010, mostly addressed access to health care, not cost or quality. It increased the population with private insurance or Medicaid, and it regulated away some of the insurance companies' worst practices. They were required to pay for 100 percent of many preventive care services, could no longer exclude clients from coverage because of preexisting conditions, and were required to cover maternity and to charge women the same premiums as men. But the ACA made little attempt to control cost. Instead, it invested in studies of new payment models. The bill created an Innovation Center within the Centers for Medicare and Medicaid Services and gave it billions of dollars to experiment with new designs. Unfortunately, after a decade, few of the new ideas have worked. The vast majority didn't save money or improve care.[37]

The experiments were various and often extraordinarily complex. That was one of their flaws, and it is also a good reason to avoid explaining them here. In general, they changed how Medicare paid for care. Instead of paying fees for services based only on the volume of care, they also accounted for quality and outcomes, the idea behind value-based payment. The concept shifts some financial risk from the payer to providers. Here's how: Under the traditional, fee-for-service model, the payer can be billed for a botched operation the same as a successful one, and then also pays for follow-up care for the patient to address the provider's own mistakes. A bad provider can make more money than a good one. Under a value-based plan, poor results yield less compensation for the provider. For example, a hospital could earn a bonus or, in rare versions, incur a penalty, depending on whether it achieved objective measures of the outcome of a procedure.

These experiments have produced disappointing results for several reasons. Some of the reasons they didn't work were peculiar to their experimental design, but others were more fundamental. Optimists point to problems that could be avoided with changes to the experimental design. For example, providers' involvement was voluntary, with a short period of commitment, which allowed them to game the system, opting in only if they expected to make more money and quitting if they didn't. A different approach would give the idea a better test, with larger incentives, longer contracts, less complexity, and mandatory involvement. With full, long-term engagement, providers would change their basic way of doing business and yield savings and better medical outcomes, according to the optimists' view.[38]

But more fundamental problems could also persist. The complexity in these arrangements arises for a reason: it is difficult to measure the quality of a doctor using statistics. Consider a parallel effort that failed, the 2001 No Child Left Behind Act, which sought to reward and punish public schools and teachers for the quality of student outcomes based on standardized tests. Test scores couldn't measure the most important qualities of teaching—knowledge, caring, communication skills, organization, patience—nor did they account for the vastly different contexts of American schools. The law became unpopular for distorting education and punishing the wrong people.[39] By the time it was repealed, a decade later, American education had gotten markedly worse compared to that in other nations.[40]

A good surgeon stays current with research, self-evaluates, listens, uses teamwork, and adheres to protocols, but changes them when necessary. We know little about how to objectively score those characteristics. The quality measures in value-based plans look at stats such as mortality, postoperative infection, unexpected return to the operating room (to fix something that went wrong), or readmission to the hospital within thirty days. Bonuses and penalties are based on these numbers, but the measures are too blunt and the bar is set too low to produce much improvement. By analogy, you can encourage excellent restaurant service with larger tips, but not if you give servers special rewards just because the food isn't poisoned.

Better, more patient-centered measures would help. For example, did the procedure allow the patient to return to treasured life activities? But those measures wouldn't address the problem of complexity (and might exacerbate it). Nor would they address the problem of procedures that were not needed in the first place or that could have been prevented with better ongoing care. Some value-based payments simply add onto an underlying fee-for-service model. The at-risk payment then only partially fixes the broken system, leaving its fundamental design intact, with misaligned incentives generating unnecessary procedures and ignoring prevention. To use another analogy, it is as if a car mechanic chose to fix a poorly running engine by adding new components rather than replacing the part that wasn't working correctly.

In those cases where tinkering with fee-for-service has worked, it drove deeper change, often in unexpected ways. The best reforms forced doctors and hospitals to think differently. As we explained in the previous chapter, we don't believe market-based reform can transform the health care system, because no real market for health care exists. But two market-based ideas, called transparency and bundling, have produced unintended benefits, because they addressed the psychology of health care providers and changed their culture.

Price transparency has made little impact on patients' buying choices, the prerequisite for business competition, for the reasons we discussed in the previous chapter—health care choices are too complex for shopping, selection of services is largely guided by physicians, and buyers are insulated from costs by insurance and middlemen. But if price transparency didn't lower prices, quality transparency has made a meaningful impact on quality of care. Patient advocates (David among them) long pushed for openness about hospital quality issues, calling for comparative grading and release of information on infection control and errors. They expected the information would move patients to choose better providers, which would drive competition for improved care. Hospitals fought transparency reforms for the same reason. But when the data came out, it was providers who paid attention, not patients. Hospital administrators and doctors studied ratings and error reports, looking at their own work and looking at their competitors' and colleagues' results. That knowledge led to serious and sustained efforts to improve. Perhaps the driver was embarrassment, pride, or a desire to be the best. Whatever it was, it helped change medical culture for the better.[41]

Bundling of care also was intended to make shopping easier and to reduce cost. In bundling programs, providers combine all the services for a hospital stay or bout of illness into a single up-front price instead of billing afterward for each examination or pill. For a knee replacement, for example, a bundle would allow you to choose the best deal in advance rather than receiving many unpredictable bills from different providers, such as the surgeon, anesthesiologist, hospital, lab, pharmacy, and so on. When Medicare tried this approach through its Innovation Center, however, it ended up paying more.[42] A review of all the experiments showed savings on lower-extremity joint replacements but mixed results for everything else.[43]

But research and experience have demonstrated that payment bundling can improve the quality of care. Jaewon Ryu studied how this happened at Geisinger and wrote about it with coauthors in the *Harvard Business Review*. Geisinger joined a network that connected medical centers to large employers, including Walmart, GE, Lowe's Home Improvement, and JetBlue, offering surgeries to their employees at set prices paid entirely by the employer. Workers would travel from around the country for cardiac, joint replacement, and spinal surgeries. To win the work from the employers, providers had to meet stiff quality and price demands. That was hard. Some hospitals needed two or three times more money than the employers were paying, and they were rejected. Geisinger and other providers that successfully joined the program had to redesign how they treated patients, developing improved teamwork, better evaluation of their conditions, concierge support for them as visitors, and careful review of cost and avoidance of waste. It took a long time to make the changes—more than a year for one procedure, Ryu wrote—and required broad involvement from staff, including the company's top leaders. But the work paid off. The surgeries came in at the planned cost, with dramatically higher quality and exceptional patient satisfaction. Working as a team to optimize the procedure had improved the outcome for patients. The improved internal systems also, incidentally, ended up reducing unnecessary procedures. Doctors at the bundled-care sites began turning down many surgeries that had been recommended by patients' home providers, prescribing less intrusive non-surgical remedies. That happened 52 percent of the time with recommendations for the most common spinal operation.[44]

We believe this idea worked because it transformed providers, at least for these procedures. These flat payments from employers remind us of Henry Kaiser paying for health care for his shipbuilding workers, leaving out the middleman of an insurance company. Providers had to adopt new ways of working together to meet the constraint of a set price, the necessity to coordinate care and share revenue, and the demand for quality, and that meant finding ways to avoid mistakes and weed out waste.

Why didn't Medicare consistently obtain savings in this model? It did in a 1998 bundling experiment for heart bypass operations at six hospitals, which demonstrated higher quality and lower cost.[45] But the agency didn't follow those lessons with its Innovation Center trials. In contrast to the clear and demanding requirements set by the private employers, Medicare issued arcane and constantly changing rules for participation. It also made the other mistakes we have already noted, with voluntary participation and inadequate financial incentives. For joint replacements, Medicare used a three-year average of costs to set the bundled price, but since costs for the procedure were falling during that time, it ended up paying an old, higher price. For cardiac surgery, complexities about knowing the severity of illness caused Medicare to pay too much.[46]

A commonality emerges among managed care innovations that have worked. Rather than adding fixes to the fee-for-service model like after-market car parts, they adopt features that change how the engine works, drawn from the success of vertically integrated health care systems. These systems align incentives for high quality, low price, and less waste, and they unify responsibility in leaders who can coordinate the complex dance of technologically advanced medical care. In this discussion, we have left out many other managed care innovations. Some work better than others, and the reasons often involve a lot more details than we want to share here. But, in general, the ideas that work tend to fall on a continuum closer to the integrated systems and further from the traditional fee-for-service model. When the health care system is paid for health, rather than for care, it performs better.

At Geisinger, innovations like these have been going on a long time. In the early 2000s, the company introduced a fixed-price cardiac operation with a ninety-day warranty and received national media attention. The gamble behind the idea was that cardiac surgery could be improved to the point that the need for follow-up care could be greatly reduced, allowing Geisinger to absorb that cost within an overall bundled price. To achieve the necessary quality leap, Geisinger's seven cardiac surgeons had to eliminate variation in how they performed the operation— they all had different styles and ways of doing things. They agreed on the forty best-practice steps for the procedure that they would always follow without fail. A single missed pre-op step meant a cancelled surgery.[47] Geisinger later expanded the approach to other procedures and aspects of the patient experience. The system even offers a lifetime guarantee on hip and knee replacements—for as long as the patient remains covered by a Geisinger health plan.[48]

Geisinger is an exceptional company, with a history and culture that have pushed it in these directions. As a payvider, it has also figured out how to make money on prevention and quality care (for example, using the lifetime guarantee to keep members in its health plan). The payvider model is a proven success that holds promise for the future. As we shall see in the next section, it is spreading, and Covid is accelerating that change.

HOW COVID IS POWERING CHANGE

Covid created a unique moment in history. It disrupted patterns of behavior that had seemed fixed and opened up futures that had seemed impossible, even in areas of life distant from health. Office buildings emptied and the purpose of cities seemed to change overnight. Business travel halted and failed to return to previous volumes, with many experts predicting it never would.[49] The role of government suddenly changed, with federal spending jumping from a fifth of the economy to a third, and new safety net payments that decreased poverty by the largest increment ever recorded.[50] Millions of people poured into the streets in the largest mass protests in our history, demanding an end to racial discrimination.[51] The president, rejected by voters for his handling of the pandemic, refused to accept defeat, and his supporters stormed the Capitol in an attempt to overturn the election.[52] Real estate and stock prices spiked amid pandemic death and economic disruption, workers became scarce while unemployment remained high, and hospitals were driven to adopt crisis standards of care to fight a preventable disease with widely available vaccines. It was a bewildering time. In this fluid moment, anything seemed possible—bad or good.

In health care, generations have come and gone with experts fully understanding the flaws in our payment system but unable to fix them. Writing in 1970, Barbara and John Ehrenreich declared that health care was in crisis because of high cost, fragmented delivery of care, lack of access by the uninsured, and deep racial inequities.[53] They were the nation's top health policy researchers at the time, frequently in the news. In 1976, Sylvia Law noted, "It is fast becoming a tradition for both popular and scholarly articles to begin with a litany of figures contrasting spiraling costs with appallingly bad American health indices," and she then cited the 7 percent of GNP that health care cost with "high" per capita spending of $324 (now 18 percent and $11,582).[54] The successful Kaiser Permanente system operated this entire time and was held up as an ideal model, but as reform efforts repeatedly failed, Kaiser came to seem like a unicorn, the unique product of an accident of history that was unlikely to recur. But perhaps now is finally the time. History seems to have become a good deal more permissive about what can happen.

Payviders had already begun to consolidate before the pandemic because of the operational and financial advantages they can achieve for owners. By combining primary care, hospitals, and insurers, they share electronic medical records effectively, capturing the totality of each patients' information, including prescriptions, labs, and surgeons' notes, all together. With that data, the large organization can start to use analytics for care management. Vertical integration also allows for a better experience as patients move through the system and, as we have explained, as the system offers prevention and other benefits upstream of the doctor's office to capture savings for the health plan. Finally, payviders can reduce the inefficiency of billing and the burnout it imposes on caregivers.[55] Americans currently spend 27 percent of our health care dollars on administration. Research indicates a simpler billing system would save 15 percent of our total spending (that's double the amount we need to cover all the uninsured).[56] The business logic of these advantages, with the benefit of "owning the whole patient," has helped justify big mergers in recent years and motivated provider organizations to start their own health plans.[57]

There is evidence that these arrangements work. Consider the Medicare Advantage program that we discussed in the previous section. An insurance company offering it can save money and provide better results by keeping seniors healthy, but the insurer still must rely on doctors and hospitals to provide care when it is needed and pay their bills in the same contentious and inefficient way as under other plans. When a vertically integrated system offers Medicare Advantage, however, it can also control the quality of medical care and coordinate data and management of patients within a single system of plan and hospital. In 2017, research at Harvard University confirmed that payviders do, indeed, get higher scores on quality from Medicare Advantage than traditional payers, including on patient satisfaction, clinical care, and response to complaints.[58] Commercial insurance customers have been happier with payviders, too, with Kaiser Permanente leading the nation in both customer and employee satisfaction.[59]

Jaewon Ryu said Geisinger has compared outcomes for its patient-members with those who are only patients or only members. "We have the data that support this," he said. "The patients do the best when we have the fully integrated experience, where they are our member, and they're using our facilities and our physicians and staff. And I think that's a function of everything being so integrated. When it's integrated, things are better coordinated. Dosage changes on your medication and boom, an outreach person from the pharmacy team reaches out and drops a new script, and you have the new pill bottle at your doorstep the next day."

Despite the advantages, however, creating a payvider organization has proved difficult. Combining a provider and payer means merging disparate cultures from far sides of the traditional battlefield between doctor and insurance company. The two have entirely different perspectives. Providers think in terms of individual patients and their immediate needs. Payers instead see patients as populations and think of their aggregate needs with analytics and actuarial calculations. Providers that start their own insurance plans have struggled to adopt the broad perspective necessary, and some have failed.

Sentara Health, a nonprofit based in Norfolk, Virginia, ultimately succeeded, creating a health plan that covers half its patients. The plan helped carry Sentara through the pandemic financially. But building a plan that could compete took fifteen years. The health system had to add a lot of new and unfamiliar capabilities and skills, had to transform its culture and operations to coordinate medical and plan operations, and had to make doctors understand that just because the in-house plan was paying, that didn't mean they should get a special deal.[60] In 2015, McKinsey consultants, looking at problems like those, and the woeful record of failures, noted that providers usually succeeded in starting health plans only in special situations such as Geisinger's or Kaiser's, with unique circumstances due to geography or history.[61]

Insurance companies have a better chance of creating a vertically integrated system by buying a provider, but it's not easy. A successful closed system, like Kaiser, requires enormous scale to provide members with all the features of contemporary medicine within its own facilities and employees, with primary care, specialists, hospitals, labs, imaging facilities, and many other parts. An open system, which owns the payer and provider, but also works with non-members, works best if the provider has enough market share to make investments in prevention and public health pay off. Geisinger's formula works in part because it serves small communities—remember, Geisinger staff knew that people who caught Covid in their communities were probably coming to their hospitals, so public health efforts at contact tracing would benefit the system. Humana reached a national scale during the HMO era of the 1990s, but its efforts backfired when its large scale came with a reputation as a bully—among doctors, the public, and other health plans—and the company ended up selling its hospitals.

But several factors have changed since the 1990s. Technology now adds to the advantages of being a payvider, creating opportunities for services and synergies that never existed before. And patients have changed. A generation after Helen Hunt's movie diatribe, most of us are accustomed to getting care from a large organization rather than a stand-alone family doctor, and we don't object to being steered where health plans want us to go rather than always getting to choose our own doctors.[62] Finally, a third option has emerged, side-stepping the need for an acquisition and merger by either a payer or a provider: partnerships that create payviders through contracts between insurance plans and health systems. Although less common, these partnership payvider organizations can produce the benefits of vertical integration without some of the challenges or risks.[63] The advantages slowly started a new trend toward vertical integration.

Then came the pandemic. It supercharged the payvider trend.

In the previous chapter, we outlined the unequal impact of Covid's financial disruptions. Small, private practices were crushed, and independent hospitals suffered serious losses, despite receiving government aid. Large provider systems did better because of their scale, but they still needed the federal bail-out. Payviders were more insulated from the financial crunch because, although Covid hurt the provider side, premiums kept flowing into the insurance plan side. And insurance companies did best of all, banking huge surpluses, because they paid far lower claims but continued to receive premiums. This financial imbalance powered rapid consolidation. As independent doctors faced financial ruin, their practices rushed to merge with large medical groups. David watched as doctors who had loathed managed care traded their treasured independence for the security of a paycheck—and saw managed care systems turning down these private practice refugees, because they would need retraining to function in team-based settings (an issue we will discuss in the next chapter). Insurance companies with fat balance sheets went shopping for struggling providers to buy.

Lawrence Prybil, the Kentucky-based health system expert we introduced in the last chapter, noted that single hospitals or small groups suffered similarly to the private practice doctor, unable to handle the weight of surging Covid cases in their local areas. Multi-state systems, by contrast, were able to balance patients, staff, and resources across regions when some areas had higher infection rates than others. Providers with their own health plans seemed to fare the best of all.

"The advantages of being part of a system were clearly powerful," Prybil said. "My sense is that this whole experience will drive consolidation more, it will continue and accelerate. It'll still take years for that process to continue. But I think that the net impact of dealing with the pandemic has been to provide additional force and motivation to pursue consolidation."

But Prybil also noted another movement, to better connect hospitals with communities and public health workers. Prybil has guided many hospital boards and leaders, in nonprofit and for-profit systems. He believes, like Jaewon Ryu at Geisinger (earlier in this chapter), that health systems' organizational missions and values are more than just words for some and that they do strive to improve their patients' and community's total health. Prybil said some hospital boards made painful, daring sacrifices during the pandemic—such as refusing to lay off staff when revenues were down—to support their communities and employees. He pointed to the famous 2019 statement by the Business Roundtable, which said the purpose of corporations should include supporting communities, not only making profit for shareholders.[64] He has worked recently with the Foundation for a Healthy Kentucky to create linkages among hospitals, businesses, community and religious organizations, and public health agencies, seeking to broaden hospitals' view of their responsibility beyond medical care to the total health of their towns and cities—even without changes in the structure of payment.

"A lot of my work for over the past decade has been to try to promote more multi-sector collaboration between the hospital community, the public health community, and the other sectors of the community," Prybil said. Covid could accelerate that process, he added. "I hope one outcome is that across the nation and certainly in the acute care provider sector—hospitals and health systems—there's a growing realization that health care delivery and public health must be viewed as two parts of one whole."[65]

Traditional health providers grow by building new facilities and attracting patients to come to them. In central Pennsylvania, Geisinger sees a new way to grow. The payvider model, and the firm's long-term community mission, have reoriented the company to work beyond its walls, blurring the distinction between health care and public health.

"I think the next chapter of Geisinger is building programs, instead of building things and expecting people to come," Ryu said. "I think our next chapter is build it and take it to the people, build it and take it further out into the communities, build it and take it into the home. Whenever you can, build it and take it into the virtual space, build it and drop it off through mail order, build it and have them seen in the clinic instead of the hospital. Build it and see them in the ER, and get them home rather than have to admit them. Build it so that even if they get admitted, they're able to go home rather than go to another institutional stay for a rehab visit. That's a lot of the mindset of what we've been looking at strategically as far as our next chapter."

For doctors and nurses, that next stage will require a new way of practicing medicine, less tied to a clinic and the traditional, hierarchical roles there, and more connected to patients' whole lives. Doctors and nurses will need flexibility, the ability to problem solve in many settings, and a willingness to tackle issues that lead to health care but are not traditionally thought of as the role of a health care provider. Geisinger and a few other institutions nationally are working to produce these new doctors and nurses. Geisinger's medical school is training young people from its communities—many from working-class families without previous college graduates—to become doctors who will serve their own towns as employees of the integrated system. It's a new kind of student body, with a new curriculum, to produce a new kind of doctor.

In the next chapter, we will learn about that work, along with the potential of this cultural change for a better, more integrated and caring way of managing our health.

Chapter 8

Training Doctors

As a human motivator, culture is often stronger than money. Culture molds who we are and what we value—almost all of us value something else more than money—and culture sets our standards for how we relate to one another, including what we owe to family, community, and nation, and what doctors and nurses owe to the patients they care for. Money may influence some people to choose a career in health care, but in our experience, most students in the health professions are motivated by deeper drives of service, caring, and a sense of purpose as healers. Often, medical education itself inserts concerns about money by loading down new graduates with enormous debts that push them to earn as much as possible—a need that helps power the volume-based approach to care that can treat patients as commodities. At the same time, the traditional model of doctor training can grind down the positive social qualities that originally brought students to medicine. Through their four years, med school students' sense of empathy measurably declines, according to research published by scientists at Thomas Jefferson University that followed them with psychological testing.[1]

The authors of that paper, led by Jefferson psychologist Mohammadreza Hojat, noted how counterproductive it is to put medical students through a system that robs them of their idealism:

> Some anecdotal reports as well as empirical studies suggest that a drastic transformation in medical students' character occurs during their medical education. When they embark on the journey to become physicians, most students are enthusiastic, filled with idealism and a genuine intention to serve those in need of help. It is ironic, though, that despite the students' initial intentions and medical school faculty's attempts to nurture human

qualities, a cynicism develops progressively during their training. For example, it has been reported that as many as three fourths of medical students become increasingly cynical about academic life and the medical profession as they progress through medical school.[2]

Medical educators have known about this problem for a long time, but, like other festering flaws in the health care system, the shortcomings of medical education grew much more obvious during the Covid crisis. This is evidence for our systemic investigation of what went wrong in the pandemic. Education lies at the heart of both strengths and weaknesses in the American health care system, so we must look there for root causes for the Covid disaster. In this chapter, we find those causes, some in unexpected places. To begin with causes discussed in earlier chapters, here are three systemic flaws that link directly to medical education: first, a lack of primary care doctors; second, a physician workforce lacking in racial and economic diversity; and, third, a culture of medical heroism that leaves doctors unable to tend to their own mental health.

To start with the first of those points, American medical education has long produced too few primary care doctors. A major reason is the cost of undergraduate medical tuition, which forces graduates to choose higher-paid specialties to repay student loans. This is a costly problem for society, because primary care is the keystone of the system. Primary care providers encourage wellness, give routine care and coordinate specialty care, and serve as the access point for patients.[3] During the pandemic, primary care proved essential, as providers worked with patients before they reached overburdened hospitals and managed their cases. But we didn't have enough primary care doctors, and they were overwhelmed. Patients who should have seen primary care doctors instead jammed emergency rooms.[4] Also, too few primary care physicians had been trained in using telemedicine, which suddenly became critically important for safety and effectiveness in seeing patients.

Second, weaknesses in medical education also worsened the tragedy of racial health inequity during the pandemic. As we discussed in chapter 4, African Americans not only were more likely to get sick from Covid but also were more likely to receive inferior care and to die. One reason is the shortage of primary care doctors: according to a recent study, if America had enough physicians for everyone in every community, we would save seven thousand lives a year, even during non-Covid times.[5] But producing that many doctors would require a huge surge in medical education, especially in primary care: for Black and Hispanic Americans to have equal access as suburban Whites, America would need another one hundred eighty thousand physicians.[6]

Beyond the numbers, however, we also learned in chapter 4 that African Americans receive inferior care because of racial bias (recall the elevated infant mortality rate for Black babies when they are delivered by White doctors).[7] Solutions, as we saw in that chapter, include training a more diverse corps of physicians, in terms of race and socioeconomic class, and nurturing the empathy and cultural understanding of all doctors. We already touched on the tendency of medical school to diminish students' empathy (and we will discuss why later). The record on diversity is at least as bad. Due to rising tuitions, medical schools are admitting fewer low-income students today than they were thirty years ago.[8] And medical schools had a higher percentage of Black male students forty years ago than they do today (the number in 2019 was just 2.9 percent).[9]

Third, Covid also battered the psyche of health care workers in ways that may leave deep damage. The pandemic exhausted doctors and nurses; exposed them to relentless, preventable death; and, in its later phase, created bizarre situations in which health care providers were threatened and harassed by the people they were trying to save. Doctors and nurses faced hostility and violence from angry patients who didn't believe Covid was real, even those deep in its grip. Some medical staff carried panic buttons and avoided going out in public in their scrubs. Many quit or retired, and those left behind faced even more stress with growing staff shortages.[10] Perhaps no educational program could have prepared a caregiver for that hell, but doctors could have been better prepared in training to seek help and rely on others, which might have made these struggles more manageable. As we discussed in chapter 6, medical schools often inculcate a myth that doctors should be heroes, able to overcome any hardships alone. Those are unhealthy attitudes for managing extreme stress and grief—it is better to be able to reach out to others for help.

The waxing and waning pandemic placed medical schools in a unique position. The stress and burnout of Covid care drove many doctors to retirement. Nurses quit, too, for the same reasons—during 2020, 60 percent of nurses said in a survey that they were considering leaving the field.[11] But even while doctors and nurses were reaching the breaking point, something wonderful happened. Young people in unprecedented numbers witnessed their important work and committed themselves to also becoming health care providers. A flood of new people applied to medical schools in 2021, citing the inspiration of Covid care and a desire to help.[12]

This is a precious resource. Will medical education handle it better than it did those who came before? Will there be enough capacity and tuition support to train all the doctors and nurses we need? Will the new students be taught in a way that retains their idealism and protects them from cynicism? Will people of color and people from low-income families come into medical professions in numbers closer to their share of the population? And will the output of schools match what is needed, with more primary care providers and doctors ready to work in coordinated health care systems as members of a team? To avoid repeating mistakes, we need change. We must not burn out these potential new doctors and nurses like those who are suffering now.

We'll investigate those points through this chapter. First, we recall David's own medical education and experience as an educator, in which he encountered both the biases that hold us back and the leadership ideas that could help create change. Next, we consider the foundations of American medical education in early twentieth-century ideology that still guides much of what educators do, partly in counterproductive ways. After that, the investigation turns to solutions, with new approaches in undergraduate medical education, which encompasses the four years after college when students earn the MD after their names. Finally, at the end of the chapter, we will look more at graduate medical education, including the phases of residency, which have another set of problems and opportunities.

A GREAT EDUCATION

David had great mentors. His father, Albert J. Nash, encouraged him constantly. Albert's own good life had rewarded an optimistic outlook. He had been born into poverty. On his first day of kindergarten on the Lower East Side of Manhattan, he couldn't understand a word the teacher was saying: Albert spoke only Yiddish. But he did well in school, and, after returning from World War II, he aced an admission exam to win a spot at Cooper Union, the top-flight New York college with free tuition, and then attended with the first class at MIT's Sloan School of Management. Later he founded a company that sold school language labs—facilities with audio equipment for learning a foreign language—and was moderately successful. The Nashes settled on Long Island with other well-off Jewish families who gathered in segregated postwar suburbs. David encountered little prejudice, because everyone in the neighborhood was Jewish and equally prosperous (this was the gilded ghetto we mentioned in chapter 2).

David's aspiration to be a doctor was not remarkable—his brother became one, too—but while still in high school he added a less common ambition: to combine medicine with business. His father characteristically encouraged the idea. In 1972, as a high school senior, David read an article that quoted Samuel P. Martin III, a medical doctor teaching at the University of Pennsylvania's Wharton School, saying he was in the business of training physician leaders. David pointed the article out to his dad—this was what he had been talking about—and Albert suggested he write a letter to Martin. David thought the idea was ridiculous. Why write to this exalted doctor in Philadelphia? But eventually he did go to his Smith Corona typewriter and pecked out a letter to Martin, who received it, called him up, and said, "I need to meet you."

The trip David made by train to Philadelphia, the first time he had been there, certainly changed his life. Martin became his mentor through his education and early career. Martin was a remarkable man, a six-foot-four-inch war hero who was also a kind and graceful southern gentleman and a brilliant clinician and scholar. In World War II, already a doctor, he had served as a captain in the Army Air Corps Medical Service, parachuting into rescues from Greenland and elsewhere in the North Atlantic. An innovator throughout his career, he moved in midlife from work as an infectious disease specialist to become an authority on leadership and health economics. He was among the first to study the financial incentives that shape health care.[13] Martin guided David through his undergraduate years at Vassar College and medical school at the University of Rochester and Brown University, planning to bring him to Wharton and add an MBA to his MD in the tuition-free Robert Wood Johnson Foundation Clinical Scholars Program.

David arrived there on a Monday in 1984 after finishing his internal medicine residency on the previous Friday night. He felt quite well educated already, but sitting with Martin at their regular breakfast, he encountered a new language and a set of ideas that he didn't understand. Martin suggested doing a "stakeholder and force-field analysis" of the challenges of improving the health care system. Before almost anyone else, Martin was talking about change management (which didn't yet have that name), examining how the health system worked and engaging with its own processes to make improvements. With his students, Martin performed autopsies of failed leadership, reviews something like our systemic analysis of the Covid failure, learning the causes of failure and the best way to avoid those issues in making positive change.

Among Martin's favorite phrases was "Process, process, process, then outcome." It was a mantra for making change from the inside. Martin believed in getting inside an organization, understanding how it functions, working with the existing power structures, and using that position to push the organization to change itself. In the decades since, David has always remained something of an internal radical, using what he learned from Martin about means and ends. In his means, David is an insider, working with the process, but in his ends, he can be a radical.

Another set of lessons helped David envision those ends, as a student, a doctor, and a teacher. Memorable moments came unexpectedly, as when David and Esther, already married as fourth-year medical students, applied for residency as a couple before the start of the traditional matching process (something that is no longer allowed but was legal in those days). They interviewed at Jefferson for their internal medicine residency, and Jefferson responded by asking them to meet with the chairman of medicine. The chairman said, "We're very interested in the two of you, but here's my question: What will happen if we put you on call on the same night and you have a marital spat?" David thanked the chairman and got up to leave. Esther looked at him like he was crazy, but clearly this was not the right place. Instead, the couple ended up at Penn's Graduate Hospital, in a then-gritty south Philadelphia neighborhood. There the chief of medicine liked the idea of a married couple working together—but when the staff learned the two new residents were already married, the revelation created shock waves of disbelief that young people today cannot comprehend.

David came back to Jefferson ten years later and stayed for thirty years. Over the decades sexist attitudes subsided as the gender of doctors equalized and as society itself changed, but disturbing problems remain. For sixteen years, David led a day of training at Jefferson's Sidney Kimmel Medical College on patient safety and quality of care, during the clerkship period in the middle of the third year, after the students had spent their first six months in clinical rotations with patients.[14] (Spending only a day on such a critical issue is another topic—we will discuss quality and safety in chapter 11.) David's daughter, Rachel, was in medical school herself, and she suggested opening the safety and quality sessions by polling the students on what they had seen during their six months in the hospital. David decided to do it. At the beginning of the day, he shooed the other professors out of the hall and asked the students—the entire 280-member third-year class—to raise their hands if they had personally been present during racist discussion about a patient during their six months in the hospital. Every hand went up. Next, he asked the women (half the class) whether they had been subjected to misogynist or inappropriate questions, comments, or behavior, in private or in front of a patient. Again, every hand. Finally, he said, "Raise your hand if you've been involved with a patient where you believed something inappropriate was going on, possibly even unsafe, and you did not say anything." Every hand went up a third time (although surveys suggested the students at that stage in their training couldn't recognize an error when they saw it).[15] And he got the same unanimous responses not only on that first day but on every day he offered the session for the next ten years.

Those raised hands signaled danger. To protect patients, team members must feel empowered to call out mistakes and inappropriate statements and acts. Racism and sexism add to an imbalance of power that silences lower-ranking members of a team (recall the concept of the authority gradient we discussed in chapter 1). Prejudice and division come into medicine from society as a whole, but the traditional system of medical education does little to defeat them. Medical education too often beats students down, pitting them in an individualistic struggle for survival rather than helping them see their commonalities and abilities to work together. Those raised hands were evidence of students' loss of empathy and idealism. Who would be idealistic after what the students had seen? Their silence was evidence they were learning to accept the unacceptable.

How do we fix this? Jefferson has prioritized addressing these issues, but change is hard and takes a long time. Cultural change can take generations. They key is education. We transmit culture by teaching. And often how we teach is even more important than the message. David had the benefit of a great start and the help of a kind and inspiring mentor who nurtured him from high school into physician leadership. Every student should receive that kind of support. But they don't, and to understand why, our investigation must look back more than a century to the roots of what it means to be a doctor in America.

A NEW FLEXNER REPORT

"Every system is perfectly designed to get the results it gets." That quotation, which we introduced in chapter 1, is especially relevant here. The American system of medical education was designed by Abraham Flexner (with the support of the Carnegie Foundation and American Medical Association), who published the Flexner Report in 1910.[16] Flexner described an ideal system of undergraduate medical education, based on a science-heavy German model and a four-year program pioneered at Johns Hopkins University, including two years of scientific training followed by two years of clinical training. He traveled to every medical school in the country to evaluate their quality, which was often low (for-profit medical schools were then common). He recommended closing many schools, and thanks to the financial support of Carnegie and the Rockefeller Foundation, his recommendations stuck, producing a complete and rapid transformation of the medical profession.[17]

It's hard to exaggerate the impact of the Flexner Report. By placing medical education on a scientific basis, it contributed to a century of discoveries that cured age-old diseases, miracles that have transformed the human condition. But Flexner also discounted the healing and caring tradition of medicine in favor of science. He believed physicians had no social role.[18] We can see these cultural beliefs enacted today in the loss of empathy felt by medical students. Medical schools built on the Flexner model winnow out students by imposing brutal demands, forcing them to compete with classmates to cram science content (much of which is obsolete by the time they start practicing). Admission favors Ivy League hotshots with high grades in chemistry and biology, who may lack the humility or life experience to become caring doctors. And the process elevates specialists as medical heroes, perpetuating a system that richly rewards the doctor who can fix the body as a broken machine but discounts the primary care physician who develops relationships with entire families and nurtures their good health over decades.

Tradition keeps this culture alive, and tradition is strong in the medical field. Doctors are trained by doctors, usually following the pedagogic concept of "see one, do one, teach one"—which ensures that the mistakes of the past are carried on to the next generation. Fifty-five-year-old doctors teach their thirty-year-old beliefs to twenty-five-year-old students. And doctors beget doctors, with one in five medical school students the child of a doctor. (That's partly because doctors can afford medical school tuition for their children, and also because they know US medical school is a great investment, with perhaps the highest net value in future earnings of any degree on Earth.[19]) In 2020, a student at Ohio State University College of Medicine in Columbus posted a dramatic film online, a horror movie depicting the overwork, isolation, and anxiety of medical school. As if to underline the profession's tradition of cynicism, doctors commenting online ridiculed the filmmaker as weak, suggested he get tougher and work harder, and said they had it worse.[20] No wonder students lose their empathy and idealism.

Flexner also helped embed racial inequity in medicine. Progressive social reformers of his period commonly equated science with racism, and Flexner's supporters overlapped with advocates and funders of eugenics, including Carnegie, Rockefeller, and William Welch, the founding dean of Hopkins. The American eugenics movement later helped inspire the Nazi Holocaust.[21] Although Flexner's family was Jewish, he based his work on an explicitly anti-Semitic book about medical education written by a German scholar.[22] In his own report, Flexner called for teaching Black doctors about hygiene, not surgery, and envisioned them as missionaries to civilize their race.[23] He called for the closure of five of the seven Black medical schools operating at the time, which did happen. The percentage of Black doctors dropped, and it didn't recover for a century[24] (Black male doctors remain almost as rare today as they were before 1910[25]). The only two Black medical schools that survived Flexner still produce the largest numbers of Black doctors today.[26]

In 2011, Thomas Duffy, a legendary clinician at Yale University Medical School, evaluated a century of Flexner's influence, writing an essay after a half-century of his own medical practice.

> The trust and respect that were extended to the profession 50 years ago have been substantially eroded. There has been a fall from grace of our vaunted profession. Physicians have lost their authenticity as trusted healers. . . . The discontent with doctor's errors, doctor's silence, doctor's experimentation, and the crass monetary orientation of the profession is legion. The profession appears to be losing its soul at the same time its body is clothed in a luminous garment of scientific knowledge. . . . This lapse has not escaped our patient population nor our critics who have richly documented the poverty of professional ideals now current in medicine. They have called for a new Flexner Report, a centennial taking stock, to address the shortcomings in medical education that have occurred in the aftermath of the original report.[27]

Of course, no single report today is likely to have the same influence as Flexner's original document, but reforms have been suggested, some fundamental and some cosmetic. David has observed the flaws in the existing paradigm in his decades as a medical educator and as the founding dean emeritus of the Jefferson College of Population Health. Forcing medical students to memorize science facts is an absurd waste. So is the Darwinian and inhumane winnowing process. Part of the problem is that most medical schools focus on an unattainable goal, which is colloquially known as producing a doctor who is a "triple threat"—a great clinician, great researcher, and great teacher. Can every doctor be a great scientist? Perhaps that was possible a century ago, but not today. Moreover, attempting to make every doctor a great scientist is destructive to the student and to the goal of producing great clinicians, which should be paramount.

As a solution, some educators have added elements to the curriculum designed to enhance medical students' understanding of the humanities, but without fundamentally changing the underlying educational system. Advocates of this approach saw Covid as an opportunity, because, they maintained, study of the humanities could help doctors reflect on the disaster and understand the historic roots of systemic racism.[28] In practice, this content more often looks like medical students taking museum field trips, writing in journals, or being strongly encouraged to attend lunchtime piano recitals. Picture, for a moment, White medical students who graduated from top universities—a typical demographic profile— listening briefly to a Chopin etude in the lobby before returning to study in a lab. Outside, mentally ill people wander homeless and residents of low-income neighborhoods die in middle age for lack of prevention and primary care. Humanities instruction is not the solution.

To change, undergraduate medical education must take away elements as well as add them. Instead of filling students with science facts, teach them to be lifelong learners who can acquire information about new discoveries as they happen. Rather than force-feeding them information in an individualistic battle for survival, surround them with colleagues in small, collaborative problem-solving groups, like the equals who practice medicine effectively in team-based clinical settings. Create a diverse student body by reducing the cost of attending and by broadening the qualities measured in admissions. Make understanding cultures and inequities a core part of the curriculum. Integrate connections with communities and with real patients from the beginning, keeping foremost the true meaning of caring. Through it all, medical students should also learn to be leaders, understanding quality measurement and improvement, how to reduce clinical variation, and how much compensation is reasonable in our society.

If this sounds revolutionary—and perhaps it is—we will show next that it is happening in a few innovative medical schools and that it works. Those schools, and others that are moving in this direction, will produce a new cadre of physicians, and with them a constituency for change. That is our best hope for breaking the bonds of tradition and remaking the culture of medicine.

TRAINING A NEW KIND OF MD

At the Geisinger Commonwealth School of Medicine, students don't memorize science information from textbooks. The school aims to teach them how to ask the right questions so they can find answers when they need them, said the president and dean, Steven Scheinman. Lectures are a thing of the past. Students receive information in the evening, through podcasts, texts, or videos, with precious class time reserved for active, small-group sessions to solve problems and teach one another. "Medical education is much more than information transfer. Medical education involves teaching them to think like physicians," Scheinman said.[29]

Along with just a few medical schools in the United States, Geisinger, based in Scranton, Pennsylvania, and founded in 2008, has adopted a new process to produce a new kind of physician (David is a member of its board). Kaiser Permanente Bernard J. Tyson School of Medicine is using a similar model in Pasadena, California, where it admitted its first students in 2020. At UC San Diego, the T. Denny Sanford Institute for Empathy and Compassion, founded in 2019 (and where David is an advisory board member), is experimenting with these new educational ideas, seeking to produce a different kind of doctor and to develop scalable practices that can be spread to other medical schools around the country.

For Geisinger and Kaiser Permanente, having an associated medical school creates the opportunity to instill new doctors with a culture that could make them more effective in their different kinds of health care systems. As we learned in the previous chapter, Geisinger is a payvider, owning a health plan that covers many of its patients, and Kaiser is a closed system, offering everything members need, including insurance and doctors on salaries. David recalls Bernard Tyson, then the CEO and chairman of Kaiser Health Plan and Hospitals, talking about the need to train doctors in a new way to work in its system, because of the difficulty of retraining doctors from the traditional mold. After Tyson died suddenly in 2019, the new medical school was named for him. These systems need doctors who can work effectively in teams, who focus on prevention and wellness rather than volume of services, whose race and economic background mirror the patient population, and who feel a connection to (and responsibility for) the communities they serve.

"The [Geisinger] system has got a financial incentive to keep patients out of the hospital, to do fewer procedures, and to focus on how well they do and on keeping them healthy," said Scheinman before he retired in 2021. "Our students have the opportunity to train in an environment in which the clinical system has been set up to keep people healthy and manage their total health, not just react when they get sick."

"There's a focus on person-centered care and community and population health," said Mark Schuster, founding dean and CEO of the Tyson school. "The approach here is that physicians work on teams with nurses and social workers and pharmacists and others. It's very much a group effort. . . . It's not a setting in which medical students learn to treat clinicians from other fields with a lack of respect."[30]

At the Sanford Institute, in San Diego, the vision is even larger—to transform medical education, based on new understanding of the neurology of empathy and compassion, and to create a new paradigm, as Abraham Flexner did in the last century.

"The overarching goal is finding ways of training young doctors to be able to hold onto their own empathy and compassion so that when they mature through their career, they've got that in hand," said William Mobley, a neurologist and distinguished professor who leads the institute as executive director. "Their resilience is there. They're always able, even in difficult situations, to listen carefully and engage the patient in a way that is really empathically and compassionately driven."[31]

For Geisinger and Tyson, the process begins in admissions and financial aid. At traditional private medical schools, admissions officers try to improve their diversity numbers by competing for a small pool of Black and Brown students who have made it through the gauntlet of elite education and who can afford tuition. Geisinger and Tyson have instead successfully enlarged the pool, gaining diversity in terms of both race and socioeconomic class and admitting large cadres of students who are their families' first college graduates. Scheinman said those students bring an important quality to the student body: they are more likely to know how it feels when a family must choose between buying prescription drugs and buying food.

"We think that there are several reasons to prefer a class that has a large number of students who are first generation in their family to go to college," Scheinman said. "One of those reasons is that their family experiences will be more like experiences of the future patients. And that dimension of economic diversity within the class is valuable not just to them and their future patients but also to the well-off kids in the class who can learn from them. A second reason is that we think that those kinds of students really value the education."

David has noticed that advantage in his own teaching: working-class students tend to be grateful, focused, and open to new ideas, and often they are humbler and more empathetic than students who arrive with perfect Ivy League pedigrees. But attending medical school now costs, on average, $250,000 at public schools and $330,000 at private schools.[32] As tuitions rise, so has the income level of students' families.[33]

Kaiser Permanente has addressed the cost problem by waiving tuition for the first five classes at the Tyson school. Tuition support comes without strings attached, and the school operates independently of the health system—the new doctors can go to work anywhere—but the gift helps fulfill Bernard Tyson's vision by increasing the pool of graduates with the kind of skills Kaiser needs. Geisinger launched a program that allows 40 percent of its students to earn tuition waivers and living stipends by working in primary care or psychiatry at Geisinger Health after they graduate—one year of tuition for each year of service. The program will help new doctors go into fields in which they are most needed without medical school debt.

But tuition isn't the only barrier keeping working-class students from going to medical school. They have to go to college first, and America's so-called meritocracy tees up college success for children from wealthy families. Those with higher incomes have access to private schools and top public schools, and many other advantages, yielding academic transcripts and test scores attractive to undergraduate college admission offices. We can see the result at Princeton University. Tuition is not a barrier at Princeton. It offers among the nation's most generous financial aid, with no tuition at all for students from families earning up to $160,000 a year. And admissions are need-blind. With that system, Princeton should be accessible and free for 83 percent of American families—but that's not how it works out. The median income of families with students at Princeton is $186,000 a year. The top 1 percent of America's wealthiest families represent 17 percent of the student body.[34] (We pick on Princeton only because it is Charles's alma mater, but the numbers are similar at other Ivy League schools.[35])

Enough college graduates want to be doctors to fill medical schools with students who have never had a bad grade. But to build a diverse student body, and to build better doctors, admissions officers need to look beyond the college transcript and scores on the MCAT (the standardized Medical College Admission Test). Geisinger and Tyson receive many tens of times more applicants than they can admit, many of them qualified on paper. But their process assumes that classroom grades and standardized tests don't measure some of the most important qualities of a potential doctor.

"Measures of academic ability, of intellectual ability, are imperfect, and the skill set of being a physician requires much more than just being really smart," Scheinman said. "You probably know many people who are brilliant, but you wouldn't want them near you as a doctor. They need good judgment. They need excellent people skills. They need a deep sense of empathy. And they need a commitment to service. And we look for all of that in admissions."

Geisinger chooses its class of 115 students out of more than seven thousand who apply. Test scores and grades screen the pool down to nine hundred who will receive an interview, but after that the school gives no more consideration to academic achievement. Instead, admission depends entirely on what interviews show about the applicant's commitment to service, life experience, and character. Each candidate faces a set of carefully designed, situational questions in one-on-one interviews. Interviewers are trained to pick up signs of empathy or dismissiveness and other cues in the applicant's behavior. To ensure the objectivity of results, each interviewer asks only a single question while the candidates rotate through a dozen short, private sessions. Some other schools also use a process of screening and Multi Mini Interviews; Geisinger is unique for applying these tools to find the special qualities it is seeking.

The Tyson school admitted only fifty students from more than ten thousand applicants for its first class, making it among the most selective in the country. (Free tuition surely was one cause of the high level of interest.) Candidates submitted portfolios showing how their qualities and interests aligned with the school's mission before their interviews.[36] The result of this holistic process became clear when the admitted students arrived, Schuster said.

"Our admissions team has been amazing at identifying students who are compassionate, energetic, committed to health equity, aware of what's going on in the world, and just really motivated," he said. "They come in with a certain specialness, a certain spirit, as so many medical students do. And we want very much to have them maintain that spirit and have it intact when they graduate. They, of course, will grow and change as everyone does. But we don't want to drum out what makes them special. We don't want to burn them out. We don't want to make them cynical. They come in with so much desire to make a difference, and we want that to be there when they graduate."

Rather than spending the first two years of training only on classroom study, students in these two medical schools begin working with patients soon after they arrive. Seeing patients lends relevance and immediacy to their book learning and provides a sense of purpose to the hard work. When students convene for case-based discussions in small groups, they have real-life experience on which to draw. Small group work also builds reflexes for treating all team members as equals, part of creating the just culture that we know helps avoid medical errors (as we discussed in chapter 1). Students receive instruction in medical quality, too, including the tools and attitudes needed to reduce errors. And community involvement begins early as well, underlining the responsibility of health care providers to keep society healthy outside the clinic's walls.

Traditional medical education trains doctors to focus on the patient in front of them and forget about what is happening outside the walls of the exam room. That concept of "one patient, one problem, one at a time" ignores the importance of social influences on a patient's health and how addressing health at the population level can benefit each of us more than looking at our problems in isolation. Covid drove home that point. Doctors couldn't do much in the exam room with patients who were already struggling to breathe, but work on masking, ventilation, and, later, vaccination did have the potential to save many thousands of lives.

The new model of undergraduate medical education also brings a focus on racial disparities and bias. Geisinger, Tyson, and the Sanford Institute at UC San Diego all integrate these issues into the curriculum, addressing them in personal as well as abstract terms. Christopher Cannavino, a pediatrician and professor at UCSD, leads Sanford's Master Clinician Program, which pairs students in the clinical years of training with mentors who help them grapple with their communication skills and bias in real-life settings.

"As they go on rounds, they'll directly observe the students as a third party and then debrief with them later in the day and talk about not only building up clinical skill sets but also how did the communication go? What's the interpersonal reaction among team members? What did you notice in terms of social determinants of health or health inequities?" Cannavino said.[37]

Even at these innovative programs, medical school is intense. There is a lot to learn. But Geisinger and Tyson don't use intensity and demanding schedules to weed anyone out. At Tyson, first-year students receive mental health counseling, supporting them in the challenge and establishing, for later in their careers, that there is nothing wrong with reaching out for help. Geisinger built weekly reflection exercises into the curriculum, with time to discuss difficult experiences, such as witnessing the death of a patient, the suffering of a child, or the commission of a medical error.

"There's a lot that we do on the wards that does train away empathy," Scheinman said. "We overwork our students and exhaust them. We show them role models of physicians who are well respected, who themselves are burned out. And so we pay a lot of attention in our student experience to encouraging resilience, encouraging ways for them to recognize signs of burnout in themselves, and how to deal with that, and paying attention to their own health throughout medical school, because that's a major cause of lack of empathy among physicians."

The Sanford Institute has explored ways to invest compassion in the traditional academic work of the first half of medical school, including cadaver dissections in first-year gross anatomy, said Lisa Eyler, a clinical psychologist and professor who directs Sanford's Center for Empathy and Compassion Training in Medical Education.

"We're including compassion practices before and during some of the more difficult dissections that the students do, and we're doing research to see how this affects their feelings towards the donor of the body and feelings in general about empathy and compassion," she said. "They did an exercise where they wrote a letter to the donor in gratitude, talking to them about what their hopes and fears were for their first year in medical school, their gratitude to the donor for being part of that journey. And then those anonymous letters were sealed and will be cremated with the donor at the end of the year."[38]

Many medical schools are modernizing and making tweaks to their traditional training, recognizing research that has shown its flaws. Some have added instruction in using technology more effectively, including how to see patients online, a topic that became urgent when the pandemic hit. (We will discuss more about how doctors use technology in the next chapter.) The model at Geisinger and Tyson has been adopted in a few other places, and pieces of it are spreading more widely, such as reduced emphasis on lectures and more focus on teamwork and lifelong learning. That's good, because Geisinger and Tyson, between them, produce only two hundred graduates a year, out of almost twenty thousand new medical doctors who graduate annually in the United States.[39] A much bigger change is needed than they can manage alone.

The Sanford Institute's research might help make that happen.

"We're looking to potentially partner with a handful of medical schools to look at the scalability of the program," said Sanford's Cannavino. "We will look how it can be adapted to the needs of each different institution so that potentially this could be a roadmap or model that all medical schools could use."

As we saw in the previous chapter, adding improved features to a fundamentally broken system can take us only so far. These innovative medical educators are instead producing a building block by training a new kind of doctor. They are using the culture-building power of education to guide their students' formation of professional identities, encouraging them to internalize, deep down, the values that could form the foundation of a better health care system.

At Geisinger, Scheinman said, earning a degree means absorbing key values as part of one's professional identity. Abraham Flexner, we suspect, would not have recognized these values as important. Scheinman can rapidly list them. New doctors should take responsibility for their patients' total wellness, not only provide a service and hand them off. They should understand the roles of team members caring for patients, including the importance of nurses, dietitians, social workers, and everyone else involved, and how the doctor's role fits in with them. They should be aware of the patient's community and cultural context, where they live, the factors challenging their health, and how well they can understand and follow instructions. After four years, the school expects graduates to incorporate such values into who they are—it even says so in the brochure sent to prospective students, which promises, "Students are continually challenged to envision and to plan for not just what kind of doctor they want to be, but also what kind of person."[40]

Scheinman said Geisinger graduates do show special qualities when they reach their next steps, in their residencies at hospitals. Surveys showed first-year graduate interns coming from Geisinger scored above graduates from other medical schools on empathy, communications skills, and that ability to work in a team.

Eyler, the psychologist at Sanford, also sees hope for the physician burnout problem. Doctors suffer in part because medical education trains them to be superhero leaders, above others and unable to admit weakness or ask for help, she said. They need compassion for themselves.

"Health care is tough, and the pandemic revealed that even more in terms of all the demands that are on physicians and how they are really called to be above the fray, but they themselves are also experiencing the stressors of the pandemic, both personally and professionally," she said. "We want to equip them not only with better skills to maintain compassion for patients under challenging situations but also to foster compassion for themselves."

We traversed several pages without mentioning the Covid pandemic, but our investigation has arrived at a fundamental cause of system failure and a solution to fix it. Minority and low-income Americans were excluded from the medical profession, at first by design and later by tradition and the structure of the educational system. When the pandemic came, health care institutions lacked awareness of the context that drove the infection because providers didn't live in those places or know much about them. In Philadelphia, a city with four medical schools, it took a Black surgeon, Ala Stanford, to deliver testing to Black neighborhoods, by grabbing supplies and a minivan and driving to the hardest-hit communities. When she did, people also lined up in the freezing cold for primary care, bringing their X-rays and pill bottles.[41] We should have had more Black doctors. We should have had more doctors who grew up in poverty. This was a failure in many parts of society, but within its roots was a failure of medical education. Doctors trained differently could have built a medical system that cared more.

WHAT'S WRONG WITH RESIDENCY

Among the most powerful documents of the pandemic was an April 2020 email from a group of forty-four residents at Elmhurst Hospital in Queens, sent to the CEO of the public NYC Health + Hospitals system that employed them. "As trainees, we are horrified and scared, paralyzed with feelings of helplessness and guilt," the trainees wrote, relating stories of watching patients die because they did not receive adequate care in overwhelmed wards staffed by inexperienced residents. The message said a fifth of the residents had considered suicide.[42]

These residents, and many others like them, had been thrown into providing complex respiratory care for Covid patients with little supervision. Some attested they had no idea what they were doing. A resident is a medical school graduate with an MD, but without enough experience to practice unsupervised. Residents work in hospitals to gain their medical licenses, much as apprentice plumbers and electricians learn their trades by doing them. Similar to a medieval guild, the medical profession makes residents pay their dues to join its ranks. They work three to eight years to gain experience with patients, with long hours and low pay, in an arrangement that is often highly profitable for hospitals. For residents, quitting isn't really an option, as doing so would mean failing residency and giving up the opportunity to be a doctor. Covid blew the lid off this flawed system by pushing it to its extremes, but the public did not express outrage. Instead, we beat on pots and pans and put up yard signs expressing gratitude. In an email response to the forty-four residents in April 2020, the CEO at NYC Health offered little to address their concerns about hurting patients, instead writing, "Thanks for reaching out. You all are heroes and I hope you feel that way because it is the only thing that can sustain you through this horrible time."[43]

The same *Wall Street Journal* article that revealed the email told other stories of residents facing patient care duties they couldn't handle. During residency, graduates work in their chosen specialty under the supervision of an attending doctor, learning by watching and then doing procedures. During the Covid crisis, residents in psychiatry, ophthalmology, podiatry, and other unrelated specialties, without experience in critical care, were suddenly thrown into wards where they had to handle technical tasks in respiratory medicine that normally require extensive training. Some reported looking up YouTube videos on their phones to learn what they should be doing. At least one patient was documented as having been killed by a ventilator set too high by a resident who did not understand how to adjust it.[44]

These events were not only the result of a crisis. Medical residency is built on a model that can create patient risk and propagate error and variations in care. Despite undeniable flaws, the system hasn't been reformed over many years, partly because residency slots, paid for by the federal government, can be a cash cow for hospitals and medical schools, especially for training in high-paid specialties. The educators' political clout and power over the fate of residents helps cement the status quo. Moreover, few members of the public understand this strange system or how it can harm them.

Here's a simplified summary of how residency works: An annual match process puts medical school graduates in residency slots at hospitals in their desired specialties. Each hospital's assigned slots are paid for by Medicare, with allocations influenced by the powerful Association of American Medical Colleges, a deans' club that spends $4.4 million a year lobbying Congress.[45] When residents arrive, as interns, they practice medicine under the supervision of attending physicians in their specialties, at first being shown how to perform procedures, later doing them on their own, and then teaching other new residents. New doctors are assumed to be ready to practice unsupervised based on the amount of time they have served and the number of procedures they have performed. For the most part, the system lacks standards addressing how to teach residents or objective measures to judge their competence. Short of egregious failure, residents pass if they put in their time.[46]

Researchers have called for reform to the process to make it safer for patients and to ensure that residents really learn what they need to know. Few hospitals even track the outcome of patient care by residents to determine whether they have done their work correctly. Many things can go wrong. The attending physician could teach flawed practices to the resident—after all, he or she learned in the same system, by watching an attending physician during residency, and that doctor may not have been using best practices either. Or the attending could lose competency over time, becoming rusty in skills or falling behind current practices while still teaching. Attending physicians often are not available at night or other off-hours times, leaving inexperienced residents to manage care without authentic supervision, even if they know they are not capable. A resident in those situations can also become overconfident and treat patients without knowing whether the work is done correctly and, short of a disaster, may never learn otherwise. Indeed, a single hospital may have different protocols for the same procedure for different residency programs. In a residency teaching system based on judgment and experience, a culture of practice can drift without reference to scientific evidence, giving rise to unexplained clinical variation and undermining a bedrock concept of quality and safety—that there should be a single best way of treating a patient in a given situation.[47]

If this situation sounds abstract, in practice it can be pretty simple. Before Steven Scheinman helped reform medical education at Geisinger, he went through residency, as did David and all doctors. He recalled learning by bad example—seeing doctors throwing tantrums, abusing nurses and other coworkers, and talking about patients when they were present, as if they were objects unable to hear.

"I saw people on the wards whose attitude towards patients was so terrible that I thought they were valuable role models for me in that they were negative role models," Scheinman said. "I wouldn't want to be anything like that person, and I'm going to watch out for signs in myself that I might turn out that way."

But that wasn't all, Scheinman said: "I also had role models of people who would be wonderful role models even now, in fact some of them still practicing. One of the people I admire most taught me to hold the patient's hand while talking to them, especially if they are hearing bad news or going through a difficult experience, and listening to their story, regardless of whether they're talking about their health at all."

As Scheinman's description points out, different people teach us different things; if tradition and judgment are the only guide to education, then we should not expect outcomes to be consistent. But, of course, we can build an educational system based on more than tradition and personal judgment. As a basic example, other fields have adopted competency testing after a required period of professional experience, such as architects and engineers, teachers, and accountants. Doctors can choose to take board exams in their specialties after residency, but they can practice independently without board certification.

Deeper change is possible, and an opportunity seemed to arise with the pandemic. The emergency disrupted hospital routines, robbing residents of hours they needed to complete time in their specialties. Some medical educators called for switching to measures of competence rather than time. Under a competency-based system, doctors would be authorized to perform procedures independently after doing them with skill and positive outcomes, rather than after a set number. Some would finish sooner than average, and others might take longer.[48]

Residency could be made safer for patients and more consistent for doctors in other ways as well. Various industries have solved similar problems by establishing standards and continuously measuring their processes and outcomes. Although that work is hard and complex, the framework guiding these transformations already exists and has worked to reduce accidents to near zero in high-risk industries such as commercial aviation or nuclear power generation.[49]

But that didn't happen. The primary reason is simple and easy to understand: This change would be hard and cost hospitals money. It is easier to pass residents based on time and numbers of procedures rather than setting competency standards, tracking outcomes, and passing only residents who prove their skill. Such a system would require additional data collection and increased supervision. That's not impossible, and Canada is already adopting a competency-based system nationally.[50] In the United States, the nonprofit Accreditation Council for Graduate Medical Education has worked toward competency standards.[51] But our medical education system lacks a central authority to mandate big changes.

Our search for root causes of the Covid failure also connects to the funding of graduate medical education—a connection that reaches back to the 1990s, when the United States last addressed how Medicare pays for residency programs. In 1994, President Bill Clinton's failed health care reform legislation called for redirecting residency funding to produce more primary care doctors—needed even then for a more just and efficient health care system, and needed desperately a quarter-century later during the pandemic. But Senator Daniel Patrick Moynihan of New York, the patron saint of medical education in the Congress (who died in 2003), helped sink Clinton's legislation partly because of that provision. Moynihan had long protected graduate education at the country's best academic medical centers because he saw the hospitals as an engine of science and innovation that could produce new cures of disease. He charged that Clinton's plan to turn out more primary care doctors would rob funding from urban New York universities, with their highly trained specialists, and that would amount to "a crime akin to the burning of the library of Alexandria." He also argued that the mandate would damage academic freedom, saying, "America could then become the country in which you could grow up to be anything you want, except a cardiologist."[52]

Moynihan was right that federally funded graduate medical education is a public good, but directing too much of that money to producing specialists in urban academic medical centers contributed to a lack of primary and preventive care, especially in low-income and rural areas, which hurt deeply during the pandemic. The carnage in Black and Brown communities reaches back, in part, to this root cause.

Financial incentives help explain why academic hospitals lobbied the federal government for this misallocation of graduate medical education funding. Medicare pays for resident salaries plus the cost of educating the residents, and hospitals then also charge for the services provided by the residents. Yet the salaries of residents are low and they are required to work many extra hours weekly to provide care. This system of payment by Medicare and by patients allows hospitals to profit from residents, especially for high-reimbursement specialty care. In contrast, primary care residents bring in less money and are less likely to practice at big hospitals.

A couple of pieces of evidence demonstrate the financial benefit of federally funded residents for hospitals. First, some hospitals have added residency slots of their own, without Medicare money supporting them. These residents cover patients who bring in reimbursements—helping the hospital bottom line even without federal funding—and indicating that federal funds are unneeded in those cases.[53] And then there was the scandal of Hahnemann University Hospital in Philadelphia, the safety-net hospital we mentioned in chapter 4. In 2019, a private equity raider dismembered the hospital financially, declared bankruptcy, and sold off the parts. Among the most valuable assets were Hahnemann's 570 residency slots. A consortium of Philadelphia hospitals bid $55 million for them. Although a judge blocked the sale—after all, the slots represented public funds—the event exposed the market value for hospitals of extracting work from students backed with Medicare training money.[54]

Normally, rather than buying slots, rich, powerful hospitals lobby to get them from the government for free. President Biden's American Rescue Plan created one thousand slots, setting off lobbying to grab this source of long-term profit at taxpayer expense.[55] The system works well for hospital profits, and it works well for doctors, who get their education paid for. Primary care doctors need that support, but do specialists such as surgeons need it? Sixty percent of surgeons are in the top 1 percent of earners in the United States.[56] In fact, doctors in general are the largest group in the 1 percent, far above the number of high earners from the financial industry or corporate world.[57] Why does federal funding reward the richest hospitals to maintain a guildlike system for the richest Americans, while low-income Americans die early for lack of inexpensive primary and preventive care? That is the system we have created—and an important cause of the Covid disaster.

These are not intractable problems. Congress could redirect funding for residency programs to produce the primary care doctors we need, rather than high-paid specialists, and to place those slots in underserved communities. Professional societies and licensing boards could set competency-based standards for residents, forcing hospitals to adopt quality and safety principles that have worked in other industries. These changes in graduate medical education, and the changes in undergraduate medical education we discussed earlier, would help address the failures made evident by the Covid disaster, and they would make Americans healthier in the future and more able to weather the next pandemic—all without spending more money.

Our health care system is unfair, and at the foundation of that unfairness is how we produce doctors. When we fix that problem, and raise up a more diverse corps of physicians trained to work for the wellness of everyone, a powerful new force will emerge for the other changes we need.

Chapter 9

The Promise and Peril of Technology

When Covid hit American hospitals in 2020 and 2021, time had run out. The United States had no national data system to track hospital capacity and manage the transfer of patients in an emergency, despite fifteen years of ineffective federal plans to build one. We cannot say how many lives were lost because of that failure. Newspapers told terrible stories of patients expiring because beds could not be found for transfers as nurses frantically called colleagues on the telephone looking for places to send them. These stories spanned the first and second years of the pandemic, with names and places that changed but the tragedy and futility repeating, in California, Oklahoma, and elsewhere.[1] Some states and cities did have strong systems to share hospital data, managing capacity within their areas, but many did not, and the federal government was partially blind, without the detailed, real-time information needed to mitigate the crisis.[2] Indeed, the *New York Times* and Johns Hopkins University became the go-to sources for up-to-date statistics on the progress of the pandemic, not the government.

Our country built and mastered the internet, and our hospitals are temples of technology, but in this crisis, when we needed parts of the health care system to communicate, our computers couldn't talk to each other. Hospitals found themselves with patients too ill to speak, about whom doctors knew almost nothing, with families absent due to the Covid hazard—and they could not obtain their records, or even look for them, because the systems were incompatible. At the best of times, 45 percent of hospitals have reported trouble simply matching the identities of patients when moving information across platforms.[3]

A generation ago, banking moved online, frictionlessly transferring money between people and companies while protecting privacy, but health care organizations continue using fax machines and CDs to move data, technology that has virtually disappeared in the rest of society.

As we dig through the wreckage of America's Covid disaster—as if sorting the scorched pieces of a crashed airliner—this technology failure stands out in our analysis of what went wrong. It is tell-tale evidence. As we have noted, hospital error investigations have much in common with probes of aviation disasters. In both, we look at the mix of technology and human factors. Communication is key. In hospital investigations, David always looks for fumbled patient hand-offs among doctors and nurses, because poor communication is a leading cause of mistakes and bad outcomes. The inability of institutions to connect digitally looks like a bigger version of that kind of error. Even before the pandemic, this issue probably cost lives. During the pandemic, we saw it magnified into a catastrophe. Examining why this situation happened—why America's hospitals are decades behind in sharing data—leads to root causes of the Covid disaster.

Organizational culture always shapes how we use technology. We introduced the concept of a just culture in chapter 1. In a just culture, everyone feels responsible for safety and is empowered to speak up to stop errors—fundamentally, issues of communication. Recently, textbooks on culture and technology gained a tragic new chapter with the disasters of the Boeing 737 MAX, which killed 346 people in 2018 and 2019. Two planes crashed when erroneous instrument readings caused a computer system to fly them into the ground, with pilots unable to understand what was happening and disengage the computer. The technology could not communicate with the human beings flying the planes. But investigators found deeper roots to the disasters in Boeing's culture. As one case study put it, "Executives, managers, and engineers at Boeing were not stumped by the complexity or unpredictability of a new technology. In a series of *decisions*, they put profits before safety, did not think through the consequences of their actions, or did not speak out loudly enough when they knew something was wrong."[4] A judge ultimately blamed a dysfunctional culture that led directly to Boeing's board of directors.[5]

Boeing is a big, complex company, but health care is eight times larger than the aviation industry, and its work is more complex and more technically advanced. Yet aviation has developed systems to correct its flaws—even cultural flaws like Boeing's—while health care remains technologically disconnected and tragically error prone. (We will have much more to say about human factors engineering and the lessons of aviation for medicine in chapter 11.)

The purpose of our investigation is to fix what is wrong, and technology also provides hope. It could address some root causes. Technological innovations are improving care by reducing variation in how doctors practice and accelerating the uptake of new research findings; helping patients change their habits to become healthier, including managing chronic diseases with fewer visits to the doctor; and extending the time and place of care to support patients wherever and whenever they need it, even making health care continuous and unbounded by clinic walls.[6] Ideas and investments are tumbling forward, often with the potential to improve lives and save money.

It is fascinating to look at why these technological innovations work and, even more, why some don't. The reasons usually go back to the health care system itself. For example, electronic health records, called EHRs, held huge promise when they were introduced in the 1990s (and they still do, and are getting better), but the technology fell short, in part, because it replicated a paper system based on an individual doctor owning a patient's chart, keeping it in a chart room, and transmitting it by fax when sending a patient to a specialist or the hospital.[7] In medicine today, teams of doctors and nurses need to share information continuously—a patient with a chronic condition could see ten providers in a year—and they need to be able to query and search for records rather than knowing who has them and waiting for them to be sent.[8] (And that process assumes they aren't waiting for an actual fax, as often happens between systems that can't communicate.)

Adding technology to a dysfunctional process can produce dysfunctional technology. Financial incentives created fragmented health care institutions, and fragmented institutions adopted fragmented information systems. In organizations driving for volume of care to bring in more money, many doctors came to see their EHR software as a brutal taskmaster, adding to their work hours and dividing them from patients—with the demands of computers a leading cause of physician burnout.[9] Doctors too often spent physical exams watching their screens as they typed rather than connecting with their patients. Evidence even

arose of EHR systems making care worse and contributing to errors—
and of doctors using paper workarounds to avoid dealing with bad systems.[10] In addition, data breaches have repeatedly exposed the records
of tens of millions of patients, undercutting the promise of privacy.[11]

Bad technology hurts, but, at a deeper level, the right technology
could go to the foundations of the health care system and rearrange how
doctors and patients relate. Think of how social media changed society.
It did much more than make communication easier; it also changed the
power relationship between leaders and the public, changed how political groups coalesce and what they believe, and even changed how teens
grow up. We may regret many of those changes, but we have to admit
the power of that single innovation to alter how society functions for
most of the seven billion people on Earth. Could a similarly powerful
new technology change health care relationships to address the flaws
exposed in the Covid crisis?

We believe the answer is yes. Telehealth is the strongest example.
During the pandemic, it was a life-saver—literally. Doctors saw patients
without being physically present, continuing their healing work during lockdowns, even when they themselves were in quarantine or sick
with Covid. But telehealth also did much more, letting doctors practice
medicine in new ways and giving patients new power and centrality in
their care.

The technology had been around for a while, with great promise, but
adoption had been slow. Doctors had resisted using it, and regulators
and payers lagged behind the times. Then Covid swept away the objections and made telehealth ubiquitous. Suddenly, patients controlled
the site of their care and who was present. They didn't have to travel,
waste time in a waiting room, or feel the vulnerability of undressing in
an exam room. Doctors gained insight into their patients' lives and the
social determinants of their health, as they saw their home surroundings
in video appointments, met family members, and picked up on the many
cues about each of our lives that are evident in our homes—whether
they are clean or cluttered, crowded or lonely, rich or poor. And care
became more available in places without enough primary care and mental health practitioners, as doctors and counselors were released from
the constraints of geography. To some degree, telehealth also reduced
the inequities of the system, although low-income communities without
broadband access were left out.

In a matter of days, the Covid crisis pushed telehealth forward by years. It even addressed problems that had contributed to the pandemic disaster by making care easier to access. Beyond the pandemic years, this technology could transform health care.

TELEHEALTH TO THE RESCUE

Judd Hollander saw Covid coming, but not everyone would listen. He is an ER doctor and senior vice president of health care delivery innovation at Jefferson Health and associate dean of strategic health initiatives at Jefferson's Sidney Kimmel Medical College. With the health system's other leaders, he began preparing for the pandemic in January 2020. He had been developing a telehealth program for more than five years and knew its potential to keep doctors working and hospitals functioning in the coming crisis. In early February, he sent an email, with Jonathan Gleason, the doctor who was Jefferson's health quality chief (introduced in chapter 2), addressing all the doctors at the system's fourteen hospitals and hundreds of office practices.

"You people need to learn how to do telemedicine in the next couple of weeks because Covid might be real and this might be the only way you can care for patients," Hollander paraphrased the email as saying. "We offered two hundred training classes during the month of February and we made it available so that if you wanted one at 3 a.m., we would do one for you, one-on-one, at 3 a.m. You know how many people took those classes in the month of February? Three. Nobody believed Covid was real or was going to be a big deal at that point in time."[12]

Hollander knew that when the wave hit, there would be no time for classes, so his team went into a film studio to record the training on video. Speaking in March 2020 at a conference in Park City, Utah, he edited his remarks to note the number of Covid cases at that moment—which increased from the beginning to the end of his talk. "It was growing in front of us," Hollander recalled. Two-thirds of the doctors in the room raised their hands when he asked, "Is this real?"

Hollander advised about telemedicine on calls with the CDC, and what he learned there increased his concern further. At home, he frantically persuaded his wife and future daughter-in-law to avoid big events, even as most people went on with life unaware. Hollander and a colleague wrote a paper on how hospitals could use telemedicine in the coming Covid crisis, which went online in the *New England Journal of Medicine* on March 11.[13] That same day, the WHO declared a pandemic, President Trump declared a health emergency and shut off travel from Europe, and the NBA canceled all games, suddenly pulling teams off the court when a player was diagnosed with Covid. Within two weeks, lockdowns had spread across the country.[14]

We all remember where we were when the United States stopped. Over the course of a week, Hollander's colleagues trained more than one thousand clinicians for telehealth. The videos allowed doctors to learn how to see patients just before they had their first visit.

"People came out of the woodwork to help us do direct-to-consumer telemedicine because they didn't have an office practice anymore," Holland said. "We shut it down and we messaged, 'Don't go to the office. Don't go to the ER. Don't go to urgent care. We don't know what this is, but we've got you covered. You can just call Jeff Connect.'"

Hollander was constantly in the media talking about telemedicine. To manage the surge and an ongoing technology integration, his technical team worked eleven days in rotations with two-hour breaks for sleep, and executives sometimes made go/no-go decisions in the middle of the night. It worked. Jefferson kept 70 percent of patient visits, with 90 percent of them online. A similar shift was happening nationally. On March 17, 2020, the Centers for Medicare and Medicaid Services relaxed rules to allow full reimbursement for telehealth visits.[15] State deregulation across the country followed, allowing doctors and mental health workers to practice across state lines without limits for the first time.[16] Telehealth jumped from around 2 percent of all doctor visits to more than 50 percent.[17] Hollander's *NEJM* paper was devoured widely and cited more than two thousand times.[18]

The advice in that paper proved correct. It said telehealth could support forward triage, allowing doctors to sort Covid cases before patients hit the ER and keeping as many as possible isolated at home, where they could be cared for remotely. Telehealth could also expand capacity by allowing doctors to cover multiple sites and spreading out the capabilities of crucial specialists. In the hospital, giving tablets to patients could allow doctors to work with them without going into their rooms, and they would help nurses cover more patients in the crisis.[19] For some patients at home with chronic conditions, the new remote systems provided better support than they had gotten before the pandemic. For the first time, they received twenty-four-hour access, home-based care, and coaching and support from professionals below the level of doctors—which all became possible with Covid's sudden relaxation of regulations and payment.[20]

These discoveries surprised Hollander less than they did other people. He had been working on telehealth at Jefferson since 2014, following a strategy (supported by Stephen Klasko, then president of the university and CEO of the health system) of trying everything at once to see what worked. Expectations were repeatedly overturned. For example, telehealth advocates thought primary care should be the place to start with pilot programs, but Hollander found that primary care doctors were initially among the least willing to change, because they valued the in-person connection with patients, and because many were older. Instead, certain specialists eagerly adopted telehealth, especially urologists. Many male patients were surprisingly willing to show their scrotums to the camera for post-vasectomy care if that meant avoiding a trip across town to do so in person. Oncologists realized some of their female breast cancer patients preferred follow-up visits online if it meant showing their breasts at home rather than in the office. Patients facing the end of their lives sometimes preferred online visits, too, Hollander said. Telehealth allowed them to receive bad news at home, surrounded by family, rather than in a sterile exam room.

Like many millions of people, Charles had his first telehealth visit with his primary care doctor in 2020 after the lockdown. His previous doctor visit, months earlier, had required a thirty-minute drive each way, fifteen minutes in the waiting room, fifteen minutes waiting in the exam room, an interaction with a nurse who took vitals and asked questions, and then responding to the same questions again, asked by the doctor. In all, the process took most of the morning. The telehealth visit omitted the taking of vitals (probably not needed so soon after the previous visit), as well as the travel, the waiting, and the redundant questions. Charles spent the entire visit face-to-face with the doctor. It lasted ten minutes. Nothing substantive was missing.

When telehealth replaces outpatient visits, technology can replace some of the physical measurements that normally happen in the doctor's office, such as taking vital signs (as we will discuss later in the chapter). But much more is possible. During Covid, systems such as

Jefferson, Northwell, and Geisinger used telehealth to move acute hospital care into patients' homes, with nurses dispatched periodically to assess them and provide oxygen and other supplies, while monitoring and meetings with doctors occurred online. The hospital at-home model has continued to spread rapidly since then, thanks to the new support of Medicare reimbursement.[21]

Many doctors liked telehealth once they tried it. Appointment no-shows were greatly reduced because patients didn't have to take off so much time for travel and waiting (and because the time to get an appointment had been cut in half).[22] Patients also were less demanding of care they didn't need, because they had spent less time and effort to see the doctor—unnecessary antibiotic prescriptions went down. Patients made fewer unnecessary trips to the emergency room, and doctors were less likely to prescribe unnecessary tests that are all too easy to order in that setting.[23] And Hollander found he gave up little with online interaction with patients. He felt he could see more rather than less.

"When you see somebody in the office, they're in the paper gown, they all look the same," Hollander said. But, as a patient, he noted, "When you see me in my house, you see my house. You know whether I'm capable of taking care of myself."

Hollander sometimes asks patients to tour their homes or looks out the window with the camera. Does an asthma patient have cats at home, dusty surroundings, or a polluted neighborhood? Are roommates of a Covid patient wearing masks? And what medicines and vitamins are in the cabinet above the sink, and which ones did the patient actually take?

"In the office, patients don't bring them. You have no idea what they're taking," Hollander said. But going through medications at home by video can yield unexpected discoveries. "They have four bottles with the same drug. A generic-name one, a brand-name one, something similar. Using the same pills. 'Did you notice they're all green and they say one hundred on them? Let's put them in one bottle, throw out the other three bottles, and only take one of these each day.'"

Hollander said doctors need training to take advantage of telehealth's strengths and avoid its pitfalls. For example, they need strategies to evaluate the body without touching it. A family member can help with a knee exam. A camera can be positioned to look down a patient's throat. And there are other tricks Hollander and his team have developed.

"We have a bunch of training videos," he said. "One of my favorite ones is the belly exam. So, when you do an abdominal exam, I can't touch you, but that doesn't mean I can't tell if you don't have something bad. And so, one of the things we do is, I will ask you to go back against the wall so that I could see from your groin on up, and ask you to jump twice. And if you just think that's stupid and you're laughing the whole time, you do not have an intra-abdominal emergency."

Young doctors tend to resist using telemedicine more than their mid-career colleagues, Hollander said, perhaps because they haven't had time to develop confidence about what information they really need during an examination. For telehealth to stick in physician culture, he believes, training must start in medical school. That is happening. Steven Scheinman, dean of Geisinger Commonwealth School of Medicine, whom we met in the last chapter, said students learn best by seeing telehealth from different perspectives, calibrating their perceptions of patients on a screen compared to real life. Geisinger students attend telehealth visits three ways: they see patients on screen while sitting at a doctor's side, they sit with patients in their homes during appointments with a doctor on screen, and they watch exams from their own screens, with the doctor and patient on video.[24]

This is a hopeful story for a quantum leap toward better, more equitable health care. Areas with mental health and physician shortages are getting more help. Adding broadband connections for low-income patients can expand care more quickly than building new clinics. And telehealth is a step toward care that centers on patients' wellness rather than providing services only after they are sick, because telehealth can break down barriers in time and space, especially when combined with coaching and continuous monitoring (as we will discuss later in this chapter). Patients and doctors have voted for these advantages by continuing to use telehealth after lockdowns ended. Telehealth numbers declined from their peak but settled at a level more than thirty times higher than before the pandemic. Telehealth especially transformed mental health and substance abuse services, with half of visits to psychiatrists now happening online.[25]

But locking in these changes depends on pandemic-level payments continuing. Medicare made telehealth payments permanent for some services, but not for others. At this writing, insurance companies were still operating under emergency rules.[26]

Before the pandemic, fee-for-service payment held back telehealth. With Medicare and most private insurance refusing to pay, health systems such as Jefferson lost revenue by adding more telehealth, Hollander said. Jefferson's leadership invested in telehealth for the advantages to patients and with the expectation that a future system of value-based payment would reward more efficient practices that promoted overall health. But most hospitals and clinics stuck with in-person medicine rather than incur a financial penalty for doing tele-health. Thus, although research showed telehealth was often better for patients, perverse economic incentives prevented its adoption. As happened at Boeing in the 737 MAX case, profits came ahead of safety or, in this case, ahead of improved patient access and outcomes.[27] Instead, large employers offered telehealth services directly to workers and as services of their plans, in order to support employees, but also to reduce overall costs by keeping employees away from doctors who would send bills to be paid.

The crash adoption of telehealth during the Covid crisis saved lives, but for those doctors and clinics who had not prepared, quality probably suffered. Not every patient or condition is appropriate for telehealth, and the technology must be ready for it to be effective—suddenly leaping into this new way of seeing patients surely produced worse care at times.[28] Indeed, evidence emerged of unscrupulous operators taking advantage of the crisis to fraudulently sell telehealth visits with unqualified doctors who had not completed their training or otherwise scam patients.[29] With all the money on the line, online operators tried to turn telemedicine into another con.

Telehealth visits normally cost as much as office visits, Hollander said, because doctors and nurses do the same work either way, and brick-and-mortar facilities still have to be paid for even if they are not being used. He added that if telehealth becomes entrenched and payment is assured, providers probably could downsize facilities, perhaps saving 15 percent. Some studies have estimated savings of 30 percent.[30] But today, hospitals investing in telehealth tend to be those that are short of in-patient capacity; hospitals paying off debt for recent expansion are mostly staying with the old, in-person model.[31]

Most of the savings from telehealth accrue to patients. Telehealth is more convenient for them, saves time and travel, and can support wellness, which also saves money for the system as a whole. Those benefits explain why payviders and vertically integrated systems (those that combine insurance and care) have led the way on telehealth, including Kaiser Permanente and Geisinger Health (discussed in chapter 7). With their responsibility for the total patient, they can capture telehealth savings through better, at-home health.

Once again, we find misaligned financial incentives as a root cause of failure in the health care system—in this case, with the slow adoption of telehealth. But the medical profession also deserves some of the blame. Some doctors resisted telehealth, we believe, because it undercut their power, moving the center of patient care more into the patient's hands. Telehealth across state lines also created competition for doctors. Indeed, after the 2020 waves of the pandemic, state medical societies and licensing boards began reimposing rules they had waived, again blocking interstate care. According to statements by licensing officials and the American Medical Association, in-state rules ensured proper oversight of doctors by local authorities, as *Kaiser Health News* reported. But oversight could be achieved without blocking interstate care. We believe the heart of the resistance came, instead, from state boards' desire to capture licensing fees and from local doctors' desire to hold on to patients they were losing to big-name providers such as Johns Hopkins Medical, which suddenly began serving tens of thousands of patients in states where it didn't have facilities.[32] Near the end of 2021, as another wave of Covid grew, half of states had ended waivers allowing telehealth by out-of-state providers, and many insurers had pulled back from paying for the services, often leaving patients stranded and at risk, especially those losing access to mental health providers.[33]

"As with most things in medicine, it's a bottom-line issue," said Harry Greenspun, a physician who is chief medical officer for the consultancy Guidehouse. "The reason telehealth has been blocked across state lines for many years related fundamentally to physicians wanting to protect their own practices."[34]

Covid hit the health care system like shock therapy, and the rapid advance of telehealth that emerged was, on balance, a positive result. We don't think this genie is going back into the bottle. Along with other, complementary technological advances, which we will discuss later, telehealth helps solve systemic flaws that the Covid disaster helped expose. It could also be one catalyst to more fundamental change, as distance medicine allows vertically integrated health care systems to grow and reach into new geographies, including Black and Brown communities that face brutal health disparities. Other catalysts are needed as well, and technology can help, as we shall see next.

BRIDGING INFORMATION GAPS

During the chaotic initial wave of Covid, in the spring of 2020, when Pennsylvania's governor, Tom Wolf, made his daily briefings, it became clear to a group of viewers in Philadelphia that they were sitting on critical information he did not have. Their nine-year-old nonprofit organization knew within minutes when Covid patients were admitted in any of hundreds of health care facilities near Philadelphia and in southern New Jersey, as well as their demographics and other key information. Wolf was relatively blind to those facts.

"They really weren't able to get detailed information yet on ethnicity, race, age of Covid patients, folks that were testing positive, and so forth, and really understanding what was happening in and around the Philadelphia region. And we had that information. We knew that," said Marty Lupinetti, the president and CEO of the nonprofit HealthShare Exchange, usually called HSX. "Within three or four days, we were sending data to the state and city that really augmented their ability to understand that level of detail."[35]

HSX was built to help health care companies share patient records from their often-incompatible information systems. But in the crisis, it was able to do much more. The city of Philadelphia and its public health authorities asked HSX to tap into its data. Hospitals in the region shared information on capacity and where patients could be transferred. HSX applied its analytic capabilities to show hot spots geographically, calculate risk scores based on patients' other health conditions, and provide information to help with contact tracing. The analysis allowed public health officials and others to see nearly in real time how racial and economic disparities were worsening the pandemic and where help was needed most.

The same story repeated in other areas of the country that have similar organizations, called health information exchanges. But the results were uneven. These home-grown nonprofits cover territories of different sizes, have different levels of support and involvement, and don't always get attention from those who need the information. Most people have never heard of them.

Health information exchanges got a starting boost from the Obama administration in the early 2010s as a solution to electronic systems that could not communicate—the same interoperability problem that left nurses in various places frantically calling on the phone to transfer Covid patients during the pandemic's surges.[36] More than seventy exchanges now exist, some covering entire states or even coalitions of states, while others stitch together smaller areas within states. The exchanges' member organizations share data through their networks, including hospitals, health systems, insurance plans, nursing homes, and clinics. Lupinetti's HSX connects more than five hundred members in Pennsylvania, New Jersey, and Delaware.[37] After a decade, the exchanges have also begun connecting among themselves, with the capacity to share information across much of the nation, and have developed regional and national partnerships.[38] But making these links is slow, complex work, entangled with myriad data standards and legal and turf issues. Creating a seamlessly connected national health network remains a dream.

Lupinetti said his organization knows how to handle the technical and privacy challenges. But the legal and political issues are harder. During the Covid crisis, public health officials needed time to negotiate data agreements that would allow sharing of information with the exchange. The ability to create a detailed picture of the emerging pandemic had to wait for signatures on those agreements.

"Part of that was to have a memo of understanding or data use agreement or some sort of rules of the road on how we were going to operate and share information," he said. "And trying to do that during a crisis or in an emergency—just very difficult."

Sometimes the reason for these problems is unclear even to those involved. Lupinetti never could unsnarl data sharing on vaccination status. The exchange could have linked data in the region's various vaccine registries to patient health records, allowing rapid verification for patients in the emergency room, outreach to the unvaccinated, and mapping of areas of low vaccine uptake. Instead, doctors had to look up names in each registry, one at a time.

That problem repeated nationally. Information systems for public health and health care do not communicate. There is no national system showing who has been vaccinated.[39] Strangely, we have created a society in which giant internet companies know almost everything about us, for the relatively frivolous purpose of targeting ads, but we rely on a patchwork of local and state nonprofit exchanges to connect health information that can save lives and improve the well-being of the public. The exchanges do good work, to the extent they are able, but we must ask why the system was built this way, with incompatible software that can be linked only a piece at a time by scores of local membership organizations.

Karen DeSalvo said a purpose lies behind these problems. She is the doctor and public health expert we met in chapter 5. She spent several years working to improve health information technology in the Obama administration, before joining Google in 2019. The firms that created EHR software made the systems incompatible by design, with data standards that recorded basic facts differently—such as gender or blood pressure—and created a medical Tower of Babel, as she called it. By keeping patients' health data proprietary, EHR companies could make money selling it, DeSalvo said—and it is extremely valuable.[40] Currently, four major EHR companies control our data, each with different segments of the health care market: Epic, Cerner, Meditech, and Allscripts.[41]

"They want to lock you in. They don't want you to be able to take your data out and move it to a new system, so they want to make it really hard for data to export," DeSalvo said. But the problem is a political one, not technical, she added. "The health care systems and the EHR companies fight this so well. They're incredible. They're incredibly sophisticated at resisting the technology implementations that would allow the kind of interoperability that [is needed]. It's technologically completely feasible; they just don't do it."

In many cases, systems don't work together to bring up information when doctors need it, and frequently cannot accurately identify patients at all, because no national standard was established to match people to their records.[42] Charles recently spent frustrating days that stretched into more than a week trying to get hospitals and doctors to exchange information about his father, who needed a surgery, in a process that required faxing numerous paper forms to nameless records clerks who could be reached no other way, not by phone or email, but who held the progress of treatment in their hands.

Strides have been made to address these problems. With government attention—including a $30 billion investment made in federal legislation in 2009—systems evolved partially from emulating the old paper records to become easier to search. The consolidation of clinics and hospitals into large, integrated health systems also aided sharing of information about patients who stay within those systems. And perhaps most important from the vantage of our systemic investigation, patients have begun to demand access to their own health records.

That last change brings us again to the heart of what went wrong when American health care failed. We lacked a culture in which patients occupy the center of medical decisions—rather than doctors, hospitals, EHR companies, or their need for profits. Giving each of us control of our own information would be a more-than-symbolic step toward creating that patient-centered culture.

"It has everything to do with power," DeSalvo said. "It's a huge, embarrassing, and frustrating issue for my profession that the medical profession, in writing, has resisted consumers having access to their records for years. It's paternalistic. The excuse usually is people can't handle the data; we need to help them. . . . Some institutions now let patients see the whole note, not just the lab tests—and, man, physicians fight that really hard. But once you can get them over it, everybody loves it."

Technology can help here, too. As computing has moved from mainframes to smartphones, the idea of creating, owning, and carrying around one's own health care information has become a real possibility. We will probably have our health records in our pockets before any smoothly operating national information network can share them between our health care providers.

THERE IS AN APP FOR THAT

Perhaps the most important piece of information for your health care is what outcome you want. The decision to seek medical attention itself depends on each patient's values and desires. Tellingly, however, today's electronic health records normally do not contain patients' advance directives, which record their preferences and whom they designate to make decisions if they are unable to do so. Instead, these documents often live in filing cabinets in lawyers' offices or stuffed with deeds and birth certificates in a safe deposit box at a bank. Covid exposed this flaw in the health care system as if uncovering a wound. Patients were separated from their families, often unable to speak, and didn't have that crucial piece of paper.

"We heard from emergency room doctors in a variety of places under incredible stress," said Jeff Zucker, a health IT entrepreneur. "We had one in particular who said her hallways were lined with gurneys. She had people backed up in the ICU. She herself spent three hours trying to locate the health care agent or identify somebody for a particular member of a family," he said. "The technology that's required to help fix our health care system does not necessarily need to be that complicated when you get to a very basic situation like that."[43]

Zucker cofounded a firm in 2007 that offers a website and smartphone app to record and communicate users' advance directives and sends the information into their medical records (he is no longer with the company). MyDirectives.com lets users record essential health information, contact information for a person entrusted to make decisions, and self-made videos telling doctors about values and desires. Doctors and ambulance drivers can access the information in the medical record from their own phones by scanning a QR code that users carry in their wallets.

The system has obvious benefits, but it isn't clear who should pay for it in our health care system. Traditionally, neither hospitals nor health insurance companies take responsibility for recording patients' values and desired outcomes for care—we're on our own in that regard. But Zucker's company found some support from value-based and Medicare Advantage plans, which are designed to make more money by improving the total health of their members. Those payers could capture the savings produced by a member's advance directive—for example, when a patient did not want expensive and futile end-of-life care. Knowing patients' values should be fundamental to value-based health care.

This payment problem is common for technology that promotes health and wellness. For example, in 2021, Cone Health, a small, nonprofit system in North Carolina, shut down an app it had invested in, which was successfully keeping diabetes patients healthier, as the *Washington Post* reported. With a value-based payment system that supported wellness, the app might have made financial sense, but a traditional payment scheme persisted for most of Cone's patients, which meant that an app that produced fewer sick diabetes patients would only reduce income for the hospital. The company withdrew support, consigning the software to be destroyed.[44] A similar fate met an app created at the Dartmouth-Hitchcock health system in New Hampshire. In trials, the software cut health care costs for people with chronic conditions by 15 percent. Dartmouth abandoned the project in 2017, selling it to a company in Sweden, where it is being used successfully in a public system with an incentive to keep people healthy.[45]

Robert Pearl has likened hospitals to Kodak, the photography company that failed to adapt to digital technology. Pearl, a plastic surgeon and best-selling author, is a professor at Stanford Medical School and former CEO of Permanente Medical Group, which cared for five million Kaiser patients. In 2020, he spoke at a population health colloquium David cochaired. The pandemic seemed to have collapsed barriers protecting doctors and hospitals from innovation and competition. It propelled a leap in technology and a surge of capital from Wall Street, promising a reordering of winners in a disrupted health care market. Local doctors would not be able to compete with distant physicians on telehealth, Pearl said. At-home care, powered by telehealth and personal health monitoring technology, would beat hospital care. "We have combustible forest, and the wind is blowing right in front of us," Pearl said.

Many of these innovations can happen if patients like them, payers reimburse them, and regulators allow them. Wearable health monitoring devices can produce records of vital signs and other indicators continuously, day and night. That much information would overwhelm a human doctor, but artificial intelligence could scan the data stream and flag health concerns. Then, when the AI tells you something might be wrong, you don't have to drive to a doctor's office. You would log on to a portal, share the data, and discuss it via text, joining a face-to-face video meeting if necessary. Should conditions warrant, your health system could create an acute care room in your home, with daily check-ins from a nurse. In this future, the hospital goes where you go. Left behind, the physical facility shrinks, as the patient becomes the center of care rather than the building.

We have the monitoring technology for this future now, but the analytical software is not ready. Doctors know what vital signs mean when taken periodically in an exam room, but we need new research to interpret numbers that are measured in daily life, around the clock. Without artificial intelligence screening that information, it would become noise, like an overactive smoke detector. This annoyance already exists for some doctors. Friends and family members with new devices can repeatedly call, panicked about high readings.

Using AI to manage these devices is new and needs more work. Some products have gone far wide of the mark, such as an Amazon wristband that, among other things, attempts to interpret users' tone of voice for cues to their health—with bizarre results.[46] But the technology is getting better. Covid rapidly advanced use of wearables. Sports teams put them on, and then workers for other businesses, to continuously track when wearers were exposed to virus carriers.[47]

Technology could disrupt the dysfunctional electronic health record industry, too, once patients fully control their own records. Many people understandably distrust big internet companies that are in the business of using and selling our information, and attempts by firms such as Google to gather up information in a national EHR have met resistance.[48] But our phones have become trusted vaults of private information, and our medical records could live there, too. Apple built an app that interfaces with clinics' EHR systems, allowing patients to download their records from many health care providers, transfer them using the phone, and keep everything in one place for their own use. Users with wearable devices can also collect information from their own bodies and store that data in the app, too.[49]

Within the hospital, technology can help doctors solve some long-standing problems. We discussed unexplained clinical variation in chapter 6. It is the disturbing phenomenon that different doctors, presented with identically situated patients, often come to very different conclusions about what to do. Besides the consequences for safety and quality of care, research shows that doctor decisions account for 80 percent of health care spending.[50] These variations produce huge cost differences around the country, but solutions have been elusive.[51] For some relatively simple physician choices, such as prescribing antibiotics or opioids, published guidelines can narrow variation, but many decisions are too complex for a cookie-cutter approach.[52] In those cases, technology can help doctors become better judges of when care is backed by scientific evidence. A system made by a company called QURE.ai simulates situations doctors face and provides feedback on their decisions to show when they deviate from evidence-based practices. In an experiment using this approach, doctors reduced unnecessary testing by more than 50 percent and improved quality scores more than 25 percent.[53]

Ultimately, making hospitals as safe as airplanes—and preventing another Covid crash—will require more innovations like these, using what we learn from deep investigation of errors to engineer human processes that will avoid their repetition. Technology can help us get there, assisting doctors to navigate medical processes that have become too complex and demanding for any individual to fully master. That will be our subject in chapter 11.

But first we must consider what we want from technology, along with what we are willing to sacrifice. We don't have a choice about whether change will happen—health care will change as technology disrupts old ways of doing things, just as Covid changed work, travel, and even how we breathe. The pandemic moved us forward in an irrevocable way. Although we can't go back, we can shape how we use health technology in the future. As this chapter has intimated, decisions about technology cannot be disentangled from power and money. We must decide who will control our information and whether our technology will promote good health or the profits of health care companies.

These thoughts lead to our next chapter, on work and employment. For seventy years, employers have paid for American health care, but they have rarely used that power to influence how the system works. Standing on the verge of this new age of health technology, with the potential for around-the-clock monitoring of our bodies, employers cannot evade their roles, for good or bad.

Chapter 10

Covid, Work, and Health

How the Covid pandemic affected you depended largely on where you worked. If you processed chickens in a factory or cooked on a line, your chances of catching and dying of the disease were far greater than if you wrote computer code or taught at a university. We discussed these differences in chapter 4, because they help explain racial inequities and the impact of the social determinants of health. But employment interacted with Covid in a second way. Where you work in America decides your access to health care. Compensation determines both whether you get health coverage and your ability to pay the deductibles that make it possible to use coverage. And there was a third link as well. Employers pay for health care as a whole system, giving them leverage to improve it. Employer health plans cover 155 million Americans, at an annual cost of over $22,000 to cover the average family, and that money sustains the health care industry.[1] A proverb says, "He who pays the piper calls the tune," but American businesses generally have evaded or failed in their responsibility to fix health care, with most executives saying it is the government's job, not theirs.[2]

Here is another root cause in our investigation of why the American health care system crashed during the pandemic, disintegrating like an airliner that missed the runway. Employers neglected their role. They manage health in the workplace, pay for coverage, and have the power to demand better from health care providers—but many remained passive, did the least they could, or failed to accept their responsibility at all. Our airplane had no pilot. Or, to make the metaphor more precise, these companies were like airlines sending us off on this journey in a rudderless aircraft, without a seatbelt, but fully fueled for high-speed flight.

Business owners and CEOs may argue they don't want responsibility for health and didn't ask for it, but this role is deeply embedded in the American economy. Health care became linked to employment seventy-five years ago, during labor shortages after World War II, when companies competed to attract workers by offering health and retirement benefits. A national health service would have been better, as in other industrialized countries, but doctors fought so-called "socialized medicine." Normally, it is impossible to make such a dramatic change against strong opposition in our democracy, because of the divided authority of checks and balances. In the United States, power is centralized in capital and decentralized in government, and businesses are better at doing big things fast.

Covid exploited America's fragmented, employer-based system. Low-income workers suffered the most. Often those classified as "essential" had the least power to demand safe working conditions and were exposed to Covid in high numbers (as we discussed in chapter 4). Pandemic job losses hit that level hardest and longest, too.[3] Some employers did what they had always done, concentrating on business rather than worker safety and health care. The welfare of low-level workers has always been at risk within some workplaces, but the crisis made those conditions impossible to ignore.

"There were some companies that probably took this very seriously. They tried to do the right thing," said Byron Scott, who has seen these issues as a physician, university teacher, nonprofit leader, and, formerly, global consultant with IBM's Watson Health. "Others just kind of did what they had to do minimally. And some, they just didn't care."[4]

But Covid has created a moment of change, one that may be as powerful as the post–World War II era when businesses first started paying for health care. Covid has remade how and where people work, the size of the labor force and the demand for workers, and the attitudes of employees and what they will accept. Many employers see their roles in a new way, too. Those changes can help remake the health care system.

"I think there's been a big sea change," Scott said. "I think there's been a big awakening in a lot of levels."

To appreciate the size of these changes, consider a few pandemic impacts that are smaller in scale but would have seemed large before.

One example: foodborne illness. Annually it kills three thousand people and sickens forty-eight million, with restaurants serving as the source of most outbreaks, and with the most common malady the vomiting and diarrhea caused by norovirus.[5] Before Covid, public health researchers confirmed what cooks and servers often said—that restaurant employees commonly came to work when they were sick with vomiting or diarrhea.[6] Considering their low wages, reliance on tips, and lack of paid sick leave, many of these workers couldn't afford to stay home (a fifth of them live in poverty).[7] The Covid crisis led many states to mandate paid sick leave and the federal government provided tax incentives to businesses that offered it.[8] A coalition of large employers and philanthropists spoke out on the issue, trying to shame businesses to offer leave and protect the public.[9] Anecdotally, many Americans seemed newly aware of how to prevent infectious disease, especially in restaurants. Then, in 2020, the CDC reported a large and unprecedented drop in foodborne illness. Those numbers were hard to interpret, with combined factors such as increased handwashing and the closure of many restaurants.[10] But new habits probably did play a part. The pandemic winter of 2020–2021 also became a season almost without influenza, demonstrating that the changes made to avoid Covid could stop other common infections.[11]

As another example of pandemic change, Scott pointed out how the new explosion of telehealth could assist both workers and employers. For workers, telehealth could be an avenue for ongoing support and monitoring of their health. For employers, it could reduce the time workers need to leave the office for doctor appointments. And for yet another example, Scott said the wide adoption of remote work would change some health insurance, as managed care plans with restricted geographic areas were rewritten to cover workers newly spread across the country.

Most dramatically, the pandemic forced employers into a role normally reserved for public health officials or elected leaders. From the early days of the pandemic, they had to decide whether to close their workplaces and for how long, whether to require masks, and how to handle social distancing. State and local officials also set rules, but they were inconsistent and sometimes not strict enough to protect workers or the public (as we discussed in chapter 5). Airlines decided how to control Covid in the air, with some leaving rows of seats open, distributing wipes, or changing how passengers got on and off, and all requiring masks and reducing food and beverage service to help passengers keep their masks on.[12] With lives on the line, employers didn't have the choice of being passive.

"If you look at our legal system, if you're not providing a safe environment for your employees, you're ultimately liable as an organization or a company," Scott said. "When you look at the perspective of ethical, moral, corporate social responsibility, they have a responsibility to their community and their employees to try to do what's right and what's best."

Later in the pandemic, with too many people refusing vaccination, employers began mandating the shot. In August 2021, United Airlines ordered all employees to get vaccinated or face termination. Early on, the airline had worked with unions to provide vaccination incentives and to build goodwill for the effort, but that had not been enough. Then, with the death of a fifty-seven-year-old pilot, CEO Scott Kirby made the decision. As he told the *New York Times*, "People are dying, and we can do something to stop that with United Airlines."[13] Other major companies followed. Large employers became a force for vaccination. Companies such as Amtrak and General Electric even confronted employees with lengthy questionnaires about their spiritual beliefs to overcome phony religious objections to vaccination.[14]

Employer vaccine mandates worked better than many commentators had predicted. In surveys, most unvaccinated workers said they would quit if their employers forced them to get the shot, but in the end, few made that choice—just 232 of United's 67,000 employees.[15] As writer and sociologist Zeynep Tufekci noted, the mandates may have been secretly welcome to some employees who had taken an anti-vax stand to comply with their political or cultural peer group. A boss's order allowed them to save face. "It may well be that some of the unvaccinated are a bit like cats stuck in a tree. They've made bad decisions earlier and now may be frozen, part in fear, and unable to admit their initial hesitancy wasn't a good idea," Tufekci wrote.[16]

President Biden also announced a vaccine mandate, using the federal government's workplace safety authority, but Republican attorneys general in twenty-six states challenged the rule, and it stalled in court while more than one thousand Americans were still dying every day. White House officials suggested businesses go ahead and carry out the mandate while waiting for a final court decision.[17] At first many did so, but late in 2021, with the legal situation murky, and worker shortages threatening operations—Amtrak at one point considered cutting service—employers backed off from mandates with the job not completed.[18] Meanwhile, the governor of Texas had issued an executive order banning vaccine mandates.[19]

The entire situation seemed to confirm the point we made earlier: In our country, with centralized capital and decentralized government, business cannot avoid its responsibility for health. Without corporate leaders requiring vaccination, it would not happen in a timely way. (And imagine the impossibility of the federal government requiring those religious questionnaires.)

Businesses changed society when they closed offices, required masks, and mandated vaccinations. They were accepting their role in health in a way they never had before. But would that new assertiveness extend to using their economic power to change the health care industry?

The economic might of employers in health care is immense, because their payments generate the profits that grow hospitals and make some doctors wealthy. Government health care (Medicare, Medicaid, military and veterans) covers 35 percent of Americans, but the government is not a generous payer, and providers complain they don't make money on those patients (this is why creating a "public option" that would allow private parties to buy into a government plan is so controversial).[20] On average, hospitals charge private payers 2.5 times more than they get from Medicare for the same services.[21] Those extra dollars represent potential savings for employers and their leverage to improve the system.

We have discussed some ways that process could work. For example, in chapter 7, we mentioned a program by large employers to demand good prices and high quality for joint replacements and other major surgeries at national centers, sending workers there from thousands of miles away. Kaiser Permanente is the original prototype of a health system created by a business, Henry Kaiser's shipbuilding company. But some other companies that have applied their economic might to reforming health care have failed. In 2018, Amazon, J.P. Morgan, and Berkshire Hathaway joined in a venture called Haven to attack health care costs and gave up only two years later. As Berkshire's Warren Buffett said, "We were fighting a tapeworm in the American economy and the tapeworm won."[22]

Haven faced the challenge—similar to all businesses—of market pressures coming from two sides. As a buyer of health care, employers face huge, concentrated health care companies that in many cities have monopolistic pricing power. As a buyer of labor, employers seek to recruit workers who like the choice and flexibility they perceive as coming from fee-for-service health plans (recall from chapter 7 how workers rebelled against HMOs in the 1990s). But most workers aren't aware of how much of their compensation goes to pay premiums for those fee-for-service plans. The tax code also plays a part. Employers benefit on their taxes from giving compensation in the form of health care instead of wages. These are major challenges, but they aren't insurmountable. Haven lacked a workable strategy and tried to do too much at one time.[23]

As we hope we have shown over many chapters, improving Americans' health requires more than health care. What we do every day matters much more than our time with doctors. Employers can protect and promote their workers' health, as they learned during the pandemic when they used masking, remote work, and vaccine mandates to take charge. Preventive health benefits are real, inexpensive, and unaffected by the market power of hospitals or insurance companies.

We also hope we have shown that reducing the cost of care and increasing its quality demands realigning the economic incentives of the system. Employers can make a difference on that problem, too, by directing their spending away from fee-for-service medicine and toward value-based plans, payviders, and closed systems.

The post-pandemic world offers a unique opportunity to make those changes happen.

THE GREAT REASSESSMENT

As the Covid crisis approached, Byron Scott was traveling in the Middle East for work. He got home to San Diego and sized up the situation with his wife, who is a mental health counselor. They decided to grab a flight to Hawaii, where they had a home, and hole up there for the coming pandemic lockdown. Living in Hawaii, she continued seeing patients via telehealth, reaching six states where she was licensed as clinical social worker. Meanwhile, he found his work broadening in a new way, as he spoke remotely to conferences he couldn't have attended physically, taught students via Zoom, and spent more time with the two boards he serves for large nonprofit medical organizations. That work, Scott found, had more meaning than what he had been doing before the pandemic, when he had been traveling heavily as a consultant. He left his corporate job in June 2020. The pandemic lockdown had closed everyone in, eliminating mobility, but, for Scott, doors seemed to be opening, showing him a new way to live and different areas of his life to prioritize.

"Covid really forced you to make some decisions about what do you do next," Scott said. "It's been good to energize and jump start, for me, and to set my next path."

Scott had started his path in life in inner-city Los Angeles. No member of his family had attended college, but Scott's mother sent him and his brother to Catholic school and the family set high expectations for his educational attainment. He attended UCLA as an undergraduate and UC San Diego for medical school. As a young doctor, he gravitated to emergency medicine, because it was about doing the right thing right away, without worrying about payment. That professional foundation, and good mentors, set him on the path to health policy and leadership, consulting, and a busy life using analytics to advise firms on their health responsibilities.

Then came Covid and its reminders of what mattered most. Millions of other people had the same experience. Commentators called it "The Great Reassessment."[24] At first, the notion that so many people—a significant portion of the population—all were reconsidering their values and direction in life seemed far-fetched, but surveys and employment data seemed to confirm a deep change was happening. A Pew Research Center study of those thrown out of work by Covid showed that a majority enjoyed being freed from their old jobs and were considering a change of occupation.[25] As the economy restarted and went into high gear, workers remained scarce, despite rising wages—the total workforce had shrunk. More workers were quitting their jobs than ever before, especially in lower-wage occupations.[26] And the change seemed to be permanent, because a huge wave of Americans had retired early, with retirements occurring at more than twice the normal rate.[27] The Great Reassessment seemed to be real.

"I think it's absolutely real," Scott said. "I think everyone, no matter what they've done in their career, their job, across demographics, across age—I think everyone's reevaluated a lot of things as a result of Covid. I think people are deciding what's important to them in terms of their time and their values and their worth."

In a positive sense, the reassessment led to workers' seeking greater meaning, such as when Scott turned more to education and volunteerism. Reporters told of corporate executives becoming school teachers or mentors for entrepreneurs and of the many who left professional or creative jobs to start their own freelance or independent businesses.[28] But more often, we suspect, reassessment meant getting away from the negative, as low-income workers decided not to return to old jobs and looked for higher pay, better working conditions, and safer workplaces.[29] The burden of the pandemic had fallen heavily on women, who reported levels of burnout far higher than those for men, as they had continued to shoulder more work at home and performed more caring roles on the job—supporting their teams in tough times—according to a report by McKinsey and LeanIn.[30] Late in the pandemic, the Pew Center found a huge increase in the number of women who wanted to leave the paid workforce entirely if they could (a change not seen in men).[31]

To some extent, companies coped with worker shortages by becoming more efficient or doing less. For example, hotel companies permanently changed their business models to offer less housekeeping during stays and fewer breakfasts and other perks, motivated at first by Covid concerns and then by the lack of chambermaids and cooks.[32] Hospitals dealt with nursing shortages with technology that allowed fewer nurses to oversee more patients.[33] But automation and efficiency couldn't bridge the shortage of blue-collar workers in lodging, bars and restaurants, food processing, trucking, delivery and package handling, construction, and many other occupations. Workers took opportunities to move up, and employers had to compete to fill entry-level jobs, offering better wages and benefits.[34] Employers with health plans for their workers broadly increased telehealth, mental health coverage, and wellness programs—more than half changed their wellness offerings.[35] McDonald's, the stereotypical employer for entry-level burger-flippers, announced higher wages, tuition benefits, 401(k) retirement contributions, and paid sick leave for the 36,500 employees in its company-owned locations.[36]

Businesses had treated health as a cost to be minimized. How much money could be saved on a health plan without alienating workers? More enlightened business leaders, especially those with expensive, skilled workers, invested significantly in wellness to avoid lost time and reduce health care claims, although, as we shall see in the next section, the bottom-line results of those programs were mixed. But many employers with low-wage workers had excluded them from benefits and didn't worry much about their health, assuming that sick workers could be easily replaced. Covid changed that calculation for some companies.

Tyson Foods is a strong example of the new role of health in business. Like the other food companies we discussed in chapter 4, Tyson's meat processing lines spread Covid rapidly early in the pandemic—in one plant, half the workers got ill at once, and Tyson plants had a total of 29,000 infections and 151 deaths, according to an October 2021 congressional report.[37] The *New York Times* reported that Tyson refused to close an Iowa pork plant amid a severe and deadly Covid outbreak in April 2020, rebuffing the local sheriff and health officials.[38] But as the pandemic wore on, Tyson adopted a new strategy, adding a chief medical officer, on-site medical facilities, and paid sick leave. In August 2021, with only half its workers vaccinated, the company mandated every employee get the shot or be fired—one of the first large companies to do so—and it soon achieved 96 percent compliance among its 60,500 workers. That was a daring move, but it paid off for Tyson, because it meant the company could count on having staff to run its plants even in hard-hit southern US communities with low vaccination rates, the *Times* reported. As a union leader pointed out, there simply weren't enough people available to risk losing them.[39]

Two trends had converged. Employers changed, taking more responsibility for the welfare of their workers and communities—often, as in the case of mask wearing and vaccination, because only they had the authority to make rules stick. And employees changed as well, demanding better and more meaningful work, with safer conditions and more caring employers. David has long written on the benefits for population health of wellness and prevention, paid sick leave, mental health care and convenient telehealth, but those improvements came slowly and incrementally due to inertia in the political process and the health care system itself. But then the pandemic made health a priority for employers and workers, igniting the incredible power and speed of the American marketplace. The change that results could benefit health far more than investments in doctors and hospitals. As a single example, think of the millions of avoided illnesses that could occur with restaurant workers receiving paid leave to stay home when they are sick.

Byron Scott said the relationship of business to health has fundamentally changed. Health is much more than simply a cost now.

"I think it comes down to the communities where employees live and work," he said. "Employers need to understand their population. Their population is their employees. And understand all those interactions where they live, how they get there, and what their extended family does—because those children or other loved ones are on their insurance plans. You need to understand all of those dynamics if you're going to be effective going forward, because things have definitely changed post-Covid."

LIVING WITH EMPLOYER-LED HEALTH

Employers already have great power over Americans' time, wealth, location, professional development, personal expression, and safety. Do we want them to control our health, too? This question means much more than it once did, because health has come to mean something more than it did when employers began paying for health coverage in the mid-twentieth century. Back then, doctor bills were like the fees we pay today for a barber or repair technician, but now, in our complex health system, that fee-for-service arrangement doesn't work well anymore. As we have seen, prevention and the ongoing maintenance of health are more important to longevity and well-being than visits to the doctor. Employers have begun taking on that work. But employer oversight of our everyday activities and decisions—essentially, the fabric of personal life—raises serious questions about our privacy and autonomy as free individuals.

Large employers have gone down this road already with employee wellness programs. The oil company BP requires employees to earn 1,000 points in its wellness program to gain enrollment in a preferred health plan with lower deductibles and better benefits. After that, an additional 1,000 points is worth a $100 gift card. Employees can earn

250 points by walking a million steps, 75 points by sleeping at least seven hours a night for twenty nights, and 25 points by meditating ten times. The program rewards participation in counseling sessions with the employee assistance program (125 points), working on retirement with a financial coach (125 points), and meeting three times with a lifestyle management coach (250 points)—and many other similar personal tasks and activities, including maintenance of serious chronic conditions. In 2021, getting a Covid vaccination was worth a whopping 500 points. Everything in the program is measured and documented, mostly using wearable technology or apps.[40]

Certainly, it seems paternalistic for an employer to measure how many hours you sleep, rewarding an early bedtime with points toward a gift card, but research shows that workers tend to ignore wellness programs without incentives.[41] That result fits with what we know about behavior. Free gym memberships generally don't increase fitness, because cost is not what keeps most of us from going to the gym—in fact, most people paying for their own gym memberships don't meet their personal expectations for actually going.[42] As Americans, we probably struggle more with these issues because of our individualism and our immersion in consumer marketing that promotes unhealthy diets and sedentary lifestyles. Most Americans probably wouldn't put up with mandatory daily calisthenics at work, as is common in Japan, a country with more communitarian values (as we discussed in chapter 3).[43] And while two-thirds of Americans said in a survey they had reduced their meat consumption, agriculture statistics indicate otherwise—we lead the world as meat eaters, consuming more than 100 kilograms each annually (more than four pounds per person per week), and that number has not gone down.[44]

America's epidemic of lifestyle diseases—including type 2 diabetes, heart disease, and obesity—has helped drive spiraling health care costs, and those costs helped drive four out of five large employers to offer wellness programs, expecting to reduce medical expenditures and improve productivity.[45] The programs often start with biomedical screening to determine what help employees need, including taking health histories and often administering blood tests, looking especially for workers with chronic conditions such as diabetes that could benefit from maintenance support.[46] But David has observed that wellness programs seem to work best supporting employees who already have healthy habits, while programs are less successful at changing the practices of those who are doing poorly. The programs are voluntary by law, so researchers studying their effectiveness must contend with selection bias and find success among willing participants who might have been on the right track already. In 2019, a rare, truly randomized study followed a program at twenty BJ's Wholesale stores, with four thousand employees, compared to a control of 140 stores, with twenty-nine thousand employees, who received no wellness program. It found modest, self-reported improvements in diet and exercise, but no overall benefit in health outcomes or work performance.[47]

That was discouraging news, but it tells us something about motivating healthy behavior. The incentives for the BJ's Wholesale workers were small—just a $25 BJ's gift card for completing a four- to eight-week module—and participation was low.[48] As with any health intervention, a dose that is too low yields an insignificant response. Instead, a program may need large incentives and intrusive electronic monitoring to make an impact. BP's program has stakes potentially worth thousands of dollars, and it inserts itself into all aspects of its employees' lives, tracking and verifying their movements, sleep, volunteerism, financial planning, and a broad range of health activities. It is powerful and intrusive, but perhaps a program needs to be that way in order to work.

Digital health devices enable these programs, and new products are pouring onto the market, building on the success of the Fitbit, which BP issues free to employees. Users wear the gadgets on the wrist, on a finger as a ring, in shoes, attached to skin, connected to phones, and even in the ears with music earbuds.[49] Monitoring from these devices can produce immense amounts of data about wearers. Science and software can't make full use of that information yet, but experts see the day coming soon when wearable devices will continuously communicate with cloud-based artificial intelligence to interpret the wearer's health all day—providing information all the time that is comparable to what we now receive only at an annual physical.[50] But who would receive that information? As the health care system exists today, your employer rather than your doctor would probably get it, because most medical practices are oriented to visits of sick patients, not wellness programs managing ongoing health.

This is a potentially disquieting future. Employers may be benevolent, but their fundamental interest in workers is for their economic production, not their health. The temptation for an employer to misuse personal health information is far greater than for a medical provider or government agency. Consider how an employer could most easily save money on an employee with unhealthy personal habits. Rather than invest in modifying the behavior, the boss could terminate the worker, and that would be legal so long as the bad habits were not caused by a disability, according to Elizabeth Brown, a law professor who has studied the programs.[51] She compiled disturbing cases in which employers used a heavy hand in their wellness programs, including firing a worker who declined to take an invasive health survey.[52] Employers provide apps to help women monitor their menstrual periods and reproduction that could expose them to discrimination over sexual activity or abortions, Brown wrote.[53] The information lacks the legal protections we have with our doctors. The Health Insurance Portability and Accountability Act (HIPAA) does not apply to digital devices gathering health information and sending it to employer wellness programs.[54] And although the programs are technically voluntary, opting out may not be possible. The incentives needed to make wellness programs effective can be large enough that, for low-income workers, refusing to participate is not a practical choice.[55]

The pandemic rapidly deepened the role of employers in their employees' health. At first, employers offered incentives for vaccination, but, as we explained, companies such as United and Tyson decided to fire workers who would not get the shot—a needed safety measure, but one that fundamentally changed the relationship of worker and boss. Physical health checks to prevent employees from spreading the virus also crossed a new threshold, potentially providing employers with a new dimension of data about their workers.[56] During the pandemic, employers began using more digital tools in health and wellness programs, including more wearable electronic monitoring, online health screenings, and support for workers at home, especially for mental health counseling.[57]

We agree with those decisions. During the Covid crisis, businesses stepped in to fill a void. America's atrophied public health establishment had failed. Medical providers, disengaged from prevention and home care, waited at emergency room doors to be overwhelmed by patients. We needed employers to require masks and vaccines and to look after their employees' mental health and wellness.

But that isn't all we need. In the post-pandemic era, we need legislation and a new social contract to protect employees' privacy and autonomy in this new world of work-based health maintenance. And we also need businesses to help fix other parts of the failed system, especially in public health and in communities, where the social determinants of health extend beyond clinics or workplaces. Ideally, we need partnerships, connecting businesses, communities, and doctors and nurses, so all can take part in addressing the health of the population as a whole. That is starting to happen. We looked at this trend from the point of view of health care providers in chapter 7. What does it look like from the perspective of business?

MUCH-NEEDED NEW PARTNERSHIPS

Despite the hardship and division our country has gone through during the pandemic—and partly because of it—businesses broadly seem to have accepted new responsibility for their role in society. We have discussed employer safety and wellness programs that aim to save money on health care and keep employees productive. But companies also are reaching outside their doors to address the social determinants of health in their communities, accepting responsibility for the neighborhoods where they operate, even if that doesn't contribute directly to their bottom line. Some corporate leaders intrinsically want to help. Others feel the push of public scoring of their environmental, social, and governance qualities, called ESG, with numbers that now inform investors when deciding whether to buy stock. And some probably follow along because social responsibility is the fashionable new trend.

"There are some companies, pre-Covid, that really have taken this whole corporate social responsibility seriously and are doing more than they have to," Byron Scott said. "They're suddenly looking at 'What can we do to invest in communities where our employees live?' . . . Covid really bore that out, and things around social justice in summer 2020, and looking at the health disparities around the country. I think if you're a large employer and in certain cities or areas where there's a huge health disparity issue, whatever you can do to help in those communities where employees live is probably the right thing to do and, in the end, could help recruit people into the organization."

In the spring of 2021, the chief medical officers of Disney, Goodyear, and IBM announced a seven-point public health roadmap with forty corporate health leaders and public health officials who had been convened by the Johns Hopkins Institute for Health and Productivity Studies.

"The coronavirus pandemic has exposed the inextricable link between healthy communities and a strong, resilient economy—and our collective failure to better prepare for this foreseeable crisis," the CMOs wrote in *Fortune*. "America's public health infrastructure needs immediate attention. Outdated public health systems and resources are no match for the virulence and lethal speed of viruses in an increasingly interconnected world. A modernized public health infrastructure will translate into healthier communities, driving lower health care costs, reducing disability payments and absenteeism, and empowering a more productive and adaptable workforce."

The plan noted that rebuilding the public health system would cost the federal government only about $4.5 billion at a time when the country was spending more than a thousand times that amount on response to the Covid crisis. But it also called for expenses that would be borne by businesses themselves, including paid sick and parental leave, child and adult day care benefits, and living wages. And in the communities where the businesses work, it called for affordable housing, safe streets for pedestrians and bikers, alcohol control, healthier food, and high-quality, universal pre-kindergarten.[58] If corporate America fought for all the changes listed in the report, they really would change public health. We're not naive enough to believe all this will happen (at least not quickly or easily), but having corporate titans sign on to ideas like these was new and encouraging.

American society, with its high-tech health system, crashed in 2020. Investigating what went wrong isn't simple, nor will the solutions be simple. Hospital and aviation investigations teach the importance of avoiding oversimplification. A complex system fails in complicated ways and solutions require detailed thought and nuance. Scott raised this point in discussing why business efforts to change health care had failed in the past, including Buffett's Haven and other efforts by tech companies including Google and Amazon, which have had limited impact so far.

"Sometimes you can try to do too much, take on too much at one time," Scott said. "It's like when you're doing a [hospital] quality improvement project, you really have to nail down what's the root cause and the issue causing the problem and not take this big picture approach. Because if you don't fix that one little thing or identify the one real problem, you're not going to get the problem solved. And then sometimes there can be multiple steps. You have to solve them sometimes one at a time or a couple at a time and not just think, 'Oh, I can boil the ocean.' . . . But I would say, we don't give up. We keep innovating. We keep figuring solutions to the obvious, known problems, and just take it a step at a time."

In the next chapter, we will look at health care quality investigations and what those detailed steps might yield as a prescription.

Chapter 11

Quality, Safety, and Investigation

Lest we forget, something remarkable happened when Covid hit the United States. Doctors and nurses performed at an extraordinary level. They adapted to impossible conditions, decoded the mystery of the disease, developed treatments, and shared those insights widely and rapidly. And they persevered. The yard signs thanking "health care heroes" disappeared as the pandemic wore on, but the heroes themselves kept caring for patients under the grinding weight of repeated, largely preventable surges, often dealing with angry patients demanding quack treatments. Through the experience, medicine learned a lot about Covid care and about how the system could adapt. New avenues of communication and collaboration cleared away barriers between hospitals, branches of medicine and even nations. Doctors truly worked together.

"Looking at what's gone on over the past eighteen months, the clinicians in the field have been spectacular," said Mary Cooper, a doctor, attorney, and professor who is director of the Health Care Quality and Safety Program at the Jefferson College of Population Health, speaking in September 2021. "The clinicians themselves have been innovative, they've been collaborative, they've been patient-centered. They have been scrupulous in following whatever the current guidelines were, which could change from week to week and month to month. And they have been extraordinarily resilient."[1]

Unfortunately, skill and heroism were not enough. Like expert pilots trying to fly a damaged plane, doctors' best efforts could not prevent a crash that left eight hundred thousand Americans dead, and counting. As we have noted through the ten previous chapters, the US health

system performed particularly poorly—disastrously so—in spite of the impressive efforts of clinicians. The problems were systemic, not individual. We've outlined many of them, including the lack of transparency that eroded the public's trust and contributed, we believe, to wide refusal of vaccines and non-pharmaceutical interventions such as masks (as we discussed in chapter 5). Doctors did a good job of communicating with one another, Cooper said, but not with the public.

"We fell down. And you can see it in the divisiveness that is occurring today, eighteen months in," she said. "The lack of any kind of message that is hopeful and that transcends all of the individualism that exists within this country is remarkable."

High-quality medical care relies on good communication and the just culture that supports it. That was missing in American society. But we have learned in hospitals, and airlines, that we can build quality intentionally, by creating a culture of transparency and conducting open and thorough investigations of errors that do occur, so that we can address their root causes. Through this book we have followed that path, investigating in the style of an aviation crash probe to learn why the American health system failed during Covid. Now, in this chapter, we complete the circle, looking at the tools themselves for improving health care quality and safety. The pandemic sheds new light here, too.

Many tools for quality and safety come directly from aviation and the study of how human beings and machines work together, called human factors engineering. There is even a movement to create a National Patient Safety Board like the National Transportation Safety Board, whose crash investigations have produced the insights that made commercial flying almost free of accidents (we will explore the NPSB idea later in this chapter).[2] By removing individual blame from the equation, NTSB investigations solve for systemic factors in what went wrong. Fixing those flaws protects future pilots from making the same mistakes.

Doctors need this protection, too. The health care system as it exists harms its practitioners. Covid helped expose this problem as well. Six months into the pandemic, half of US health care workers reported being burned out and 38 percent reported anxiety and depression.[3] Even before Covid, health care workers were suffering much higher levels of burnout, depression, and suicidal thinking than people in other occupations, and research showed the system itself was producing

those feelings in previously healthy people—students entering medicine were less likely to be depressed or suicidal than their peers in the general population.[4] After working in health care, however, their mental health tended to suffer, with doctors more than twice as likely to die by suicide as average Americans.[5] And while burnout doesn't equal depression—it is caused by workplace conditions and is not a mental illness—it is associated with more medical errors (not to mention headaches, insomnia, severe injury, type 2 diabetes, coronary heart disease, gastrointestinal and respiratory concerns, musculoskeletal discomfort, and all-cause mortality).[6]

We suspect Covid's epidemic of physician burnout did harm the quality of care and increase errors—but we cannot know, because the Center for Medicare and Medicaid Services and other organizations suspended most quality tracking when the pandemic hit. Given the circumstances, CMS had no choice: in the crisis, hospitals needed to direct resources to patients, not the often-cumbersome process of fulfilling quality measurement obligations. Quality measures generally require manual handling of data and are treated as added administrative processes separate from care. The results can show up as long as a year after the care is given, much too late to complete a feedback loop for improvement—a process we know helps us hone our ability in any skilled endeavor, from flying a plane to placing a catheter in a major vessel in the body (called a central line). As a pair of Johns Hopkins health quality experts pointed out, a well-functioning quality measurement system would automatically draw data from hospital information systems to give doctors immediate feedback on their performance. A system like that could have continued functioning in the background during the Covid crisis, and it could even have produced real-time information on the relative worth of varying new treatments protocols as they were developed.[7]

Hospitals did report on infections in the second half of 2020, and that data showed a huge jump. Infections related to central lines were 47 percent higher compared to a year earlier, and three other kinds of hospital infections went up steeply, too. These are important markers of quality, and extensive efforts by public health agencies and hospitals had reduced them significantly over the previous five years.[8] The reasons for the bad 2020 statistics were obvious—we know doctors were under extreme stress and were improvising during Covid surges—but that also demonstrates the weakness of the system, which should be able to function safely even when attention is distracted due to other issues.[9]

Why does this matter? Because many hundreds of Americans lose their lives daily due to avoidable medical harm. Medical mistakes were the third-most-common cause of death, after cancer and coronary disease, until Covid knocked them down to fourth. The best recent estimate says about 250,000 lives are lost every year—and that may be an underestimate, because we don't have a system to accurately count these deaths.[10]

When David began practicing medicine, the American Medical Association routinely denied the existence of medical errors as a major problem, calling them isolated incidents. Only after the news media highlighted a series of shocking deaths caused by errors in the mid-1990s did the problem receive serious attention from national institutions.[11] Betsy Lehman's case broke the dam. She was a thirty-nine-year-old health columnist for the *Boston Globe*, the mother of two young children, killed in 1995 by a massive overdose of chemotherapy drugs at the Dana Farber Cancer Institute. Five top doctors had signed off on the erroneous dose. When Lehman protested that something was wrong, staff ignored her. And the true cause of her death was only discovered three months later during an unrelated review of records.[12] In 1999, the National Academy of Medicine (then called the Institute of Medicine) used Lehman's story to begin its landmark study on the issue, *To Err Is Human*, which estimated forty-eight thousand to ninety-eight thousand Americans were dying annually from hospital errors, based on the fragmentary data then available.[13] That report started the movement for quality and safety that continues today, based on systemic changes rather than individual blame.

Unfortunately, progress has been slow and uneven in the two decades since. This is a hard problem. Medicine cannot be simplified: errors often involve long chains of causation that are difficult to identify and can be fixed only by deep, thoughtful work. In the search for a single solution for errors, we have gone down some paths that didn't get us to the destination. Checklists had their day—they were borrowed from aviation—especially after Atul Gawande's bestselling *Checklist Manifesto* in 2009.[14] But evidence of checklist benefits were mixed, and they created the side effect of burnout-inducing bureaucracy, without taking into account the abstract and flexible nature of good medical thinking.[15]

Robert Wears and Kathleen Sutcliffe blamed the general failure of the safety and quality movement—so many are still dying—on medical middle management systems that co-opted it, producing bureaucracy and ineffective activity, but that did not call on experts in engineering and psychology who had already brought safety advances to other industries.[16] From the hospital bedside, the bureaucratic approach feels like measurement mania, with ever more uninformative, box-checking measures imposed on clinicians, who ultimately feel overwhelmed and ignore the exercise as senseless busywork.

It now seems clear that there must be many solutions. We need cultural change, including transparency, equality among members of medical teams, and organizational and leadership focus on safety. We need human factors engineers to design machines and systems that anticipate potential errors and prevent them. And we need systemic change in each of the domains we have already discussed—properly aligned financial incentives in medicine, doctors trained as safety-oriented team members, technology designed to support that work rather than generate profits for technology companies, and the leadership that should come from employers, as they take up their responsibility as the funders of the system.

All these issues converge on health care quality and safety. Yes, the system crashed during Covid like an airliner with a design flaw, but the signs of the coming crash were evident prior to the pandemic in the terrible toll of deaths due to errors. When we address these problems, we will save lives, ease the psychological burden of health care work, and control the cost of health care by reducing unnecessary care and doing more procedures right the first time. The task is large and complex, but the good news is that we now understand the problems and we have effective solutions—as we will learn in the balance of this chapter.

HUMAN FACTORS ENGINEERING

Hospital investigations should start as soon as possible after an error, because memories change each time we tell our stories. Oren Guttman, an anesthesiologist, leads this work at Jefferson Health, as enterprise vice president for high reliability and patient safety. Most often, he said, it turns out that people are not the problem.

"The very first thing is to get to the people, quickly, download the information from them, and make sure we care for them, because they've usually been traumatized by the events," Guttman said. "Our approach is really understanding how the operating system didn't meet the high professional standards of the people who use them. . . . What are the holes and the vulnerabilities in the system which exceeded human capability and capacity and ultimately led to operator error?"[17]

Guttman said engineers design medical equipment to be used as they imagine work will be done in the hospital, but often a wide gap exists between that imagined work process and what actually happens in the clinic. Health care workers span the gap by adjusting their processes to meet the needs of the machines, but doing so incurs a cognitive load to manage the workaround—and all of us have only so much room in our minds to concentrate on multiple tasks. When we overwhelm those mental limits, operator errors happen.

"We want to know how the work is performed for a few reasons," Guttman said. "Usually when we see the difference between what is imagined and what is actually performed, that gap elucidates tremendous amounts of insight into how the system is actually broken. And usually the humans involved are sources of innovation and they're probably protecting the patients. It's probably amazing that it doesn't fail more often."

Complex electronic medical record systems notoriously miss the mark, demanding mental energy that should be devoted to patients.

"The example with the EMR—it should be easy to find information," Guttman said. "I shouldn't have to go through five clicks to find something, and because you made it five clicks in—you have to click, click, click, click, click to finally find it—no one is going to do it, and now you have all these errors."

Human factors engineering finds ways to build machines that partner positively with human capabilities. It reverses the paradigm of people learning how to use machines; instead, machines should be built to work with people. The prototypical example comes from aviation and was shared with us by Jonathan Gleason, the doctor we met in chapter 2 who was Jefferson's chief quality and safety officer during the pandemic. During World War II, pilots returning from missions in B-17 bombers repeatedly landed without lowering the aircrafts' wheels. Why? Pilots came in exhausted after long flights and perhaps controlling damaged planes. To lower the wheels, they had to operate a lever that was identical to a nearby lever for the flaps. Sometimes, on landing, they activated the flaps instead of the wheels. One solution would have been additional training, accountability, and building a greater culture of safety among the pilots. But airmen found a better solution—namely, putting a rubber band on the lever, so the pilot could identify the correct control by its feel, Gleason said. That resolved the problem simply and without adding to the pilot's cognitive burden.

A similar example happened during the pandemic, as nurses administered vaccinations. As soon as the FDA approved the Pfizer-BioNTech vaccine dose for children ages five to eleven, in October 2021, reports began pouring in of accidents in which children that age received the dose for patients twelve and older, or adults received the pediatric dose—this error happened thousands of times. An investigation showed the labeling on the vaccine vial was potentially confusing, but the manufacturer had color-coded caps to prevent mix-ups: purple for adult doses and orange for children. Why didn't that work? Nurses necessarily discarded the cap when preparing the first dose in a syringe, leaving only the confusing labeling as a clue. After the syringes were separated from the vials, no labeling remained to prevent a mistake. Investigators came up with a set of solutions to prevent the mistakes: labeling syringes, bringing the vial to the patient, verifying the patient's age and name multiple times, and documenting every step.[18] A better solution would have changed the labeling, perhaps by color-coding the vials rather than their caps.

Gleason said the goal of human factors engineering in the hospital should be to make mistakes impossible. At Jefferson, a nurse noted that an intravenous infusion pump could administer two drugs at the same time that should never be given together. Rather than further train nurses to avoid that problem, Gleason said the machine could be redesigned so it would never give the drugs together. In another example, the hospital addressed the hazard posed by MRI machines, which have powerful magnets—in a famous 2001 case, a six-year-old New York boy was killed by an oxygen tank the size of a fire extinguisher that flew toward the huge magnet and smashed his skull, and many similar accidents have happened.[19] At Jefferson, a medical device containing a small amount of metal was nudged too close to a machine during cleaning and the magnets pulled it in violently (no one was hurt). Protocols had required the device to be kept at a safe distance from the machine, and one solution would have been to give additional training to the cleaning crew. Instead, the hospital bolted the device to the wall so that accident would be impossible.

These are simple, understandable examples, but much more is possible. With digitization of health care rapidly advancing, technology could prevent complex errors and augment human mental capabilities. Gleason pointed out that a doctor who wants to give a drug no longer writes out a prescription on a piece of paper that passes through many hands; instead, she enters it in an electronic system that passes the information onward through various other systems to the pharmacist, who hands the drug to the patient. Those electronic systems can be built with safeguards—for example, Guttman said, they could prevent overprescription of opioids. Artificial intelligence systems could help with diagnosis, reminding doctors of the list of possibilities to rule out when faced by a given set of symptoms, or comparing an electrocardiogram to a database of billions of past cases to provide the probability of myocardial infarction (or heart attack). Those tools exist, Guttman said, but they need to be embedded in the workflow of health care delivery.

"Health care is a complex interaction between humans and machines," Gleason said. "Machines are our tools and our partners, and the future will be human-machine teaming."[20]

In this brave new world, improving the skills of doctors and nurses is not enough, Gleason said. Better training, communication, and culture cannot alone make hospitals safe.

"We are now in a socio-technical environment and a social approach to safety is insufficient," he said. "It's always been insufficient, but Covid showed definitely how insufficient it is. Now we have the opportunity, because of the socio-technical environment, to use human factors engineers to account for human capabilities and limitations to quantitatively design systems that will produce better results, regardless of whether or not you've got a great culture or a poor culture, or whether you've got a strong human performer or a weak human performer. We can use those systems to account for those capabilities and limitations to produce excellent outcomes, regardless of those factors."

This vision is appealing, but it remains far distant. As we noted in chapter 9, science hasn't kept up with technology. Continuous wearable health monitors can turn out vast rivers of data, but neither doctors nor computer programs know how to interpret it. The technology also needs to be better. Rather than aiding health care workers, technology too often has divided them from patients and added to their workload. And creating a productive human-machine team would require a leap for the health care establishment, which has resisted technological improvements that threaten profits or power relationships (recall the slow adoption of telehealth before Covid and other examples in chapter 9).

This movement also faces a problem of scale. When an airplane crashes and NTSB investigators find a design flaw, pulling all copies of that model out of operation and fixing them is a relatively straightforward process. But each of America's six thousand hospitals is different, and many safety incidents have characteristics unique to their setting. To really emulate aviation, each hospital would have to be treated as its own model of airplane. But we are far from having enough resources to address every issue at that level of expertise, and likely we never will. Gleason estimates that America has only about fifty clinically informed human factors engineers.

He suggests a National Patient Safety Board could help span the gap in capabilities. The NPSB could look at the most common or severe safety threats, spreading the skills of the few experts available to hospitals across the country. The NPSB proposal was advanced by the Jewish Healthcare Foundation in Pittsburgh and has attracted other supporters. Sponsors contemplate a stand-alone organization that would receive vast streams of health care data for analysis by disinterested experts. Patterns of problems could lead to non-binding recommendations for improvement to all hospitals. But the plan depends on the willingness of hospitals to release data, the availability of expertise for the analysis, and voluntary uptake of the recommendations by health care providers—all issues the NTSB does not face in its aviation investigations. Despite these limitations, there is a lot of room for improvement, so it might work. As former NTSB chairman Christopher Hart told the *Wall Street Journal*, medicine has generally ignored the issue of human-machine interaction, a choice he likened to "teaching people to drive better on icy roads, but not doing anything about the icy roads."[21]

In fact, both approaches are essential. Aviation safety is a powerful metaphor for medical safety—we have used it heavily, perhaps to the edge of reader patience—but it has limits. In aviation, standardization and technology can nearly eliminate accidents, because airplanes and runways are standard. Checklists can make sure nothing is missed in the cockpit before take-off. In medicine, checklists help only with routine tasks, not nuanced decisions about care. Gleason noted that expert panels of doctors disagree on standards of care in complex areas of medicine such as cardiology and oncology. And standardization alone cannot produce patient-centered care, because every patient is different. Should you get a cancer-screening mammogram? It depends on your values and goals. Experts may say the harm of unnecessary biopsies is not worth the benefit for your age group, but perhaps you have valid personal reasons why that potential harm would be worthwhile for you. In an ideal system, an empathetic doctor would work through those issues with a woman based on her goals, with a nuanced understanding of the cost and benefits, and a sense of the resources of the system.

Medicine is not science. It is a human endeavor for caregiving. As we will explore in the next section, the quality of care depends on how people work together as well as the technology they use.

TRANSPARENCY AND COMMUNICATION

In 1999, the report *To Err Is Human* set off a deep cultural change in medicine, moving doctors and hospitals toward transparency and humility. Mary Cooper reminded us how far we have come from the attitudes that prevailed when she received her MD from Temple University in 1985.

"As clinicians, especially those of us in the older generation, we were not necessarily trained to be transparent," she said. "We were trained to be the expert and to pat people on the head and say to them, 'This is what you should do,' without giving them any evidence or the reasoning behind it. That's just how we were all trained. But the world is different now."

Today, patients often research their own conditions on the internet, they want to hear their doctors' level of certainty about their diagnosis, and they insist on understanding their treatment and participating in decisions about it. Those are all good changes that improve the quality of care. Patients know more about their bodies than anyone else, and only they know the values and goals that should guide their desired outcomes. Doctors get better results by teaming with patients, nurses, and all the others involved in care, because many minds and perspectives contribute to better decisions and follow-through than any single, godlike physician who controls everything.

Before the safety and quality movement—and the publication of *To Err Is Human*—doctors and hospitals usually hid their errors (and often they still do). They feared malpractice litigation, often assuming that injured patients would seek huge paydays and that apologies would be used against them in court. When the Academy of Medicine exposed the truth about how many people were being harmed, those attitudes began to change.

"People were shocked to know of those numbers, and that led to us, as a profession, opening those doors, taking off that weight of silence, and saying, when we make mistakes, we're going to be forthright with you and share those mistakes, with the hope that all of us can make it better for the next time, for the next person, for the next process, for the next outcome," Cooper said. "And so the transparency movement in medicine really arose out of the safety movement in medicine."

The truth is that most families whose loved one is harmed by a medical error don't want to go to court. They want their loss promptly recognized with an apology, to have the problem fixed to protect others, and to receive reasonable compensation for their legitimate costs.[22] Hospital programs that take this approach rather than hiding mistakes and preparing for lawsuits have reduced malpractice claims and payments.[23] However, research shows that liability and the fear of lawsuits do not lead to improved health care outcomes.[24]

Human nature explains this seeming paradox that admitting error is less expensive than hiding it. Victims of adverse events who receive a prompt and honest apology, and caring support, can forgive. Researchers have found that monetary compensation generally is not high on their list of priorities. But when a harmed patient meets a hospital's wall of silence, they naturally assume the physician or facility did something wrong and lacks the honor or respect to admit it. "The resultant anger leads to the kinds of lawyer commercials seen on television and a desire, not merely for compensation, but for punishment of the 'perpetrators,'" wrote David Meyers, a Maryland emergency room physician.[25]

The state of Pennsylvania led the movement toward openness in 1986, with legislation that requires tracking of infections and other hospital quality data, as well as liability protection for health care institutions if they disclose mistakes and address them. In 1991, using data generated by the new law, David (and colleagues) wrote a paper that showed the unequal mortality rates for coronary bypass surgery at five Philadelphia teaching hospitals. In a sign of the attitudes of those times, the *New England Journal of Medicine* turned down the paper because an editor thought it could be libelous.[26] Instead, the *Journal of the American Medical Association* published it, and the paper became widely cited.[27] In 1994, a landmark paper by Harvard University's Lucian Leape got a similar response at the *NEJM* before helping transform the field.[28]

In 2001, the University of Michigan pioneered a program to acknowledge patient harm, disclose and communicate it to patients and families, and compensate them for costs—for example, covering day care for a mother who had to spend extra time in the hospital.[29] In 2012, the federal Agency for Healthcare Research and Quality put out a model program for hospitals called CANDOR (the acronym is for Communication and Optimal Resolution), to move beyond the "deny and defend" model of responding to incidents of patient harm and toward transparency and correction of the underlying problems. Part of the program emphasizes the need to change hospital culture, from the CEO downward, and to train doctors to admit mistakes and apologize honestly—something that doesn't come naturally to many of us.[30]

In chapter 1, we described the pain of meeting with families of harmed patients. The physician for Betsy Lehman, the *Globe* columnist who died due to a drug error in 1995, and another patient harmed by the same error, told a reporter about meeting with their families at the time. He said, "Those two meetings, which took place within hours of each other, were the saddest individual occurrences I remember. I looked into their eyes and all I could see was abject grief and misery. It was the kind of misery that was penetrating."[31] The shame and regret of the incident led to vigorous investigation, and the ripples of that response are still felt today in the safety and quality movement in medicine. That's the power of honesty and transparency.

In 2001, the National Academy of Medicine published a follow-up report, adding solutions to the problems identified in *To Err Is Human.* The new report, *Crossing the Quality Chasm*, recommended improvements in payment models, education, technology, and dissemination of clinical knowledge. That list overlays neatly on the chapters of this book, written more than twenty years later. And among the report's most powerful recommendations was transparency.

"At times, today's health care system appears to put a premium on secrecy," the authors wrote. "In the future health care system, the rule should be: Have no secrets. Make all information flow freely so that anyone involved in the system, including patients and families, can make the most informed choices and know at any time whatever facts may be relevant to a patient's decision making."[32]

During Covid, our national health system as a whole didn't follow that rule, as Cooper pointed out. Although we know that patients want to hear about uncertainties from their doctors, public advice on Covid was full of absolutes. More transparent statements would have acknowledged the unknowns and explained the reasons behind contradictions—contradictions such as the instructions at one time to engage in lockdowns and sanitize mail and groceries, and at another time to do none of those things. Yes, the science changed and balancing interests raised different priorities. But trusting the public with information about those considerations at the time could have made changes of course less costly to trust.

"Covid kind of encapsulated that, because all the decision making was out in public all the time," Cooper said. "But if we didn't bring honesty and integrity to that decision making process, then understandably people got frustrated with us."

Leading hospitals in the safety and quality movement have convened patient-family advisory councils and opened their ears to the communities where they operate, but Covid public health edicts came from the top down, Cooper noted. Today, medicine is abandoning the patriarchal model of physician-centered care, recognizing the importance of patients as partners in setting their own goals, but management of Covid did not respect differences in populations in that same way. Cooper noted that residents of dense urban areas and sparsely populated rural regions would naturally feel differently about the disease.

"Extrapolating it to the larger situation with Covid, is recognizing that different people have different perceptions," she said. "We need to address each of those. We have to go to each person as they come to us, not as we want them to be."

Late in the second year of the pandemic, America seemed to have broken into pieces. Rather than bringing us together, the crisis had increased our divisions. Views that once would have seemed fringe or even psychotic were adopted by some elected leaders, including wild conspiracy theories and insistence on the use of treatments without evidence of efficacy, such as the deworming medication ivermectin. Certainly, the health system cannot take full blame for the madness, which was also driven by bad actors on the internet seeking profit or political gain. But full transparency from the start would have helped.

The good news, however, is that the health system also improved and made quality advances during the pandemic, as we will explore next.

MAKING HEALTH CARE A SYSTEM

The word *system* is ill suited to the fragmented and conflicting group of organizations, institutions, and individuals responsible for our health. The word implies a mechanism that works according to some design or intention, but the US health system grew up organically in an environment of market and political competition, educational traditions, and expediency. Even within a single hospital, tensions pull along different axes, with varying economic forces; the wills of independent physicians and insurance companies; the factors of worker gender and class; and patients' racial, spiritual, and social backgrounds. Rather than a system, health care often looks more like an arena.

The shock of Covid forced hospitals and health care as a whole to become more of an actual system. Virtually every hospital activated an incident command structure during the pandemic. The incident command system is an organizational response to crisis originated by California firefighters in the 1970s. It became commonplace in all emergency management agencies even before it was mandated by the federal government in 2004. The concept brings together the headquarters of every organization managing an incident into a single command post with unified responsibilities and immediate communication and coordination among players. In essence, incident command forces a unified system into existence.[33]

In 2005, Hurricane Katrina demonstrated how bad disaster response could be. We learned about the public health aspects of the chaos from Karen DeSalvo in chapter 5, who stepped in as a doctor to improvise care on the streets of New Orleans. A 2006 National Research Council

Report documented the organizational pathologies from Katrina that are common in disasters—the maladies an incident command system is intended to address. The failings included insufficient response, confusion regarding authority, resource shortages and misallocation, poor communication among organizations and with the public, failures in leadership, and inequities in providing assistance.[34] For our purposes, it is interesting to note that all these same problems afflict the health system—they are the same issues we have discussed throughout the book. During Covid, faced with crisis, health care organizations adopted the incident command system and performed as more rationally coordinated units.

In chapter 6, Northwell Health CEO Mike Dowling described how his doctors also formed a system-wide medical committee to make all clinical decisions during the Covid crisis. Jonathan Gleason said Jefferson Health set up a similar task force in Philadelphia. A clinical committee is a leadership and communication tool to create standards of care and to reduce variations in how patients with the same diagnosis are treated. It has the potential to improve quality and reduce unnecessary treatment by narrowing physicians' choices in similar circumstances. Clinical committees do have limitations, as experts may disagree on treatment standards. And patients should be at the committee table, too, bringing community values to the discussion. These committees are an important step in creating a true system of health care.

The Covid response also benefited from what hospitals had learned over the past decade from other industries with high-reliability practices, including aviation, nuclear energy, and amusement parks, Cooper said. They used huddles, which give small teams a chance to quickly share information and make decisions collaboratively on the floor. And they had hand-off structures to make sure that information would be given accurately and completely when responsibility for a patient was transferred between caregivers. These skills reduce the risk of errors at any time. During the crisis they probably expanded teams' capabilities to handle heavy loads of patients.

Beyond the realm of what was already known, Cooper said the global health system showed qualities in the Covid response that originally had been described by complexity science. As clinicians shared experiences, new insights emerged from many people's ideas. Discovery went into overdrive. Traditionally, understanding and developing treatments for a disease takes many years, as individual researchers devise hypotheses, write grants for studies, perform clinical trials, and publish their work in peer-reviewed journals. Faced with a crisis causing thousands of deaths a day, doctors short-cut that process, sharing their observations on blogs and floating their ideas on pre-press servers. Doctors in the United States treated overseas colleagues on the internet as equals in these exchanges, as they often had failed to do in the past, Cooper said. Helpful treatments emerged rapidly from this process that kept patients alive and conserved resources. Cooper saw this emergence as similar to a feature of complex systems, a phenomenon in nature in which order can arise without individual design, such as the gathering of a weather system or schooling of a group of fish.

"An example," Cooper said, "is the notion that rather than putting everybody on ventilators as their oxygen levels dropped, to keep them on external oxygen at a high level and to essentially rotate them, 'prone them,' it's called. Turn them so that they were on their knees and essentially their lungs were draining from the back. And that, plus high levels of oxygen, kept a lot of people off of ventilators. There were no randomized clinical trials done on that. People started talking about it, people started using it. They saw results. They started spreading it to other colleagues around the country and within probably two months, three months, it became standard of care."[35]

An influential 2001 paper by two well-known health quality scientists advanced the idea of health as a complex, self-organized system. Paul Plsek and Trisha Greenhalgh argued against a mechanistic concept of health or top-down systemic control of the health care enterprise, saying those were outmoded metaphors for a field with unmanageable complexity controlled by many groups of autonomous practitioners. Instead, they called on models from physics, biology, and financial markets, in which self-organizing systems develop and find solutions, often in unexpected ways, and sometimes with results superior to the ability of any individual within the system.

"There is an insoluble paradox between the need for consistent and evidence-based standards of care and the unique predicament, context, priorities, and choices of the individual patient," Plsek and Greenhalgh wrote. "Whereas conventional reductionist scientific thinking assumes that we shall eventually figure it all out and resolve all the unresolved issues, complexity theory is comfortable with and even values such inherent tension between different parts of the system."[36]

These ideas bring us across the spectrum of thought on how to "fix" health care. Engineers would find ways to build machines based on deep, detailed research about how we work in the hospital to make errors impossible, working within health systems managed for error detection and clinical standardization, and with leadership accountable to patients for safety and quality. At the other end of the spectrum, complexity theorists—and doctors sharing ideas with distant colleagues on the internet—would explode the whole idea of standards with a fluid system that advances through constant communication and innovation.

In fact, we see the need for both. We can imagine a health system in which the minds of brilliant clinicians are freed to develop innovative treatments in cooperation with distant colleagues, partnering with nurses and patients. And we can also imagine how the tools of quality and safety would empower those great minds, by protecting them from avoidable errors and from situations in which technology would overrun their mental capability to safely provide care. We can further imagine economic incentives that would encourage both those goods, an educational system that would provide the skills and values needed, the technology that would enable it with communication and artificial intelligence, and the employers who would gladly pay the bills for a safer and more efficient system that results.

Nothing in this vision is in conflict. All the strands tie together. They go back to the just culture, in which every member of the health care team can speak up freely, and to the values of the patient who is respected and honored as the center of the entire enterprise. We will trace each of those connections in the final chapter, along with how the strands themselves extend far beyond hospital walls to the entire society that is the context for our health.

Covid devastated the health system. Through immeasurable grief and loss, we saw clearly what was wrong and how the flaws we already knew about had become the seeds of disaster. This was our catastrophic airplane crash.

But we also learned a lot about how to do better. We should keep the way clinicians communicated freely across disciplines and international borders to find treatments. We should keep the insights about unifying oversight of clinical decisions. And we should keep the remote care technology that allowed doctors to triage patients before they filled the emergency room.

"I think it'll be a shame if everybody goes back to the way we were doing it," Cooper said. "I'm out talking to people and really encouraging them to learn from their experiences this past year and a half and do something new. Don't go back."

We are counting on that advice. In the final chapter, we will consider how that new, better system will look—and the tools to get us there.

Chapter 12

Our Preliminary Report and Recommendations

The NTSB doesn't rush plane crash investigations. Final reports sometimes come out years after the last funeral.[1] As we write today, dying continues from the Covid crash, and this book cannot be a final report, either. In December 2021, the omicron variant exploded with lightning-fast doubling of infections across the globe. We have learned through two years of pandemic shock not to make predictions, and we won't. However, even the NTSB releases preliminary reports, designed to capture urgent messages from the wreckage to keep others safe in the here and now. We also know more than enough to interpret the health disaster in front of us and to give urgent warnings to limit future tragedies—in fact, we and many others knew enough to recommend changes before the virus infected its first victim.

In chapter 7, we cited books much like this one that were written fifty years ago, by Barbara and John Ehrenreich and others, exposing flaws we are still talking about—the fragmented health care system, its excessive cost and lack of universal access, and the ignored social determinants of health and racial inequities. David has spent much of his career studying these issues and pushing for solutions from within academic medicine. Not enough happened. Then the Covid disaster hit, and these fatal flaws harmed millions of people, altering how society sees the health system and the potential for change.

Before Covid, American health care wore a protective facade of technological and clinical superiority that shielded it from public outrage. Technological white magic does exist. David received its blessings as we were writing this chapter, when a family member received rapid, effective treatment for a stroke, emerging unscathed from an episode that a generation ago would likely have been fatal. Even with thanks for that blessing, however, we could not forget that this medical miracle happened because David's family member lived in a favored zip code—near a top-rated suburban hospital—and in an income bracket with excellent health coverage. Those factors favor only a select group of Americans, and, through the pandemic years, their numbers have shrunk. A survey by the Gallup consultancy and the nonprofit West Health found that, by late 2021, the number of Americans reporting they skipped medical care due to cost had jumped by three-fold, to 30 percent.[2]

That survey began with an open-ended question—before respondents could think about the topic or otherwise be influenced—asking for three top-of-mind words or phrases describing the US health care system. In 2019, most people answered from the pre-Covid frame of American exceptionalism, thinking of the technological prowess of our system. About half said either "the best in the world" or "among the very best." Two years later, late in 2021, the same opening question elicited different answers. "Expensive" and "broken" were the most frequent responses. Combined with "unfair," "overpriced," and "complicated," these negative words were offered in two-thirds of answers. More than half of respondents said the last time they had personally received medical care was not worth the money, and virtually everyone agreed—including more than 90 percent of both Republicans and Democrats—that the cost of health care was too high. Large majorities of both parties also agreed that they expected nothing to be done to fix the problem.[3]

We are living through a time of profound darkness and pessimism. One of the repeated lessons of the pandemic has been that, however bad things seem at the moment, they can always get worse. But the potential for positive change in the health system hasn't been as great in a lifetime. We have hit bottom, a breaking point that forces the recognition of the need for change. The Gallup survey shows that the public understands. Within the health system, professionals know more deeply. Doctors' and nurses' struggles with despair and exhaustion have driven a giant career migration into coordinated systems that can support them better. Provider organizations straining to stay afloat are forming new partnerships and consolidating into more effective arrangements with better-aligned incentives. We foresee no top-down, universal solution, and we don't expect a government fix, but the pandemic itself is driving substantive changes through the system that will make a difference.

In this chapter, in the style of a preliminary accident report on the Covid crash, we will review key evidence of the fatal flaws that we have written about in greater depth in the preceding chapters, illustrated by scenes from current life in America, including the leadership failures, cultural factors, racial inequities, public health weaknesses, and the provider crisis. Next, we will review recommendations informed by those findings, with interlocking solutions, including realigning financial incentives, medical education, technology, the role of employers, and the safety and quality movement, which connects them all.

At the darkest time we can least afford despair and surrender. Now, while the pain is fresh, we should look carefully into root causes and address them.

LEADERSHIP AND CULTURE

In the autumn of 2021, a poisonous brew of fear and hatred boiled over in city council and school board meeting rooms all over the United States, bringing never-before-seen animosity to the most personal level of community decision making. It happened at meetings that had always been peaceful and dull, including of the Central Bucks County School Board, in a middle-class suburb north of Philadelphia. There, the chief medical officer of Doylestown Hospital, commenting on the value of masks, faced uncontrolled rage as parents leaped to their feet and shouted directly in his face, forcing him to withdraw. Anti-mask parents speaking to the board equated masks to Holocaust gas chambers and alleged that the government and the local hospital intended vaccines to hurt or paralyze children for their own financial benefit. Similar disruptions and demonstrations happened around the country (including the convulsions in Alaska that we mentioned in chapter 3).[4]

Often, these civic explosions combined attacks on infection controls, opposition to anti-racist instruction in schools, and misuse of Holocaust imagery and other anti-Semitic themes. A reporter in Bucks County noted that the same people who opposed children wearing masks also opposed teaching them about systemic racism, which some asserted did not exist. And most were strong supporters of former President Trump.[5]

The video of the Doylestown doctor being shouted down reminded us of Trump's campaign rally on November 2, 2020, when he implied that Covid was a political creation intended to hurt his reelection and that it would disappear soon after the Election Day, and he encouraged the crowd as it chanted, "Fire Fauci."[6] As White House health advisor, Anthony Fauci needed a security detail from early in the pandemic, with security added later to protect his daughters as well.[7] Trump also used anti-racism as a political weapon, issuing an executive order to halt diversity training at federal agencies.[8]

As we argued in chapter 3, however, blaming Trump alone for Covid denial is too easy. His message found an avid audience. After he lost reelection, he was banned from social media platforms, but opposition to public health measures continued, especially in conservative states, where vaccination rates remained low and mask mandates were rare.[9] Late in 2021, when Trump urged followers to get boosters, his audience booed him and polls showed his voters were unpersuaded.[10] It wasn't all about Trump. Conservative media and politicians originated ideas that spread into local meetings where conflict erupted, but the receptivity to those ideas came from a deeper source than everyday politics, in a cultural identity based on individualism and disbelieving science.

Science, of course, doesn't need us to believe in it in order to be true. When the pandemic refused to go away, reality put terrible pressure on people still in denial. Covid deaths were much higher in Republican-leaning states with low vaccination rates and little use of masks—in the second half of 2021, death rates were three times higher in counties that had voted for Trump.[11] Attacking doctors in these circumstances, although irrational, made some emotional sense, as rage for these preventable tragedies transferred to the nearest authority figures. The abuse landed on the doctor from Doylestown, as it did on medical workers in many hospitals, who faced anger from patients whose own decisions had led to their illnesses. In the mythology of American medicine, the doctor as superhero could solve any problem. Now the hero doctor image was inverted. Some health care workers tried to hide their occupations in public. The hero had become a scapegoat.

In December 2021, Covid hammered Rhode Island, with a surge that exceeded all those that had come before. Laura Forman, chief of emergency medicine at Kent Hospital in Warwick, told an NPR interviewer that the hospital was running out of beds, pillows, IV pumps, and staff. Of the many dead, she noted, all were unvaccinated.[12]

"There are literally days—many days—when we are trying to find a place to move a patient who has died so that we can make room for a sick patient coming in, and to do that day in and day out is excruciatingly painful, and to know that this could all be prevented if people were willing to get a couple of shots in the arm is demoralizing," Forman said. "We are all risking our lives every day to take care of people who are unwilling to get a couple of shots to protect all of us."[13]

RACE, SOCIAL DETERMINANTS, AND PUBLIC HEALTH

During the spring and summer of 2020, the streets of hundreds of cities and towns filled with people of all races protesting police violence against African Americans. The stress and suffering of the initial Covid wave, with so many Black deaths, had exploded like a breached boiler when a Minneapolis cop murdered George Floyd. The moment was disorienting and sometimes scary, but these expressions of resistance to systemic racism were overdue. We marched as well. In the sad history of the pandemic, the movement for racial equity was one good outcome.

Then, one night in October 2020, after the summer of protests had ended, a twenty-seven-year-old Black man in West Philadelphia, Walter Wallace Jr., had a mental health episode at home. His family called 911 for help.[14] As usually happens in the United States in mental health crises, the police were dispatched to handle the call.[15] American prisons would be mostly empty without people who have mental health problems, and 10 to 25 percent of prisoners are seriously mentally ill.[16] Philadelphia police had been sent to the family's house for these calls before, and the officers who responded knew Wallace was mentally ill, but they were not equipped to deal with a patient having an episode and lacked non-lethal means to handle potential violence, such as tasers. Wallace approached with a knife, and they killed him with fourteen shots.[17]

Protesters poured into the streets. As night fell, a police car was set on fire, and violence broke out between police and protesters. On subsequent nights, looting ripped through the city and protests spread to other cities. A curfew was declared, and National Guard troops deployed.[18] Damage was deep, not only to property but also to the city's psyche, its reputation, and the connections between citizens and their government. A year later, the City of Philadelphia agreed to pay Wallace's family $2.5 million and to equip officers with tasers.[19] But the fundamental issues remained.

Suppose Philadelphia—and other American cities—had adequate mental health care for everyone, in clinics rather than prisons, and dispatched mental health professionals rather than police when a person had a crisis. Too expensive? Compared to what? Major American cities burned in the night because of this one case, and a man died. He was one of many—more than one in four people killed by police in the United States are mentally ill.[20] Nationally, perhaps a million mentally ill adults live in prisons, which in Pennsylvania costs about $48,000 per person per year.[21]

This tragic, frustrating case gathered up the strands of structural racism, the social determinants of health, and the inadequacy of the public health system. Wallace lived in one of the low-income, majority-Black neighborhoods we discussed in chapter 4, where life expectancies are much shorter and health services much harder to come by than in White neighborhoods or the suburbs. We know how to address the problems that shorten lives there, with public health and essential health care (including mental health) and, going more deeply and lastingly, with education that provides real opportunity; safe, affordable housing; and affordable, nutritious food.

Too expensive? Again, compared to what? In chapter 7, we presented the extraordinary fact that the United States devotes a quarter of our vast health care spending for diabetes care, far more than the value of all the food produced by every farm and fishing boat in the nation. Surely, we would save money if we diverted some of that medical spending to providing healthy food, helping prevent type 2 diabetes and stabilizing those who have it—especially in neighborhoods like the area where Walter Wallace lived, where 19 percent of residents have diabetes and where healthy foods are scarce.

Here is another way to look at the social conditions affecting any man living in Wallace's Philadelphia neighborhood: Plenty of people there have heart disease, but if medical science could cure all heart disease, that would add four years to life expectancy globally.[22] However, a man living at Wallace's address in West Philadelphia could gain four times as much time on Earth by moving five miles east to City Center—that would increase his life expectancy by seventeen years.[23] He would have access to good food, a healthier physical environment, doctors and mental health counselors, safe housing, recreation facilities, quality education, and street trees that create cooler summer temperatures, and he would be less likely to be shot by the police (or by anyone else).[24] Of course, that move wouldn't be possible for a man with Wallace's income—he worked as an Uber Eats driver—because the White-majority City Center neighborhood would be too expensive.

Covid brought out the brutal unfairness of these disparities by killing many more people in neighborhoods such as Walter Wallace's. As we explained in chapter 4, that happened because of where people worked, where they lived and with how many people, and poor health engendered by their living circumstances; in addition, it was because they had less access to medical care and because African Americans received less effective medical care, making them more likely to die once they were in the hospital.

Today, every doctor knows about the social determinants of health, and some acknowledge a responsibility to address these issues outside the clinic. To emphasize that duty, Donald Berwick has called them, instead, the "moral determinants of health." Berwick, a doctor and policy expert, focused on patient safety as leader of the Institute for Healthcare Improvement. In the pandemic, he used that forum to call on hospitals to address food and housing security; immigration, corrections, and prison health; climate change; voting rights; education; early-childhood support; and elderly loneliness—in addition to health coverage. All, he said, are part of the moral imperative that shapes us as human beings.[25]

"If the moral law within dictated that the shared goal was health, and if logic counseled that science should be the guide to investing and that the endeavor must be communal, not just individual, then the list above would be a clear and rational to-do list to get started on well-being," Berwick wrote. "Healers are called to heal. When the fabric of communities upon which health depends is torn, then healers are called upon to mend it."[26]

Perhaps it seems naive to call on the inner moral guide of hospital leaders to address inequities that have lasted since as long as any of us has been alive. Most health care organizations make money from sick people and have little incentive to make these cost-effective investments in public health. But Covid may be changing that situation, too, as the status quo becomes unsustainable and people working in the field look for a better way. Health care providers were tested by the Covid crisis, and many failed. We may be more ready for change than ever before.

PROVIDERS IN CRISIS

In December 2021, the *Wall Street Journal* published a heartbreaking story by Anna Wilde Mathews about a talented primary care doctor in Bellingham, Washington, whom the paper had followed for twenty-one months.[27] The story told of various patients in Christine Hancock's Medicaid clinic, including one whom she had helped recover from addiction, another she supported through isolation as an elder, and a third she stabilized with serious mental illness and diabetes. Hancock's skill and caring as a doctor constantly showed. She made extraordinary sacrifices to keep these patients on track over two pandemic years, working many extra hours while also managing her young children, who were at home due to school and day care shutdowns. During her daughter's fifth birthday party, she was paged seven times. Hancock wrote in her journal, "I'm barely able to wrap my mind around what I need to do for tomorrow, let alone how I'm going to shepherd my kid through the rest of his kindergarten year . . . and not commit any medical errors in the process."[28]

The burdens on Hancock were impossible. Many of her patients died. Mathews's story became one of defeat, an incredible effort that failed, with casualties of Covid who were killed not directly by the virus but indirectly, due to isolation, social disruption, and an overburdened medical system. This hero-doctor story was a story of heroic tragedy. In a year when doctors, nurses, and other medical professionals were asked to do more than anyone could, it portrayed the deep hardship many faced, as well as the futility and loss that became a recurrent theme of the Covid years. Many of these professionals just couldn't take it anymore. By October 2021, half a million health care workers had left the field, leaving nursing homes, clinics, and hospitals with open positions they could not fill.[29]

But David read this newspaper story differently. It wasn't really about Covid at all. Most of the work Hancock had been called on to do should have been done by nurses, social workers, counselors, long-term care attendants, and other workers with particular skills. A well-functioning system would have given the load to a team rather than putting an impossible burden on one woman. Someone trained to work in substance abuse would have gone to the recovering addict's home to check on him when he missed appointments; a home health worker would have brought meals, cheer, and care to the isolated elder; and a mental health worker would have intervened with the diabetic patient suffering from schizoaffective disorder—then they might not have died. Hancock and her patients were victims not of Covid but of a system missing critical parts that dumped everything on a lone, overwhelmed primary care doctor. In fact, these problems had been around for a long time before Covid made them so obvious. They had been around as long as underpaid, undersupported primary care doctors had tried vainly to solve social determinants of health that were the responsibility of the larger health system and society at large.

Many doctors failed during Covid because they could not live up to impossible, superhuman expectations. That wasn't new to Covid, either. Doctor burnout and high rates of suicide have destroyed careers and lives for many years. We know how to address this problem: teamwork. Doctors working in a team of equals don't have to be heroes. If the system works correctly, they can go home to their families at night. But to support these teams, we need large, coordinated health systems structured as health-promoting organizations. A team of professionals in a big system can support patients with a range of unique, shared skills, a deep bench for backup, and a broad geographic span to flex during a crisis. In chapter 6, we looked at the strength of these large systems and the better care they were able to give during Covid. Doctors trained to work in those integrated systems could take off their superhero capes without quitting medicine. A team role is healthier for patients and healthier for the doctors themselves.

Covid financially crushed doctors in individual private practice, and they quit in droves to join large, coordinated systems where they could collect steady paychecks. Individual hospitals and small health systems of a few sites met much the same fate, driving consolidation and mergers. The fee-for-service business model, which seemed so attractive as a way to make money—delivering more care and sending more bills, regardless of outcome—became an anchor pulling down hospitals and private practice doctors, as complex Covid patients failed to pay their way and the usual bread-and-butter of elective procedures fell away. These trends moved the entire system in the right direction, toward integration and teamwork.

Although size helped during the pandemic, however, big consolidated systems generally do not provide better care and have not solved important quality problems, such as variations in care provided by different doctors or at different sites, or the one-quarter of care that is unneeded. With their market power, they can dictate prices, which generally have little relation to the cost of services provided or to their value for patients—prices are set in opaque negotiations with insurance companies and vary wildly between patients. A deeper change is needed, tying compensation to the quality and outcome of care and rewarding providers for enhancing the health of their patients rather than doing more procedures. As we shall see in the next section, the pandemic pushed forward those changes, too.

SOLUTIONS

In the first half of the book, we investigated flaws in the health system exposed by the Covid crash, grouping them into five chapters: leadership failure, culture, racial inequities and the social determinants of health, weakness in public health, and the crisis for providers. In the second half, we considered solutions (and additional, related flaws) in properly aligning providers' financial incentives, training doctors, applying technology, mobilizing employers, and addressing quality and patient safety. That's a lot to take in. In this section, we'll try to summarize and simplify these ideas.

To begin, let's imagine a health system that would have been more resilient to the Covid threat, one that we could realistically picture in the context of American culture. After that, we'll consider five groups of solutions that could produce such a system, while avoiding the fatal flaws we have identified throughout this book.

First, the system would be dedicated to health. It would invest resources where the health and well-being of people could be most improved. We know the largest factors in our health are life circumstances and habits—the social determinants of health—rather than health care and hospitals. If spending on pollution control or delivering healthy meals saves more lives than an equal amount spent on cardiac surgery, we should reallocate resources to do the greater good. And, yes, a market economy can support such a system if economic incentives align with the health of the population rather than only fixing problems for certain individuals.

With a health system like that, a pandemic virus would encounter a healthier population less vulnerable to disease.

The system would be fair. Everyone would have an equal chance at a healthy, productive life, regardless of their race, social class, income, or geography. Health care providers taking care of patients would look like them and understand and respect them. African Americans would get the same quality of care as White patients. Low-income workers would have safe places to do their jobs and would receive paid leave when they got sick.

If we lived within that system, many fewer people would have died from Covid, because we would have equalized the level of safety and care toward that enjoyed by middle-class White Americans, who suffered much less.

The system would remove walls between public health and health care. Brilliant doctors, expert at fixing broken bodies and curing disease, would focus more on preventing those injuries and illnesses from ever occurring. Big, rich organizations dedicated to healing would also be responsible for public health, along with agencies connected geographically and technologically in a vast safety net protecting Americans.

A system like that would have seen Covid coming and would have protected us more effectively with transparent communication, frequent and early testing, and efficiently distributed vaccines.

The system's healers would be guided by their patients' individual values, working toward outcomes addressing the totality of their health and well-being with whatever tools would be most effective—even if the best tool did not involve medicine. More health care would happen at home, using technology to center care on where the patient is most comfortable. High-reliability organizations serving our health would constantly measure how they met patient goals, continuously improving their culture, processes, and technology to eliminate errors and get each patient toward their hoped-for outcome. Medical records would belong to each of us and be immediately available whenever we needed them.

A system like that would have cared for Covid patients more successfully.

The culture of the health system would be just. Health workers would relate as equals in teams. Patients and their families would be respected as team members, too. And society would be more just, with greater equality among people, and no one left behind and rendered valueless in the eyes of caregivers because they lacked the ability to pay.

In a just system, no safety-net hospital would have been abandoned to being overwhelmed by Covid patients. And perhaps, in a just culture, the voices of experts and scientists would be more respected, reducing the deadly power of demagogues and con men.

If the health system we've just described sounds utopian, that is only because we're inured to one that is so profoundly broken. The system we've described is the minimum we should accept, especially in a nation of our spectacular wealth and health spending. No greater effort is needed for this change, because we are already making a herculean, unsustainable effort to hold up the system that is not serving us well. Grasping the scale of our current effort is difficult. In America's past, its biggest, most world-changing technical efforts—the Manhattan Project to build the atomic bomb and the Apollo program to put humans on the Moon—each consumed, at peak, 0.4 percent of US gross domestic product.[30] In 2020, health care cost forty-nine times more in GDP terms, consuming 19.7 percent of all our output.[31] Would addressing our nation's housing problems be too expensive as a way to improve health? We already spend more on health care than every dollar allocated to housing every American.[32] Far from being utopian, we believe the health system we have described would save enormous amounts of money and produce far better health for Americans—as well as giving us better lives.

But who would have the power to create this new health system, and how would they do it? We discussed in chapter 10 the difficulty of dramatic change in our political system, and that's as true as it has ever been. Fortunately, Americans don't need to wait for Congress. The transformation of the health care system has already begun, and Covid has accelerated it. Change will come from many, distributed decision makers as they come to understand their own power and the opportunity that exists to repair newly obvious flaws. Here are some of the interlocking solutions that can help reassemble our health system—this huge, amorphous conglomeration of disconnected pieces—into a real system of health that serves Americans.

Realigning Financial Incentives

We must begin paying the health system to produce good health rather than procedures and services. This works. Payviders and vertically integrated systems do change their way of doing business, focusing more on prevention and maintenance of health rather than waiting for people to get sick—because it profits them to do so (see chapter 7). Medicare Advantage has shown how aligning incentives can save money for the government, earn more money for insurance companies, and produce healthier and more satisfied clients.

Educating Doctors

At the foundation of a new health system, we will need physicians with professional identities and skills compatible with being equal team members, drawing salaries rather than being business owners and working not as mechanics but as facilitators of their patients' total well-being (see chapter 8). We also need their mix of race and class to reflect that of the population. And we will need them to grow into skilled practitioners without losing their empathy and compassion for their patients, and for themselves.

Applying Technology

Hospitals are temples of technology—something like old mainframe computers that filled rooms—but the world today moves on mobile devices, cloud computing, and sensors that communicate all around us. Health care organizations fought the disruptive influence of this kind of technology, protecting their own power and profits, but the explosion of telehealth during the pandemic began to change that equation, giving patients new access to care and centrality in how it is delivered (see chapter 9). As we create a new health system, technology can help.

Mobilizing Employers

Those paying for the health system have the power to change it. They can take over day-to-day responsibility for the health of their employees, get involved in politics and civic affairs in their communities to address inequities and social determinants, and vote with their dollars to support vertically integrated health care providers (see chapter 10). Covid made business managers into public health managers, as they were forced to make decisions about infection control policies. They have been part of the health system for generations, and now they have the means and awareness to make it better.

Addressing Quality and Safety

Each of the other solutions listed previously connects to the movement for medical quality and patient safety, which is about designing better health care upward from the smallest details and across the culture of the entire system (see chapter 11). Until Covid came along, the tragic failure of the health system to protect patients—with errors killing a quarter million a year—was the most profound indicator of its dysfunction. The tools of the quality and safety movement are powerful levers for change.

This point brings us back, for a final time, to aviation crash investigations. The drive to make commercial aviation safe, and virtually end fatal accidents, required careful study of each systemic problem and feedback to engineers and pilots to correct it. And then it required something else we haven't discussed as much: the will to apply those new practices faultlessly, every time, and permanently.

David recently boarded the last flight of the day from Philadelphia to Florida, at the end of an exhausting workday, on a plane that had just arrived from Dallas. As the aircraft pulled back from the gate, an engine warning light illuminated in the cockpit. The pilots brought the plane back to the gate and a mechanic checked the problem. Apparently, a software glitch had caused the light to go on. The plane pulled back again to leave, but the light went back on. No doubt the pilot was tired, and certainly the passengers were tired and grumpy, but no choice had to be made—the flight certainly would not depart with that light on. Everyone got off the plane while the airline found another one for the flight. David arrived in Florida in the wee hours of the morning. He was safe, as were the other passengers and the flight crew.

Perhaps that seems like an unremarkable story. It's a story about a plane that didn't crash, like every other airliner aloft that day. But it is remarkable, because it came about due to years of intense, unrelenting effort and a standard of safety that allowed no exceptions. After looking at how accidents happened, aviators established processes to prevent them, and they never deviated, even when everyone was tired and unhappy.

Now consider what was happening at the same time in health care. Eighteen health care organizations across the country canceled their vaccination mandates, giving hospital staff discretion to accept much higher risk of contracting and spreading Covid to patients.[33] That was worse than a plane flying with a warning light on. It was like making the preflight checklist optional. Imagine a copilot saying, "I don't feel like doing the checklist today. Let's just take off." That would be absurd. And that's why it is just as safe to fly to Florida late at night or on the weekend, but it is not as safe to get hospital care during those times.[34]

Covid taught us how to fix the fatal flaws in the health system. In fact, those who were paying attention already knew. Here is our preliminary report on the Covid crash. Now it is time to implement the findings. Those of us who work in the health care field should take the first steps. Our organizations have grown so large that we have immense economic and political might in our communities. We can begin making the changes recommended here tomorrow—as employers, community members, and caregivers. We have no excuses anymore.

WHEN THE DYING STOPS

At this writing, we don't know when the Covid pandemic will end. The rapid evolution and transmission of the virus are fundamentally unpredictable. At some indefinite point, the disease will become endemic and, in some sense, a part of life. Everything that doesn't kill us eventually does. We cannot predict when that moment will arrive or even be sure we will recognize it when it happens. But perhaps we can imagine what the world will be like afterward.

We are fairly certain this will not be the last novel pathogen to challenge our species. Our connected economy and technology have shrunk the globe to put us all within weeks of the most dangerous of pathogenic mutations, as we learned when the omicron variant of Covid went from discovery to dominance in less than a month. Another new virus could be even worse, and we need to be ready. Understanding and addressing the fatal flaws in our health system can save countless lives at the best of times, and investing in the good health of everyone in our communities will make us more resistant to disease. Creating a health system that provides good care to all would also strengthen us in the face of a viral disaster.

But a potential hazard stands in the way. As the Covid threat retreats to the background, Americans may forget what we learned. As we saw in chapter 2, the lessons of the 1918 flu pandemic were misinterpreted for ninety years until scientists exhumed frozen victims and read forgotten records to tell the true story of what had happened—and how to avoid repetition of that catastrophe (America's failure to heed those lessons has been another large part of our story). We must not repeat that mistake of collective amnesia and misinterpretation, because we probably don't have a century to prepare for the next pandemic.

The last two years have passed like a nightmare for our country and for many Americans, who lost loved ones, careers, or their mental health, or even contracted long Covid and don't know when they will return to full function, if ever. The world last endured such universal, global suffering in World War II. As the war ended, few wished to think about their experiences or discuss what they had been through, as Ian Toll describes in *Twilight of the Gods*, the final book in a trilogy about the Pacific war.

Veterans insisted on remembering and honoring those who had paid the ultimate price—but with that exception, in 1945 and 1946, they were not much interested in hearing about it. Their attention was directed to the future, not the past. Ben Bradlee, who had served in destroyers in the Pacific and would become editor-in-chief of the *Washington Post*, wrote that the postwar zeitgeist had left little space for wartime reminiscences: "In 1946, who cared what you did in the war? I thought that people who sat around and talked about their war were terrible bores." Only gradually, with time and perspective, did he begin to understand how formative an experience the war had been, for himself and his entire generation.[35]

That was almost eighty years ago (and was itself eighty years after the end of the US Civil War). What happened next? Eventually, the war became recognized as the twentieth century's central event and source of cultural mythology. Out of it came an explosion of social and political change and technological progress: the end of colonialism, the rise of the civil rights movement, the Cold War, the space race, computers, and the beginning of modern health care. The convulsion of the war broke lose the floodgates of change, for good and bad. In that postwar era of vigor and fluidity, the world we have lived in for the last eighty years was born.

We should not underestimate the opportunity contained in a moment like that, which could be repeated in the moment that is coming. We will be creating the post-Covid world. We must remember our lessons. If we do, we can grasp this chance to build a system that supports the true good health of us all, with justice, equity, and compassion.

Notes

INTRODUCTION

1. Rebekah Rollston and Sandro Galea, "COVID-19 and the Social Determinants of Health," in *American Journal of Health Promotion* 34(6) (June 19, 2020): 687–89, https://journals.sagepub.com/doi/full/10.1177/0890 117120930536b.

2. Jon Kamp, Robbie Whelan, and Anthony DeBarros, "U.S. Covid-19 Deaths in 2021 Surpass 2020's," in *Wall Street Journal*, November 20, 2021, https://www.wsj.com/articles/u-s-covid-19-deaths-in-2021-surpass-2020-11637426356.

3. Johns Hopkins University and Medicine, "Mortality Analyses," Johns Hopkins Coronavirus Resource Center, 2021, https://coronavirus.jhu.edu/data/mortality.

4. Salma M. Abdalla et al., "Claiming Health as a Public Good in the Post-COVID-19 Era," in *Development* 63 (2020): 200–204, https://doi.org/10.1057/s41301-020-00255-z.

5. Sandro Galea, *The Contagion Next Time* (Oxford: Oxford University Press, 2021).

6. Sandro Galea, *Well: What We Need to Talk about When We Talk about Health* (Oxford: Oxford University Press, 2019).

CHAPTER 1

1. For consistency, all Covid mortality data is taken as of December 2021 from Johns Hopkins University, "Coronavirus Resource Center," https://coronavirus.jhu.edu/.

2. Covid deaths from Jane Spencer and Christina Jewett, "Lost on the Front Line: Tracks Health Workers Who Died of COVID-19," *Kaiser Health News*, April 8, 2021, https://khn.org/news/article/us-health-workers-deaths-covid-lost-on-the-frontline/. Average annual deaths (157–353) from K. A. Sepkowitz and L. Eisenberg, "Occupational Deaths among Healthcare Workers," *Emerging Infectious Diseases* 11, no. 7 (2005): 1003–8, doi:10.3201/eid1107.041038.

3. Health care spending as a percent of GDP from the US Centers for Medicare and Medicaid Services: https://www.cms.gov/Research-Statistics-Data-and-Systems/Statistics-Trends-and-Reports/NationalHealthExpendData/NationalHealthAccountsHistorical. Military spending as percent of GDP from the World Bank: https://data.worldbank.org/indicator/MS.MIL.XPND.GD.ZS.

4. John Nance, interview by Charles Wohlforth, October 28, 2020.

5. Hilary Waldman, "CCMC Could Lose License," *Hartford Courant*, September 17, 2005, https://www.courant.com/news/connecticut/hc-xpm-2005-09-17-0509170874-story.html.

6. James Reason, "Human Error: Models and Management," *BMJ: British Medical Journal* 320, no. 7237 (March 18, 2000): 768–70, https://www.ncbi.nlm.nih.gov/pmc/articles/PMC1117770/.

7. John Nance, *Why Hospitals Should Fly: The Ultimate Flight Plan to Patient Safety and Quality Care* (Bozeman, MT: Second River Healthcare, 2008).

8. Tyson K. Cobb, "Wrong Site Surgery—Where Are We and What Is the Next Step?" *Hand* 7 (2012): 229–32, https://www.ncbi.nlm.nih.gov/pmc/articles/PMC3351519/pdf/11552_2012_Article_9405.pdf.

9. Earl Conway and Paul Batalden, "Like Magic? ('Every System Is Perfectly Designed . . .')," Institute for Healthcare Improvement, August 21, 2015, http://www.ihi.org/communities/blogs/origin-of-every-system-is-perfectly-designed-quote.

10. Johns Hopkins University, "Coronavirus Resource Center."

11. Dan Diamond, "Feuds, Fibs and Finger-Pointing: Trump Officials Say Coronavirus Response Was Worse Than Known," *Washington Post*, March 29, 2021, https://www.washingtonpost.com/health/2021/03/29/trump-officials-tell-all-coronavirus-response/.

12. Rebecca Masters et al., "Return on Investment of Public Health Interventions: A Systematic Review," *Journal of Epidemiology and Community Health* 71, no. 8 (August 1, 2017): 827–34, https://doi.org/10.1136/jech-2016-208141.

13. Christina Morales, Allyson Waller, and Marie Fazio, "A Timeline of Trump's Symptoms and Treatments," *New York Times*, October 4, 2020, https://www.nytimes.com/2020/10/04/us/trump-covid-symptoms-timeline.html.

14. James A. Levine, "Poverty and Obesity in the U.S.," *Diabetes* 60, no. 11 (November 1, 2011): 2667–68, https://doi.org/10.2337/db11-1118.

15. John D. Birkmeyer et al., "The Impact of the COVID-19 Pandemic on Hospital Admissions in the United States," *Health Affairs* 39, no. 11 (November 1, 2020): 2010–17, https://doi.org/10.1377/hlthaff.2020.00980.

16. Steven H. Woolf et al., "Excess Deaths from COVID-19 and Other Causes, March-April 2020," *JAMA* 324, no. 5 (August 4, 2020): 510, https://doi.org/10.1001/jama.2020.11787.

17. Birkmeyer et al., "The Impact of the COVID-19 Pandemic on Hospital Admissions in the United States."

18. Pauline W. Chen, "Where Have All the Hospital Patients Gone?" *New York Times*, October 20, 2020, sec. Well, https://www.nytimes.com/2020/10/20/well/where-have-all-the-hospital-patients-gone.html.

19. William H. Shrank, Teresa L. Rogstad, and Natasha Parekh, "Waste in the US Health Care System: Estimated Costs and Potential for Savings," *JAMA* 322, no. 15 (October 15, 2019): 1501, https://jamanetwork.com/journals/jama/article-abstract/2752664.

20. Elliott M. Antman and Eugene Braunwald, "Managing Stable Ischemic Heart Disease," *New England Journal of Medicine* 382, no. 15 (April 9, 2020): 1468–70, https://doi.org/10.1056/NEJMe2000239.

21. Martin Makary and Michael Daniel, "Medical Error—the Third Leading Cause of Death in the US," *BMJ* 353 (2016): i2139, http://doi.org/10.1136/bmj.i2139.

CHAPTER 2

1. Rick Ruggles, "Seven New Mexico Hospitals Swamped to Point of 'Crisis Standards' Designation," *Santa Fe New Mexican*, December 9, 2021, https://www.santafenewmexican.com/news/local_news/seven-new-mexico-hospitals-swamped-to-point-of-crisis-standards-designation/article_a9a57e78-58fa-11ec-8dda-53fd55d95320.html.

2. Johns Hopkins University, "Coronavirus Resource Center," Johns Hopkins Coronavirus Resource Center, https://coronavirus.jhu.edu/.

3. Centers for Disease Control and Prevention, "1918 Pandemic (H1N1 Virus)," Centers for Disease Control and Prevention, June 16, 2020, https://www.cdc.gov/flu/pandemic-resources/1918-pandemic-h1n1.html.

4. Ann H. Reid et al., "Origin and Evolution of the 1918 'Spanish' Influenza Virus Hemagglutinin Gene," *Proceedings of the National Academy of Sciences* 96, no. 4 (February 16, 1999): 1651–56, https://www.pnas.org/content/96/4/1651.

5. Edwin O. Jordan, *Epidemic Influenza: A Survey* (Chicago: American Medical Association, 1927), http://hdl.handle.net/2027/spo.8580flu.0016.858.

6. Alex Navarro, interview by Charles Wohlforth, April 22, 2021.

7. Howard Markel et al., *A Historical Assessment of Nonpharmaceutical Disease Containment Strategies Employed by Selected U.S. Communities during the Second Wave of the 1918–1920 Influenza Pandemic* (Washington, DC: US Department of Defense/Defense Threat Reduction Agency, January 31, 2006).

8. Leviticus 13.

9. Marty Cetron, interview by Charles Wohlforth, May 3, 2021.

10. Howard Markel et al., "Nonpharmaceutical Interventions Implemented by US Cities During the 1918–1919 Influenza Pandemic," *JAMA* 298, no. 6 (August 8, 2007): 644, https://doi.org/10.1001/jama.298.6.644.

11. Centers for Disease Control and Prevention, *Interim Pre-Pandemic Planning Guidance: Community Strategy for Pandemic Influenza Mitigation in the United States—Early, Targeted, Layered Use of Nonpharmaceutical Interventions* (Atlanta, GA: Centers for Disease Control and Prevention, February 2007), https://www.cdc.gov/flu/pandemic-resources/pdf/community_mitigation-sm.pdf.

12. Dan Barry and Caitlin Dickerson, "The Killer Flu of 1918: A Philadelphia Story," *New York Times*, April 4, 2020, https://www.nytimes.com/2020/04/04/us/coronavirus-spanish-flu-philadelphia-pennsylvania.html.

13. Esther Nash, interview by Charles Wohlforth, March 9, 2021.

14. World Health Organization, "Ebola Virus Disease," World Health Organization, February 23, 2021, https://www.who.int/news-room/fact-sheets/detail/ebola-virus-disease.

15. Bruce Meyer, interview by Charles Wohlforth, March 26, 2021.

16. Centers for Disease Control and Prevention, "First Travel-Related Case of 2019 Novel Coronavirus Detected in United States," January 21, 2020, https://www.cdc.gov/media/releases/2020/p0121-novel-coronavirus-travel-case.html.

17. World Health Organization, "Naming the Coronavirus Disease (COVID-19) and the Virus That Causes It," World Health Organization, February 11, 2020, https://www.who.int/emergencies/diseases/novel-coronavirus-2019/technical-guidance/naming-the-coronavirus-disease-(covid-2019)-and-the-virus-that-causes-it.

18. Rachel Nash, interview by Charles Wohlforth, April 5, 2021.

19. Centers for Disease Control and Prevention, "In-Hospital Mortality among Hospital Confirmed COVID-19 Encounters by Week from Selected Hospitals," May 17, 2021, https://www.cdc.gov/nchs/covid19/nhcs/hospital-mortality-by-week.htm.

20. Christopher M. Petrilli et al., "Factors Associated with Hospital Admission and Critical Illness among 5279 People with Coronavirus Disease 2019 in New York City: Prospective Cohort Study," *BMJ* 369 (May 22, 2020): m1966, https://doi.org/10.1136/bmj.m1966.

21. Jane Spencer and Christina Jewett, "'Lost on the Front Line': Tracks Health Workers Who Died of COVID-19," *Kaiser Health News*, April 8, 2021, https://khn.org/news/article/us-health-workers-deaths-covid-lost-on-the-frontline/.

22. Ibid.

23. Dan Diamond, "Feuds, Fibs and Finger-Pointing: Trump Officials Say Coronavirus Response Was Worse Than Known," *Washington Post*, March 29, 2021, https://www.washingtonpost.com/health/2021/03/29/trump-officials-tell-all-coronavirus-response/.

24. Eric Klinenberg, "We Need Social Solidarity, Not Just Social Distancing," *New York Times*, March 14, 2020, sec. Opinion, https://www.nytimes.com/2020/03/14/opinion/coronavirus-social-distancing.html.

25. Eric Klinenberg, *Heat Wave: A Social Autopsy of Disaster in Chicago*, second edition (Chicago: University of Chicago Press, 2015).

26. Alisa Chang and Eric Klinenberg, "What a 1995 Heat Wave May Teach Us about Responding to the Coronavirus Outbreak," NPR, March 31, 2020, https://www.npr.org/2020/03/31/824730922/what-a-1995-heat-wave-may-teach-us-about-responding-to-the-coronavirus-outbreak.

27. Robert Costa and Philip Rucker, "Woodward Book: Trump Says He Knew Coronavirus Was 'Deadly' and Worse Than the Flu While Intentionally Misleading Americans," *Washington Post*, September 9, 2020, https://www.washingtonpost.com/politics/bob-woodward-rage-book-trump/2020/09/09/0368fe3c-efd2-11ea-b4bc-3a2098fc73d4_story.html.

28. Michael C. Bender and Rebecca Ballhaus, "How Trump Sowed Covid Supply Chaos. 'Try Getting It Yourselves,'" *Wall Street Journal*, August 31, 2020, sec. US, https://www.wsj.com/articles/how-trump-sowed-covid-supply-chaos-try-getting-it-yourselves-11598893051; Melanie Evans and Michael Siconolfi, "U.S. Strategic Stockpile of Medical Supplies Is Outmatched by Coronavirus," *Wall Street Journal*, March 23, 2020, sec. US, https://www.wsj.com/articles/u-s-strategic-stockpile-of-medical-supplies-is-outmatched-by-coronavirus-11584990542.

29. Gina Kolata, "In a First, *New England Journal of Medicine* Joins Never-Trumpers," *New York Times*, October 7, 2020, sec. Health, https://www.nytimes.com/2020/10/07/health/new-england-journal-trump.html.

30. Editors of *NEJM*, "Dying in a Leadership Vacuum," *New England Journal of Medicine*, October 7, 2020, https://doi.org/10.1056/NEJMe2029812.

31. David Leonhardt, "U.S. Covid Deaths Get Even Redder," *New York Times*, November 8, 2021, https://www.nytimes.com/2021/11/08/briefing/covid-death-toll-red-america.html.

32. Alexandra Ellerbeck, "The Health 202: Here's How the U.S. Compares to Other Countries on the Coronavirus Pandemic," *Washington Post*, April 12, 2021, https://www.washingtonpost.com/politics/2021/04/12/health-202-here-how-us-compares-other-countries-coronavirus-pandemic/.

33. Ryan Basen, "COVID Patients' Crackpot Theories Take Toll on Healthcare Workers," *MedPage Today*, November 19, 2020, https://www.medpagetoday.com/infectiousdisease/covid19/89796.

34. Keri N. Althoff et al., "Antibodies to SARS-CoV-2 in All of Us Research Program Participants, January 2–March 18, 2020," *Clinical Infectious Diseases*, no. ciab519 (June 15, 2021), https://doi.org/10.1093/cid/ciab519.

35. Feliz Solomon and Wilawan Watcharasakwet, "Thailand Once Shut Out Covid-19 but Is Now Pivoting to Living with It," *Wall Street Journal*, June 19, 2021, sec. World, https://www.wsj.com/articles/thailand-once-shut-out-covid-19-but-is-now-pivoting-to-living-with-it-11624107310.

36. David Willman, "The CDC's Failed Race against Covid-19: A Threat Underestimated and a Test Overcomplicated," *Washington Post*, December 26, 2020, https://www.washingtonpost.com/investigations/cdc-covid/2020/12/25/c2b418ae-4206-11eb-8db8-395dedaaa036_story.html.

37. Shawn Boburg et al., "Inside the Coronavirus Testing Failure: Alarm and Dismay among the Scientists Who Sought to Help," *Washington Post*, April 3, 2020, https://www.washingtonpost.com/investigations/2020/04/03/coronavirus-cdc-test-kits-public-health-labs/.

CHAPTER 3

1. Aaron Blake, "The Most-Vaccinated Big Counties in America Are Beating the Worst of the Coronavirus," *Washington Post*, December 4, 2021, https://www.washingtonpost.com/politics/2021/12/04/big-counties-are-proving-how-vaccination-works/.

2. Stephanie Nolen, "I Am Living in a Covid-Free World Just a Few Hundred Miles from Manhattan," *New York Times*, November 18, 2020, sec. Opinion, https://www.nytimes.com/2020/11/18/opinion/covid-halifax-nova-scotia-canada.html.

3. Rebecca Kanthor, "Revisiting Wuhan a Year after the Coronavirus Hit the City," *The World from PRX*, January 21, 2021, https://www.pri.org/stories/2021-01-21/revisiting-wuhan-year-after-coronavirus-hit-city.

4. For consistency, all Covid mortality data is taken as of December 2021 from Johns Hopkins University, "Coronavirus Resource Center," Johns Hopkins Coronavirus Resource Center, December 14, 2021, https://coronavirus.jhu.edu/.

5. Richard Glover, "10 Reasons for Australia's Covid-19 Success Story," *Washington Post*, sec. Opinion, March 15, 2021, https://www.washingtonpost.com/opinions/2021/03/15/10-reasons-australias-covid-19-success-story/.

6. Bojan Pancevski, "Finland and Norway Avoid Covid-19 Lockdowns but Keep the Virus at Bay," *Wall Street Journal*, November 18, 2020, sec. World, https://www.wsj.com/articles/finland-and-norway-avoid-covid-19-lockdowns-but-keep-the-virus-at-bay-11605704407.

7. Philip Bump, "The Two Halves of the Pandemic," *Washington Post*, December 1, 2021, https://www.washingtonpost.com/politics/2021/12/01/two-halves-pandemic/.

8. Centers for Disease Control and Prevention, "Estimated Disease Burden of COVID-19," May 19, 2021, https://www.cdc.gov/coronavirus/2019-ncov/cases-updates/burden.html.

9. Brian Neelon et al., "Associations between Governor Political Affiliation and COVID-19 Cases, Deaths, and Testing in the U.S.," *American Journal of Preventive Medicine* 61, no. 1 (July 1, 2021): 115–19, https://doi.org/10.1016/j.amepre.2021.01.034.

10. Olga Shvetsova et al., Public Health Policies as a Link between Governor Political Affiliation and COVID-19 Outcomes: Response to Neelon et al., unpublished. Also: Julie VanDusky-Allen and Olga Shvetsova, "How America's Partisan Divide over Pandemic Responses Played Out in the States," *The Conversation*, May 12, 2021, http://theconversation.com/how-americas-partisan-divide-over-pandemic-responses-played-out-in-the-states-157565.

11. Olga Shvetsova, interview by Charles Wohlforth, July 1, 2021.

12. Karen DeSalvo, chief health officer, Google Health, interview by Charles Wohlforth, April 16, 2021.

13. Amy Quinn, "Chaos, Anxiety, Frustration—but No Appointment for a Vaccine," *NJ.com*, January 16, 2021, sec. Opinion, https://www.nj.com/opinion/2021/01/chaos-anxiety-frustration-but-no-appointment-for-a-vaccine-opinion.html.

14. Liz Hamel et al., "KFF COVID-19 Vaccine Monitor: September 2021," *KFF*, September 28, 2021, https://www.kff.org/coronavirus-covid-19/poll-finding/kff-covid-19-vaccine-monitor-september-2021/.

15. Morgan Krakow and Annie Berman, "Alaska Used to Lead the Nation in COVID-19 Vaccinations. Six Months in, the State Has Fallen Behind," *Anchorage Daily News*, June 11, 2021, sec. Alaska News, https://www.

adn.com/alaska-news/2021/06/10/alaska-used-to-lead-the-nation-in-covid-19-vaccinations-six-months-later-the-state-has-fallen-behind/.

16. Zaz Hollander, "Impossible Choices Inside Alaska's Inundated Hospitals," *Anchorage Daily News*, September 17, 2021, https://www.adn.com/alaska-news/2021/09/17/impossible-choices-inside-alaskas-inundated-hospitals/.

17. Michelle Theriault Boots and Emily Goodykoontz, "Jewish Leaders Decry Use of Holocaust Symbolism to Protest Anchorage Mask Ordinance," *Anchorage Daily News*, September 30, 2021, https://www.adn.com/alaska-news/anchorage/2021/09/30/a-direct-disrespect-jewish-leaders-decry-use-of-holocaust-symbolism-to-protest-anchorage-mask-ordinance/.

18. Gary Fineout, "Poll Shows DeSantis on Solid Ground as Democrats Try to Find Openings," *Politico*, May 12, 2021, sec. Politico Florida, https://politi.co/3uKdt1Z.

19. Nolan M. Kavanagh, Rishi R. Goel, and Atheendar S. Venkataramani, "County-Level Socioeconomic and Political Predictors of Distancing for COVID-19," *American Journal of Preventive Medicine* 61, no. 1 (July 2021): 13–19, https://doi.org/10.1016/j.amepre.2021.01.040.

20. David A. Graham, "It's Not Vaccine Hesitancy. It's COVID-19 Denialism," *The Atlantic*, April 27, 2021, sec. Ideas, https://www.theatlantic.com/ideas/archive/2021/04/its-not-vaccine-hesitancy-its-covid-denialism/618724/.

21. Barton Swaim, "Politics: The Experts and the Pandemic," *Wall Street Journal*, December 18, 2020, sec. Arts, https://www.wsj.com/articles/politics-the-experts-and-the-pandemic-11608331377.

22. Ibid.

23. Kathyrn R. Fair et al., "Estimating COVID-19 Cases and Deaths Prevented by Non-Pharmaceutical Interventions, and the Impact of Individual Actions: A Retrospective Model-Based Analysis," *MedRxiv* pre-print, June 24, 2021, 2021.03.26.21254421, https://doi.org/10.1101/2021.03.26.21254421.

24. Leah C. Windsor et al., "Gender in the Time of COVID-19: Evaluating National Leadership and COVID-19 Fatalities," *PLOS ONE* 15, no. 12 (December 31, 2020): e0244531, https://doi.org/10.1371/journal.pone.0244531.

25. Leah Windsor, interview by Charles Wohlforth, April 22, 2021.

26. Geert Hofstede, "Dimensionalizing Cultures: The Hofstede Model in Context," *Online Readings in Psychology and Culture* 2, no. 1 (December 1, 2011), https://doi.org/10.9707/2307-0919.1014.

27. Geert Hofstede, "The 6 Dimensions Model of National Culture," 2021, https://geerthofstede.com/culture-geert-hofstede-gert-jan-hofstede/6d-model-of-national-culture/.

28. Hofstede, "Dimensionalizing Cultures," 11.

29. Charles Wohlforth, *The Fate of Nature: Rediscovering Our Ability to Rescue the Earth* (New York: Thomas Dunne Books/St. Martin's Press, 2010).

30. Ian Duncan et al., "Medicare Cost at End of Life," *American Journal of Hospice & Palliative Care* 36, no. 8 (August 2019): 705–10, https://doi.org/10.1177/1049909119836204.

31. Claude Fischer, "Paradoxes of American Individualism," *Sociological Forum* 23, no. 2 (June 2008), https://doi.org/10.1111/j.1573-7861.2008.00066.x.

32. Leana Wen, interview by Charles Wohlforth, March 26, 2021.

33. Rose Rudd et al., "Increases in Drug and Opioid Overdose Deaths—United States, 2000–2014," *Centers for Disease Control and Prevention Morbidity and Mortality Weekly Report* 64, no. 50 (January 1, 2016): 1378–82, https://www.cdc.gov/mmwr/preview/mmwrhtml/mm6450a3.htm.

34. Centers of Disease Control, National Center for Health Statistics, "Drug Overdose Deaths in the U.S. Top 100,000 Annually," Media release, https://www.cdc.gov/nchs/pressroom/nchs_press_releases/2021/20211117.htm.

35. US Attorney's Office, District of New Jersey, "Opioid Manufacturer Purdue Pharma Admits Guilt in Fraud and Kickback Conspiracies," United States Department of Justice, November 24, 2020, https://www.justice.gov/usao-nj/pr/opioid-manufacturer-purdue-pharma-admits-guilt-fraud-and-kickback-conspiracies.

36. Leana S. Wen, "Opinion: The CDC Is Missing a Critical Opportunity to Get Americans Vaccinated," *Washington Post*, March 8, 2021, https://www.washingtonpost.com/opinions/cdc-recommendations-vaccinated-masks-limited/2021/03/08/a05353ac-804e-11eb-9ca6-54e187ee4939_story.html.

37. Associated Press, "Warp-Speed Spending and Other Surreal Stats of COVID Times," *US News & World Report*, March 13, 2021, sec. Health News, //www.usnews.com/news/health-news/articles/2021-03-13/warp-speed-spending-and-other-surreal-stats-of-covid-times.

38. Jerome H. Kim et al., "Operation Warp Speed: Implications for Global Vaccine Security," *The Lancet Global Health* 9, no. 7 (July 1, 2021): e1017–21, https://doi.org/10.1016/S2214-109X(21)00140-6.

39. Jason Beiriger and David B. Nash, "Testing Testimonial," *Population Health Management*, April 16, 2021, https://doi.org/10.1089/pop.2021.0056.

40. Ibid.

41. Brad Smith, "CMS Innovation Center at 10 Years—Progress and Lessons Learned," *New England Journal of Medicine* 384, no. 8 (February 25, 2021): 759–64, https://doi.org/10.1056/NEJMsb2031138.

42. "UnitedHealth Group," *Fortune*, June 2, 2021, https://fortune.com/company/unitedhealth-group/fortune500/.

CHAPTER 4

1. Demographics from the US Census Bureau, QuickFacts, Queens County (Queens Borough), New York, April 1, 2020, https://www.census.gov/quickfacts/fact/table/queenscountyqueensboroughnewyork/POP645219; languages from City of New York, "Top Languages Spoken at Home," online factsheet, https://www1.nyc.gov/assets/planning/download/pdf/data-maps/nyc-population/acs/top_lang_2015pums5yr_nyc.pdf.

2. Eric Bressman, "Safety Net: Reflections on the Elmhurst Experience," *NEJM Journal Watch*, May 19, 2020, https://blogs.jwatch.org/general-medicine/index.php/2020/05/safety-net-reflections-on-the-elmhurst-experience/.

3. David A. Ansell, MD, *The Death Gap: How Inequality Kills* (Chicago: University of Chicago Press, 2021), x.

4. John Scholsberg, Linsey Davis, and Sabina Ghebremedhin, "Philadelphia Doctor Takes to Streets to Help Black Communities Get Tested for COVID-19," ABC News, April 29, 2020, sec. Coronavirus Health & Science, https://abcnews.go.com/US/philadelphia-doctor-takes-streets-black-communities-tested-covid/story?id=70405257.

5. Queen Muse, "How Ala Stanford Became a Champion for the Health of Black Philadelphians amid COVID," *Philadelphia Magazine*, August 8, 2020, https://www.phillymag.com/healthcare-news/2020/08/08/ala-stanford-black-doctors-covid-19-consortium.

6. Schlosberg et al., "Philadelphia Doctor Takes to Streets."

7. Sandra Brooks, interview by Charles Wohlforth, April 13, 2021.

8. Victor Fiorillo and Gabby Houck, "*Good Morning America* Told Ala Stanford the City Named a Street after Her. It Didn't," *Philadelphia Magazine*, April 14, 2021, https://www.phillymag.com/news/2021/04/14/ala-stanford-street-philadelphia/.

9. W. E. Burghardt Du Bois, *The Philadelphia Negro: A Social Study* (Philadelphia: University of Pennsylvania, 1899), 1, 295–97.

10. Ibid., 160.

11. Apoorva Mandavilli, "Editor of *JAMA* Leaves after Outcry over Colleague's Remarks on Racism," *New York Times*, June 1, 2021, https://www.nytimes.com/2021/06/01/health/jama-bauchner-racism.html.

12. Digital Scholarship Lab, University of Richmond, "Mapping Inequality: Redlining in New Deal America," *American Panorama*, 2021, https://dsl.richmond.edu/panorama/redlining/. The quote from the Philadelphia map is located at https://dsl.richmond.edu/panorama/redlining/#loc=5/39.1/-94.58.

13. Digital Scholarship Lab, University of Richmond, "Mapping Inequality."

14. Sun Jung Oh and John Yinger, "What Have We Learned from Paired Testing in Housing Markets?" *Cityscape* 17, no. 3 (2015): 15–60, https://www.jstor.org/stable/26326960.

15. Ann Choi, Olivia Winslow, and Arthur Browne, "Long Island Divided," *Newsday*, November 17, 2019, sec. Long Island, https://projects.newsday.com/long-island/real-estate-agents-investigation/.

16. David Elesh, "Deindustrialization," *The Encyclopedia of Greater Philadelphia*, 2017, https://philadelphiaencyclopedia.org/archive/deindustrialization/.

17. District Performance Office, "District Scorecard," The School District of Philadelphia, June 4, 2021, https://www.philasd.org/performance/programsservices/school-progress-reports/district-scorecard/.

18. Ajay Chaudry et al., *Poverty in the United States: 50-Year Trends and Safety Net Impacts*, Office of the Assistant Secretary for Planning and Evaluation, US Department of Health and Human Services, March 2016, https://aspe.hhs.gov/sites/default/files/private/pdf/154286/50YearTrends.pdf.

19. Atheendar S. Venkataramani, Rourke O'Brien, and Alexander C. Tsai, "Declining Life Expectancy in the United States: The Need for Social Policy as Health Policy," *JAMA* 325, no. 7 (February 16, 2021): 621–22, https://doi.org/10.1001/jama.2020.26339.

20. Raj Chetty et al., "The Association Between Income and Life Expectancy in the United States, 2001–2014," *JAMA* 315, no. 16 (April 26, 2016): 1750–66, https://doi.org/10.1001/jama.2016.4226.

21. Ezekiel J. Emanuel et al., "Comparing Health Outcomes of Privileged US Citizens with Those of Average Residents of Other Developed Countries," *JAMA Internal Medicine* 181, no. 3 (March 1, 2021): 339–44, https://doi.org/10.1001/jamainternmed.2020.7484.

22. Martin Luther King Jr., *Letter from Birmingham Jail* (London: Penguin Classics, 2018).

23. Hans Kellner, "Heat Vulnerability Index Highlights City Hot Spots," City of Philadelphia, July 16, 2019, https://www.phila.gov/2019-07-16-heat-vulnerability-index-highlights-city-hot-spots/.

24. Drew Shindell et al., "The Effects of Heat Exposure on Human Mortality throughout the United States," *GeoHealth* 4, no. 4 (2020), https://doi.org/10.1029/2019GH000234.

25. Advocacy Department, "Facts: Bridging the Gap, CVD and Health Equity," American Heart Association, 2015.

26. Monika M. Safford et al., "Number of Social Determinants of Health and Fatal and Nonfatal Incident Coronary Heart Disease in the REGARDS Study," *Circulation* 143, no. 3 (January 19, 2021): 244–53, https://doi.org/10.1161/CIRCULATIONAHA.120.048026.

27. Du Bois, *The Philadelphia Negro*, 158.

28. Philadelphia Department of Public Health, and Drexel University Urban Health Collaborative, "Close to Home: The Health of Philadelphia's Neighborhoods," Philadelphia Department of Public Health, July 31,

2019, https://www.phila.gov/media/20190801133844/Neighborhood-Rankings_7_31_19.pdf.

29. Du Bois, *The Philadelphia Negro*, 163.

30. *New York Times*, "Coronavirus in the U.S.: Latest Map and Case Count," https://www.nytimes.com/interactive/2021/us/covid-cases.html.

31. Farida B. Ahmad et al., "Provisional Mortality Data—United States, 2020," *Centers for Disease Control, Morbidity and Mortality Weekly Report* 70 (April 9, 2021): 519–22, https://doi.org/10.15585/mmwr.mm7014e1.

32. Sarah Miller, Laura R. Wherry, and Bhashkar Mazumder, "Estimated Mortality Increases during the COVID-19 Pandemic by Socioeconomic Status, Race, and Ethnicity," *Health Affairs* 40, no. 8 (August 1, 2021): 1252–60, https://doi.org/10.1377/hlthaff.2021.00414.

33. Jonathan Gleason et al., "The Devastating Impact of Covid-19 on Individuals with Intellectual Disabilities in the United States," *NEJM Catalyst Innovations in Care Delivery*, March 5, 2021, https://catalyst.nejm.org/doi/full/10.1056/CAT.21.0051.

34. Sharon Otterman, "'I Trust Science,' Says Nurse Who Is First to Get Vaccine in U.S.," *New York Times*, December 14, 2020, sec. New York, https://www.nytimes.com/2020/12/14/nyregion/us-covid-vaccine-first-sandra-lindsay.html.

35. Nambi Ndugga, Latoya Hill, and Samantha Artiga, "Latest Data on COVID-19 Vaccinations by Race/Ethnicity," *KFF*, August 4, 2021, https://www.kff.org/coronavirus-covid-19/issue-brief/latest-data-on-covid-19-vaccinations-race-ethnicity/.

36. Rodney E. Rohde and Ryan McNamara, "US Is Split between the Vaccinated and Unvaccinated—and Deaths and Hospitalizations Reflect This Divide," *The Conversation*, July 22, 2021, http://theconversation.com/us-is-split-between-the-vaccinated-and-unvaccinated-and-deaths-and-hospitaliza-tions-reflect-this-divide-164460.

37. "Coronavirus in the U.S.: Latest Map and Case Count."

38. Miller et al., "Estimated Mortality Increases."

39. David A. Asch et al., "Patient and Hospital Factors Associated with Differences in Mortality Rates among Black and White US Medicare Beneficiaries Hospitalized with COVID-19 Infection," *JAMA Network Open* 4, no. 6 (June 17, 2021), https://doi.org/10.1001/jamanetworkopen.2021.12842.

40. Elizabeth Arias et al., "Provisional Life Expectancy Estimates for 2020," Centers for Disease Control and Prevention, July 2021, https://doi.org/10.15620/cdc:100392.

41. Liz Hamel et al., "KFF COVID-19 Vaccine Monitor: September 2021," *KFF*, September 28, 2021, https://www.kff.org/coronavirus-covid-19/poll-finding/kff-covid-19-vaccine-monitor-september-2021/.

42. Yea-Hung Chen et al., "Excess Mortality Associated with the COVID-19 Pandemic among Californians 18–65 Years of Age, by Occupational Sector and Occupation: March through November 2020," *PLOS ONE* 16, no. 6 (June 4, 2021), https://doi.org/10.1371/journal.pone.0252454.

43. Amy Maxman, "Inequality's Deadly Toll," *Nature* 592 (April 29, 2021): 674–80, https://www.nature.com/immersive/d41586-021-00943-x/index.html.

44. Charles A. Taylor, Christopher Boulos and Douglas Almond, "Livestock Plants and COVID-19 Transmission," *PNAS* 117, no. 50: 31706–15, https://doi.org/10.1073/pnas.2010115117.

45. Serina Chang et al., "Mobility Network Models of COVID-19 Explain Inequities and Inform Reopening," *Nature* 589, no. 7840 (January 2021): 82–87, https://doi.org/10.1038/s41586-020-2923-3.

46. Jan Mutchler, "Nearly Two-Thirds of Older Black Americans Can't Afford to Live Alone without Help—and It's Even Tougher for Latinos," *The Conversation*, November 17, 2020, https://theconversation.com/nearly-two-thirds-of-older-black-americans-cant-afford-to-live-alone-without-help-and-its-even-tougher-for-latinos-146913.

47. Sara Rimer, "Blacks Carry Load of Care for Their Elderly," *New York Times*, March 15, 1998, sec. U.S., https://www.nytimes.com/1998/03/15/us/blacks-carry-load-of-care-for-their-elderly.html.

48. Rebecca J. Gorges and R. Tamara Konetzka, "Factors Associated with Racial Differences in Deaths among Nursing Home Residents with COVID-19 Infection in the US," *JAMA Network Open* 4, no. 2 (February 10, 2021), https://doi.org/10.1001/jamanetworkopen.2020.37431.

49. Du Bois, *The Philadelphia Negro*, 163.

50. Ansell, *The Death Gap*, 197.

51. Brad N. Greenwood et al., "Physician–Patient Racial Concordance and Disparities in Birthing Mortality for Newborns," *PNAS* 117, no. 35 (September 1, 2020): 21194–200, https://doi.org/10.1073/pnas.1913405117.

52. Janice Sabin, "How We Fail Black Patients in Pain," *AAMC*, January 6, 2020, https://www.aamc.org/news-insights/how-we-fail-black-patients-pain.

53. Fenit Nirappil, "A Black Doctor Alleged Racist Treatment before Dying of Covid-19: 'This Is How Black People Get Killed,'" *Washington Post*, December 4, 2020, sec. Health, https://www.washingtonpost.com/health/2020/12/24/covid-susan-moore-medical-racism/.

54. Ansell, *The Death Gap*, xix–xx.

55. Ibid., 194.

56. David Ansell, interview by Charles Wohlforth, August 2, 2021.

57. Asch et al., "Patient and Hospital Factors."

58. Melanie Evans, Alexandra Berzon, and Daniela Hernandez, "Some California Hospitals Refused Covid-19 Transfers for Financial Reasons, State Emails Show," *Wall Street Journal*, October 19, 2020, sec. Investigations,

https://www.wsj.com/articles/some-california-hospitals-refused-covid-19-transfers-for-financial-reasons-state-emails-show-11603108814.

59. Kristina Fiore, "Is a Residency Program an Asset to Be Sold?" *MedPage Today*, September 20, 2019, https://www.medpagetoday.com/special-reports/exclusives/82292.

60. Maria Cramer, "Philadelphia Hospital to Stay Closed after Owner Requests Nearly $1 Million a Month," *New York Times*, March 27, 2020, sec. U.S., https://www.nytimes.com/2020/03/27/us/coronavirus-philadelphia-hahnemann-hospital.html.

61. Nina Feldman, "Why the Head of the Black Doctors COVID-19 Consortium Decided to Get Vaccinated," *WHYY*, December 16, 2020, https://whyy.org/articles/why-the-head-of-the-black-doctors-covid-19-consortium-decided-to-get-vaccinated/.

62. Diana Schow, Elisa J. Sobo, and Stephanie McClure, "US Black and Latino Communities Often Have Low Vaccination Rates—but Blaming Vaccine Hesitancy Misses the Mark," *The Conversation*, July 7, 2021, http://theconversation.com/us-black-and-latino-communities-often-have-low-vaccination-rates-but-blaming-vaccine-hesitancy-misses-the-mark-163169.

63. Aallyah Wright, "Republican Men Are Vaccine-Hesitant, but There's Little Focus on Them," Pew Charitable Trusts, April 23, 2021, https://pew.org/3xh75RF.

64. David A. Ansell et al., "Health Equity as a System Strategy: The Rush University Medical Center Framework," *NEJM Catalyst* 2, no. 5 (May 2021), https://doi.org/10.1056/CAT.20.0674.

CHAPTER 5

1. Institute of Medicine Committee for the Study of the Future of Public Health, *The Future of Public Health* (Washington, DC: National Academies Press, 1988), https://www.ncbi.nlm.nih.gov/books/NBK218224/.

2. Dora Costa, "Health and the Economy in the United States, from 1750 to the Present," *Journal of Economic Literature* 53, no. 3 (September 2015): 503–70, https://doi.org/10.1257/jel.53.3.503.

3. Robert M. Kaplan and Arnold Milstein, "Contributions of Health Care to Longevity: A Review of 4 Estimation Methods," *Annals of Family Medicine* 17, no. 3 (May 1, 2019): 267–72, https://doi.org/10.1370/afm.2362.

4. Rebecca Masters et al., "Return on Investment of Public Health Interventions: A Systematic Review," *Journal of Epidemiology and Community Health* 71, no. 8 (August 1, 2017): 827–34, https://doi.org/10.1136/jech-2016-208141; Timothy T. Brown, "Returns on Investment in California County

Departments of Public Health," *American Journal of Public Health* 106, no. 8 (August 1, 2016): 1477–82, https://doi.org/10.2105/AJPH.2016.303233.

5. David J. Hunter, "The Complementarity of Public Health and Medicine: Achieving 'the Highest Attainable Standard of Health,'" *New England Journal of Medicine* 385, no. 6 (August 5, 2021): 481–84, https://doi.org/10.1056/NEJMp2102550.

6. Jason D. Buxbaum et al., "Contributions of Public Health, Pharmaceuticals, and Other Medical Care to US Life Expectancy Changes, 1990–2015," *Health Affairs* 39, no. 9 (September 1, 2020): 1546–56, https://doi.org/10.1377/hlthaff.2020.00284.

7. Centers for Medicare and Medicaid Services, "National Health Expenditure Data," December 16, 2020, https://www.cms.gov/Research-Statistics-Data-and-Systems/Statistics-Trends-and-Reports/NationalHealthExpendData/NationalHealthAccountsHistorical.

8. Caroline Au Yeung and Robert Hest, "Exploring Public Health Indicators with State Health Compare: State Public Health Funding," State Health Access Data Assistance Center, May 2020, https://www.shadac.org/sites/default/files/State%20Public%20Health%20Funding_May%202020.pdf.

9. For state-level employee losses, see Association of State and Territorial Health Officials, "New Data on State Health Agencies Shows Shrinking Workforce and Decreased Funding Leading up to the COVID-19 Pandemic," https://astho.org/Press-Room/New-Data-on-State-Health-Agencies-Shows-Shrinking-Workforce-andDecreased-Funding-Leading-up-to-the-COVID-19-Pandemic/09-24–20/; for local-level employee losses, see Kellie Hall, Nathalie Robin, and Kari O'Donnell, "The 2018 Forces of Change in America's Local Public Health System," National Association of County and City Health Officials Voice, *NACCHO Voice*, November 20, 2018, https://www.naccho.org/blog/articles/the-2018-forces-of-change-in-americas-local-public-health-system.

10. Karen DeSalvo et al., "Public Health COVID-19 Impact Assessment: Lessons Learned and Compelling Needs," *NAM Perspectives*, April 7, 2021, https://doi.org/10.31478/202104c.

11. J. Mac McCullough, "Declines in Spending Despite Positive Returns on Investment: Understanding Public Health's Wrong Pocket Problem," *Frontiers in Public Health* 7 (June 18, 2019): 159, https://doi.org/10.3389/fpubh.2019.00159.

12. Anna Maria Barry-Jester et al., "Pandemic Backlash Jeopardizes Public Health Powers, Leaders," Kaiser Health News, December 15, 2020, https://khn.org/news/article/pandemic-backlash-jeopardizes-public-health-powers-leaders/.

13. Anne Schuchat, "What I Learned in 33 Years at the C.D.C.," *New York Times*, June 10, 2021, sec. Opinion, https://www.nytimes.com/2021/06/10/opinion/anne-schuchat-cdc-retirement.html.

14. DeSalvo et al., "Public Health COVID-19 Impact Assessment."

15. Karen DeSalvo, interview by Charles Wohlforth, April 16, 2021.

16. Center for Countering Digital Hate, *The Disinformation Dozen* (London: CCDH, March 21, 2021), https://www.counterhate.com/disinformationdozen; and Tom Buchanan, "Why Do People Spread False Information Online? The Effects of Message and Viewer Characteristics on Self-Reported Likelihood of Sharing Social Media Disinformation," *PLoS ONE* 15(10): e0239666, https://doi.org/10.1371/journal.pone.0239666.

17. Katie Rogers et al., "Trump's Suggestion That Disinfectants Could Be Used to Treat Coronavirus Prompts Aggressive Pushback," *New York Times*, April 24, 2020, https://www.nytimes.com/2020/04/24/us/politics/trump-inject-disinfectant-bleach-coronavirus.html.

18. Thomas R. Marshall, "The 1964 Surgeon General's Report and Americans' Beliefs about Smoking," *Journal of the History of Medicine and Allied Sciences* 70, no. 2 (April 2015): 250–78, https://doi.org/10.1093/jhmas/jrt057.

19. Theodore R. Holford et al., "Tobacco Control and the Reduction in Smoking-Related Premature Deaths in the United States, 1964–2012," *JAMA* 311, no. 2 (January 8, 2014): 164–71, https://doi.org/10.1001/jama.2013.285112.

20. Padraic O'Malley, Jethro Rainford, and Alison Thompson, "Transparency during Public Health Emergencies: From Rhetoric to Reality," *Bulletin of the World Health Organization* 87 (September 1, 2009): 614–18, https://doi.org/10.2471/BLT.08.056689.

21. O'Malley et al., "Transparency during Public Health Emergencies."

22. Zeynep Tufekci, "5 Pandemic Mistakes We Keep Repeating," *The Atlantic*, February 26, 2021, sec. Ideas, https://www.theatlantic.com/ideas/archive/2021/02/how-public-health-messaging-backfired/618147/.

23. Amy Maxmen, "Why Did the World's Pandemic Warning System Fail When COVID Hit?" *Nature* 589, no. 7843 (January 23, 2021): 499–500, https://doi.org/10.1038/d41586-021-00162-4.

24. Zeynep Tufekci, "Why Did It Take So Long to Accept the Facts about Covid?" *New York Times*, May 7, 2021, sec. Opinion, https://www.nytimes.com/2021/05/07/opinion/coronavirus-airborne-transmission.html.

25. World Health Organization, "Weekly Epidemiological Update on COVID-19–11 May 2021," WHO, May 11, 2021 https://www.who.int/publications/m/item/weekly-epidemiological-update-on-covid-19---11-may-2021.

26. Roxanne Khamsi, "A Lack of Transparency Is Undermining Pandemic Policy," *Wired*, November 16, 2020, https://www.wired.com/story/a-lack-of-transparency-is-undermining-pandemic-policy/.

27. CNN, "CNN's Facts First Searchable Database," https://www.cnn.com/factsfirst/politics/factcheck_e58c20c6-8735-4022-a1f5-1580bc732c45.

28. Khamsi, "A Lack of Transparency"; on temperature checks, see Roni Caryn Rabin, "Fever Checks Are No Safeguard against Covid-19," *New York Times*, September 13, 2020, sec. Health, https://www.nytimes.com/2020/09/13/health/covid-fever-checks-dining.html.

29. Amanda Mull, "The Logic of Pandemic Restrictions Is Falling Apart," *The Atlantic*, November 25, 2020, sec. Health, https://www.theatlantic.com/health/archive/2020/11/pandemic-restrictions-no-logic/617204/.

30. DeSalvo et al., "Public Health COVID-19 Impact Assessment."

31. Michelle Fiscus, "Tennessee's Former Top Vaccine Official: 'I Am Afraid for My State,'" *The Tennessean*, July 12, 2021, sec. Health, https://www.tennessean.com/story/news/health/2021/07/12/covid-19-tennessee-fired-vaccine-official-michelle-fiscus-fears-state/7945291002/.

32. Hunter, "The Complementarity of Public Health and Medicine."

33. Centers for Disease Control and Prevention, "New CDC Data Finds Adult Obesity Is Increasing," CDC, September 17, 2020, https://www.cdc.gov/media/releases/2020/s0917-adult-obesity-increasing.html.

34. David M. Cutler, Edward L. Glaeser, and Jesse M. Shapiro, "Why Have Americans Become More Obese?" *Journal of Economic Perspectives* 17, no. 3 (September 2003): 93–118, https://doi.org/10.1257/089533003769204371.

35. Meredith Wadman, "Why COVID-19 Is More Deadly in People with Obesity—Even If They're Young," *Science*, September 8, 2020, https://www.science.org/content/article/why-covid-19-more-deadly-people-obesity-even-if-theyre-young.

36. Michael Lerner, "Going Dry," National Endowment for the Humanities, September 2011, https://www.neh.gov/humanities/2011/septemberoctober/feature/going-dry.

37. National Safety Council, "Car Crash Deaths and Rates," https://injuryfacts.nsc.org/motor-vehicle/historical-fatality-trends/deaths-and-rates/.

38. D'vera Cohn et al., "Gun Homicide Rate Down 49% Since 1993 Peak; Public Unaware," Pew Research Center, May 7, 2013, https://www.pewresearch.org/social-trends/2013/05/07/gun-homicide-rate-down-49-since-1993-peak-public-unaware/.

39. Alec MacGillis, "What Philadelphia Reveals about America's Homicide Surge," ProPublica, July 30, 2021, https://www.propublica.org/article/philadelphia-homicide-surge?token=tg74b8VQrqWdM-PFRUNWBD84ZpaGuM3h.

40. Ibid.

41. Ibid.

42. National Association of Home Builders, "Housing's Contribution to Gross Domestic Product," https://www.nahb.org/news-and-economics/housing-economics/housings-economic-impact/housings-contribution-to-gross-domestic-product, accessed December 22, 2021.

43. Jaana Remes et al., "Prioritizing Health: A Prescription for Prosperity," McKinsey & Company, July 8, 2020, https://www.mckinsey.com/industries/healthcare-systems-and-services/our-insights/prioritizing-health-a-prescription-for-prosperity.

CHAPTER 6

1. Northwell Health, "Fact Sheet February 2021," Northwell Health, February 2021, https://www.northwell.edu/sites/northwell.edu/files/2021-02/Fact-Sheet-February-2021.pdf.

2. Michael Dowling, interview by Charles Wohlforth, May 27, 2021.

3. Debbie McGoldrick, "New Memoir by Michael Dowling Matches *Angela's Ashes* for Biting Truth and Insight," Irish Central, December 21, 2020, https://www.irishcentral.com/opinion/debbiemcgoldrick/review-michael-dowling-after-the-roof-caved-in.

4. Michael J. Alkire, Doug Miller, and Beth Cloyd. "PINC AI Data Shows Hospitals Paying $24B More for Labor amid COVID-19 Pandemic," Premier Inc., October 6, 2021, https://www.premierinc.com/newsroom/blog/pinc-ai-data-shows-hospitals-paying-24b-more-for-labor-amid-covid-19-pandemic.

5. Alexandra Alter and Elizabeth A. Harris, "'A Publisher's Worst Nightmare': How Cuomo's Book Became a Cautionary Tale," *New York Times*, August 10, 2021, sec. Books, https://www.nytimes.com/2021/08/10/books/cuomo-book-penguin-random-house.html.

6. Michael Schwirtz, "The 1,000-Bed *Comfort* Was Supposed to Aid New York. It Has 20 Patients," *New York Times*, April 2, 2020, sec. New York, https://www.nytimes.com/2020/04/02/nyregion/ny-coronavirus-usns-comfort.html.

7. Danielle Ofri, "The Business of Health Care Depends on Exploiting Doctors and Nurses," *New York Times*, June 8, 2019, sec. Opinion, https://www.nytimes.com/2019/06/08/opinion/sunday/hospitals-doctors-nurses-burnout.html.

8. Urmimala Sarkar and Christine Cassel, "Humanism before Heroism in Medicine," *JAMA* 326, no. 2 (July 13, 2021): 127–28, https://doi.org/10.1001/jama.2021.9569.

9. Michael A. Rosen et al., "Teamwork in Healthcare: Key Discoveries Enabling Safer, High-Quality Care," *American Psychologist* 73, no. 4 (2018): 433–50, https://doi.org/10.1037/amp0000298.

10. Andis Robeznieks, "Physician Survey Details Depth of Pandemic's Financial Impact," American Medical Association, October 28, 2020, https://www.ama-assn.org/practice-management/sustainability/physician-survey-details-depth-pandemic-s-financial-impact.

11. Christopher Rowland, "Diagnosis for Family Doctors: Less Money, Greater Hardship, and Patients on Video," *Washington Post*, September 8, 2020, https://www.washingtonpost.com/business/2020/09/08/family-doctors-financial-crisis-coronavirus/.

12. Laura Dyrda, "70% of Physicians Are Now Employed by Hospitals or Corporations," *Becker's ASC Review*, July 1, 2021, https://www.beckersasc.com/asc-transactions-and-valuation-issues/70-of-physicians-are-now-employed-by-hospitals-or-corporations.html.

13. Zachary Iscol, "What I Saw at the Javits Center's Covid-19 Hospital," CNN, May 8, 2020, https://www.cnn.com/2020/05/08/opinions/javits-centers-covid-19-hospital-iscol/index.html.

14. Ira Nash, "Big Challenges Require Large-Scale Solutions— as the COVID-19 Pandemic Is Proving," *Modern Healthcare*, April 4, 2020, https://www.modernhealthcare.com/opinion-editorial/big-challenges-require-large-scale-solutions-covid-19-pandemic-proving.

15. Lawrence Prybil, interview by Charles Wohlforth, August 19, 2021.

16. Melanie Evans and Alexandra Berzon, "Why Hospitals Can't Handle Covid Surges: They're Flying Blind," *Wall Street Journal*, September 30, 2020, sec. US, https://www.wsj.com/articles/hospitals-covid-surge-data-11601478409.

17. Russell Gold and Melanie Evans, "Why Did Covid Overwhelm Hospitals? A Yearslong Drive for Efficiency," *Wall Street Journal*, September 17, 2020, sec. US, https://www.wsj.com/articles/hospitals-for-years-banked-on-lean-staffing-the-pandemic-overwhelmed-them-11600351907.

18. Ibid.

19. Leonard L. Berry et al., "The High Stakes of Outsourcing in Health Care," *Mayo Clinic Proceedings* (August 16, 2021), https://doi.org/10.1016/j.mayocp.2021.07.003.

20. Nancy D. Beaulieu et al., "Changes in Quality of Care after Hospital Mergers and Acquisitions," *New England Journal of Medicine* 382, no. 1 (January 2, 2020): 51–59, https://doi.org/10.1056/NEJMsa1901383.

21. Femke Atsma, Glyn Elwyn, and Gert Westert, "Understanding Unwarranted Variation in Clinical Practice: A Focus on Network Effects, Reflective Medicine and Learning Health Systems," *International Journal for Quality in Health Care* 32, no. 4 (June 2020): 271–74, https://doi.org/10.1093/intqhc/mzaa023.

22. Joseph P. Newhouse et al., *Variation in Health Care Spending: Target Decision Making, Not Geography* (Washington, DC: National Academies Press, 2013), https://www.ncbi.nlm.nih.gov/books/NBK201637/.

23. William P. Luan et al., "Large Spending Variations Found among Military HMO Enrollees: A Look Using Compulsory Patient Migration," *Institute for Defense Analyses*, January 9, 2019, http://dx.doi.org/10.13140/RG.2.2.22515.37920.

24. Sanjaya Kumar and David B. Nash, *Demand Better! Revive Our Broken Healthcare System* (Bozeman, MT: Second River Press, 2010), 111–14.

25. Chris Outcalt, "'He Thought What He Was Doing Was Good for People,'" *The Atlantic*, August 13, 2021, sec. Politics, https://www.theatlantic.com/politics/archive/2021/08/health-care-sherman-sorensen-pfo-closures/619649/.

26. Elliott M. Antman and Eugene Braunwald, "Managing Stable Ischemic Heart Disease," *New England Journal of Medicine* 382, no. 15 (April 9, 2020): 1468–70, https://doi.org/10.1056/NEJMe2000239.

27. Sarah Kliff, Josh Katz, and Rumsey Taylor, "Hospitals and Insurers Didn't Want You to See These Prices. Here's Why," *New York Times*, August 22, 2021, sec. The Upshot, https://www.nytimes.com/interactive/2021/08/22/upshot/hospital-prices.html.

28. Rajender Agarwal, Olena Mazurenko, and Nir Menachemi, "High-Deductible Health Plans Reduce Health Care Cost and Utilization, Including Use of Needed Preventive Services," *Health Affairs* 36, no. 10 (October 1, 2017): 1762–68, https://doi.org/10.1377/hlthaff.2017.0610.

29. Michael Chernew et al., "Are Health Care Services Shoppable? Evidence from the Consumption of Lower-Limb MRI Scans," Working Paper, Working Paper Series (National Bureau of Economic Research, July 2018), https://doi.org/10.3386/w24869.

30. Eric Pace, "Milton Roemer, H.M.O. Advocate, Dies at 84," *New York Times*, January 14, 2001, sec. U.S., https://www.nytimes.com/2001/01/14/us/milton-roemer-hmo-advocate-dies-at-84.html.

31. Associated Press, "Warp-Speed Spending and Other Surreal Stats of COVID Times," *US News & World Report*, March 13, 2021, sec. Health News, https://www.usnews.com/news/health-news/articles/2021-03-13/warp-speed-spending-and-other-surreal-stats-of-covid-times.

32. David Lenihan, "The Covid-19 Relief Bill Created 1,000 More Residency Slots for New Doctors. Wealthy Hospitals Should Be Last in Line to Get Them," *STAT*, June 25, 2021, https://www.statnews.com/2021/06/25/new-residency-slots-wealthy-hospitals-last-in-line/.

33. Karyn Schwartz and Anthony Damico, "Distribution of CARES Act Funding among Hospitals," *KFF*, May 13, 2020, https://www.kff.org/health-costs/issue-brief/distribution-of-cares-act-funding-among-hospitals/.

34. Centers for Medicare and Medicaid Services, "National Health Expenditure Data Fact Sheet," December 16, 2020, https://www.cms.gov/Research-Statistics-Data-and-Systems/Statistics-Trends-and-Reports/NationalHealthExpendData/NHE-Fact-Sheet.

35. Alex Spanko, "Medicaid's Share of Nursing Home Revenue, Resident Days Hits Record High as Medicare Drops to Historic Low," *Skilled Nursing News*, December 11, 2019, https://skillednursingnews.com/2019/12/

medicaids-share-of-nursing-home-revenue-resident-days-hits-record-high-as-medicare-drops-to-historic-low/.

36. Will Englund and Joel Jacobs, "How Government Incentives Shaped the Nursing Home Business—and Left It Vulnerable to a Pandemic," *Washington Post*, November 27, 2020, https://www.washingtonpost.com/business/2020/11/27/nursing-home-incentives/.

37. Public Policy Institute, "COVID-19 Nursing Home Resident and Staff Deaths: AARP Nursing Home Dashboard," AARP, September 15, 2021, https://www.aarp.org/ppi/issues/caregiving/info-2020/nursing-home-covid-dashboard.html.

38. Priya Chidambaram et al., "Is the End of the Long-Term Care Crisis within Sight? New COVID-19 Cases and Deaths in Long-Term Care Facilities Are Dropping," *KFF*, February 24, 2021, https://www.kff.org/policy-watch/is-the-end-of-the-long-term-care-crisis-within-sight-new-covid-19-cases-and-deaths-in-long-term-care-facilities-are-dropping/.

39. Maggie Flynn, "48 States Saw Nursing Home Occupancy of 80% or Worse as 2021 Dawned—with Census as Low as 56%," *Skilled Nursing News*, January 25, 2021, https://skillednursingnews.com/2021/01/48-states-saw-nursing-home-occupancy-of-80-or-worse-as-2021-dawned-with-census-as-low-as-56/.

CHAPTER 7

1. The Center for Rural Pennsylvania, "Demographics—County Profiles," https://www.rural.palegislature.us/county_profiles.cfm.

2. Geisinger, "Geisinger: An Evolution of Caring," https://www.geisinger.org/about-geisinger.

3. Geisinger, "Learn about Fresh Food Farmacy," https://www.geisinger.org/freshfoodfarmacy/learn-more

4. Kathleen Kassel and Anikka Martin, "Ag and Food Sectors and the Economy," USDA Economic Research Service, October 12, 2021, https://www.ers.usda.gov/data-products/ag-and-food-statistics-charting-the-essentials/ag-and-food-sectors-and-the-economy/; and Mathew C. Riddle and William H. Herman, "The Cost of Diabetes Care—An Elephant in the Room," *Diabetes Journal* 41 (2018): 929–32, https://care.diabetesjournals.org/content/41/5/929.full-text.pdf.

5. Tamara Baer et al., "How Healthcare Payers Can Expand Nutrition Support for the Food Insecure," McKinsey & Company, November 24, 2021, https://www.mckinsey.com/featured-insights/food-security/how-healthcare-payers-can-expand-nutrition-support-for-the-food-insecure.

6. Alec Kurtz et al., "Long-Term Effects of Malnutrition on Severity of COVID-19," *Nature Scientific Reports* 11 (2021):14974, https://doi.org/10.1038/s41598-021-94138-z.

7. Baer et al., "How Healthcare Payers Can Expand."

8. Seth A. Berkowitz, "Association between Receipt of a Medically Tailored Meal Program and Health Care Use," *JAMA Internal Medicine* 179, no. 6 (2019):786–93, doi:10.1001/jamainternmed.2019.0198.

9. Jaewon Ryu, interview by Charles Wohlforth, April 14, 2021.

10. Geisinger, "Leadership Team," https://www.geisinger.org/about-geisinger/leadership/leadership-team/jaewon-ryu.

11. The Harris Poll, "Harris Poll: Only Nine Percent of U.S. Consumers Believe Pharma and Biotechnology Put Patients over Profits; Only 16 Percent Believe Health Insurers Do," January 17, 2017, https://theharrispoll.com/only-nine-percent-of-u-s-consumers-believe-pharmaceutical-and-biotechnology-companies-put-patients-over-profits-while-only-16-percent-believe-health-insurance-companies-do-according-to-a-harris-pol/.

12. Emily Clark, Jennifer Rost, and Anna Stolyarova, "Innovation and Value: What Payer-Led Managed-Care Models May Look Like," McKinsey & Company, December 2, 2021, https://www.mckinsey.com/industries/healthcare-systems-and-services/our-insights/innovation-and-value-what-payer-led-managed-care-models-may-look-like.

13. Harold Brubaker, "Jefferson Completes Acquisition of Health Partners Insurer from Temple Health," *Philadelphia Inquirer*, November 1, 2021, https://www.inquirer.com/business/health/jefferson-completes-acquisition-health-partners-hpp-temple-20211101.html.

14. Gunjan Khanna, Ebben Smith, and Saum Sutaria, "Provider-Led Health Plans: The Next Frontier—or the 1990s All Over Again?" McKinsey & Company, 2015, https://healthcare.mckinsey.com/sites/default/files/Provider-led%20health%20plans.pdf.

15. Linda Hasco, "Here Are Pa.'s 20 Largest Employers, and the Biggest Employers in Each County," *PennLive*, April 20, 2018, sec. Pennsylvania Real-Time News, https://www.pennlive.com/news/erry-2018/04/eb7d0c4952761/pas_top_20_employers_and_the_t.html.

16. George B. Moseley, "The U.S. Health Care Non-System, 1908–2008," *AMA Journal of Ethics* 10, no. 5 (May 1, 2008): 324–31, https://doi.org/10.1001/virtualmentor.2008.10.5.mhst1-0805.

17. Ibid.

18. Jesse Pines et al., "Kaiser Permanente–California: A Model for Integrated Care for the Ill and Injured," Center for Health Policy at Brookings, May 4, 2015, https://www.brookings.edu/wp-content/uploads/2015/04/050415EmerMedCaseStudyKaiser.pdf.

19. Kaiser Permanente, "Kaiser Permanente 2019 Annual Report," https://healthy.kaiserpermanente.org/static/health/annual_reports/kp_annualreport_2019/.

20. Khanna et al., "Provider-Led Health Plans."

21. BusinessWire, "Amazon Hiring 75,000 Employees across Fulfillment and Transportation, with Average Starting Pay of Over $17 per Hour and Sign-On Bonuses of Up to $1,000," May 13, 2021, https://www.businesswire.com/news/home/20210513005366/en/Amazon-Hiring-75000-Employees-Across-Fulfillment-and-Transportation-With-Average-Starting-Pay-of-Over-17-Per-Hour-and-Sign-On-Bonuses-of-Up-To-1000.

22. Moseley, "The U.S. Health Care Non-System."

23. Linda Peeno, "Managed Care Ethics: The Close View," National Coalition of Mental Health Professionals and Consumers, May 30, 1996, https://web.archive.org/web/20080601094042/http://www.nomanagedcare.org/DrPeenotestimony.html.

24. Marshall Fine, "Hollywood's Newest Villain: HMOs," *Los Angeles Times*, July 3, 1998, https://www.latimes.com/archives/la-xpm-1998-jul-03-ca-264-story.html.

25. Milt Freudenheim, "Humana Bets All on Managed Care," *New York Times*, May 20, 1993, sec. Business, https://www.nytimes.com/1993/05/20/business/humana-bets-all-on-managed-care.html.

26. Adam Clymer, "The Health Care Debate: The Overview; National Health Program, President's Greatest Goal, Declared Dead in Congress," *New York Times*, September 27, 1994, sec. U.S., https://www.nytimes.com/1994/09/27/us/health-care-debate-overview-national-health-program-president-s-greatest-goal.html; US House of Representatives, "Majority Changes in the House of Representatives, 1856 to Present," US House of Representatives History, Art, and Archives, 2021, https://history.house.gov/Institution/Majority-Changes/Majority-Changes/.

27. Moseley, "The U.S. Health Care Non-System."

28. Meredith Freed et al., "Medicare Advantage in 2021: Enrollment Update and Key Trends," *KFF*, June 21, 2021, https://www.kff.org/medicare/issue-brief/medicare-advantage-in-2021-enrollment-update-and-key-trends/.

29. Jeannie Fuglesten Biniek et al., "Medicare Advantage in 2021: Star Ratings and Bonuses," *KFF*, June 21, 2021, https://www.kff.org/medicare/issue-brief/medicare-advantage-in-2021-star-ratings-and-bonuses/.

30. Eva DuGoff et al., "Quality, Health, and Spending in Medicare Advantage and Traditional Medicare," *American Journal of Managed Care* 27, no. 9 (September 2021): 395–400, https://doi.org/10.37765/ajmc.2021.88641.

31. Baer et al., "How Healthcare Payers Can Expand."

32. Sachin Jain, "Medicare for All? The Better Route to Universal Coverage Would Be Medicare Advantage for All," *Modern Healthcare*, January 7, 2021,

https://www.modernhealthcare.com/opinion-editorial/medicare-all-better-route-universal-coverage-would-be-medicare-advantage-all.

33. Centers for Medicare and Medicaid Services, "Medicare and Medicaid Programs: Policy and Regulatory Revisions in Response to the COVID-19 Public Health Emergency," Federal Register, April 6, 2020, https://www.federalregister.gov/documents/2020/04/06/2020-06990/medicare-and-medicaid-programs-policy-and-regulatory-revisions-in-response-to-the-covid-19-public.

34. Courtney Harold Van Houtven and Walter D. Dawson, "Medicare and Home Health: Taking Stock in the COVID-19 Era," Commonwealth Fund, Issues Brief, October 21, 2020, https://doi.org/10.26099/kq2n-1s19.

35. DuGoff et al., "Quality, Health, and Spending in Medicare Advantage."

36. Freed et al., "Medicare Advantage in 2021."

37. Brad Smith, "CMS Innovation Center at 10 Years—Progress and Lessons Learned," *New England Journal of Medicine* 384, no. 8 (February 25, 2021): 759–64, https://doi.org/10.1056/NEJMsb2031138.

38. Rachel M. Werner et al., "The Future of Value-Based Payment: A Road Map to 2030," Penn LDI, February 17, 2021, https://ldi.upenn.edu/our-work/research-updates/the-future-of-value-based-payment-a-road-map-to-2030/.

39. Lily E. García and Otha Thornton, "'No Child' Has Failed," *Washington Post*, February 13, 2015, sec. Opinions, https://www.washingtonpost.com/opinions/no-child-has-failed/2015/02/13/8d619026-b2f8-11e4-827f-93f454140e2b_story.html.

40. Megan Carpentier, "No Child Left Behind Has Been Unsuccessful, Says Bipartisan Report," *The Guardian*, August 9, 2016, sec. Education, https://www.theguardian.com/education/2016/aug/09/no-child-left-behind-bill-unsuccessful-report-us-schools.

41. David B. Nash, "'Sunshine Is the Best Disinfectant,'" *American Health & Drug Benefits* 10, no. 4 (June 2017): 163–64, https://www.researchgate.net/publication/33685618_Sunshine_is_the_Best_Disinfectant.

42. Smith, "CMS Innovation Center at 10 Years."

43. Rajender Agarwal et al., "The Impact of Bundled Payment on Health Care Spending, Utilization, and Quality: A Systematic Review," *Health Affairs* 39, no. 1 (January 1, 2020): 50–57, https://doi.org/10.1377/hlthaff.2019.00784.

44. Jonathan R. Slotkin et al., "Why GE, Boeing, Lowe's, and Walmart Are Directly Buying Health Care for Employees," *Harvard Business Review*, June 8, 2017, https://hbr.org/2017/06/why-ge-boeing-lowes-and-walmart-are-directly-buying-health-care-for-employees.

45. Centers for Medicare and Medicaid Services, "Medicare Participating Heart Bypass Center Demonstration," May 4, 2021, https://innovation.cms.gov/medicare-demonstrations/medicare-participating-heart-bypass-center-demonstration.

46. Smith, "CMS Innovation Center at 10 Years."

47. Reed Abelson, "In Bid for Better Care, Surgery with a Warranty," *New York Times*, May 17, 2007, sec. Business, https://www.nytimes.com/2007/05/17/business/17quality.html.

48. Geisinger, "Lifetime Hip and Knee Guarantee," https://www.geisinger.org/patient-care/conditions-treatments-specialty/lifetime-hip-and-knee.

49. Hannah Sampson, "Will Business Travel Ever Be the Same?" *Washington Post*, August 4, 2021, sec. Travel, https://www.washingtonpost.com/travel/2021/08/04/business-travel-recovery-pandemic/.

50. US Office of Management and Budget and Federal Reserve Bank of St. Louis, "Federal Net Outlays as Percent of Gross Domestic Product," Federal Reserve Bank of St. Louis (FRED, Federal Reserve Bank of St. Louis, 2021), https://fred.stlouisfed.org/series/FYONGDA188S; Heather Long and Amy Goldstein, "Poverty Fell Overall in 2020 as Result of Massive Stimulus Checks and Unemployment Aid, Census Bureau Says," *Washington Post*, September 14, 2021, sec. Economy, https://www.washingtonpost.com/business/2021/09/14/us-census-poverty-health-insurance-2020/.

51. Larry Buchanan, Quoctrung Bui, and Jugal K. Patel, "Black Lives Matter May Be the Largest Movement in U.S. History," *New York Times*, July 3, 2020, sec. U.S., https://www.nytimes.com/interactive/2020/07/03/us/george-floyd-protests-crowd-size.html.

52. Summer Lin, "Why Did Trump Lose? His Own Top Pollster Blames COVID, More in Newly Released Report," McClatchy Washington Bureau, February 2, 2021, sec. Politics & Government, https://www.mcclatchydc.com/news/politics-government/article248943964.html.

53. Barbara and John Ehrenreich, *American Health Empire: Power, Profits, and Politics* (New York: Vintage Books, 1970), 3–18.

54. Sylvia A. Law, *Blue Cross: What Went Wrong?* (New Haven, CT: Yale University Press, 1976), 1; Centers for Medicare and Medicaid Services, "National Health Expenditure Data Historical," December 16, 2020, https://www.cms.gov/Research-Statistics-Data-and-Systems/Statistics-Trends-and-Reports/NationalHealthExpendData/NationalHealthAccountsHistorical

55. Peter Orszag and Rahul Rekhi, "The Economic Case for Vertical Integration in Health Care," *NEJM Catalyst* 1, no. 3 (June 2020), https://doi.org/10.1056/CAT.20.0119.

56. Aliya Jiwani et al., "Billing and Insurance-Related Administrative Costs in United States' Health Care: Synthesis of Micro-Costing Evidence," *BMC Health Services Research* 14, no. 1 (November 13, 2014): 556, https://doi.org/10.1186/s12913-014-0556-7.

57. Orszag and Rekhi, "The Economic Case for Vertical Integration."

58. Garret Johnson, Zoe M. Lyon, and Austin Frakt, "Provider-Offered Medicare Advantage Plans: Recent Growth and Care Quality," *Health Affairs* 36, no. 3 (March 1, 2017): 539–47, https://doi.org/10.1377/hlthaff.2016.0722.

59. Faith Adams and William Willsea, *The US Health Insurers Customer Experience Index, 2018*, Forrester, June 19, 2018, https://www.forrester.com/report/The-US-Health-Insurers-Customer-Experience-Index-2018/RES142622.

60. Howard Kern, "So You Want to Start a Health Plan? A Look at Sentara's Integrated Model—and President and CEO Howard Kern's Advice," *Becker's Hospital Review*, November 9, 2020, https://www.beckershospitalreview.com/strategy/so-you-want-to-start-a-health-plan-a-look-at-sentara-s-integrated-model-and-president-ceo-howard-kern-s-advice.html.

61. Khanna et al., "Provider-Led Health Plans."

62. Ibid.

63. Zachary N. Goldberg and David B. Nash, "The Payvider: An Evolving Model," *Population Health Management*, October 2021, 528–30, http://doi.org/10.1089/pop.2021.0164.

64. Business Roundtable, "Business Roundtable Redefines the Purpose of a Corporation to Promote 'An Economy That Serves All Americans,'" August 19, 2019, https://www.businessroundtable.org/business-roundtable-redefines-the-purpose-of-a-corporation-to-promote-an-economy-that-serves-all-americans.

65. Lawrence Pybil interview by Charles Wohlforth, August 19, 2021.

CHAPTER 8

1. Mohammadreza Hojat et al., "The Devil Is in the Third Year: A Longitudinal Study of Erosion of Empathy in Medical School," *Academic Medicine: Journal of the Association of American Medical Colleges* 84, no. 9 (September 2009): 1182–91, https://doi.org/10.1097/ACM.0b013e3181b17e55.

2. Ibid.

3. Leiyu Shi, "The Impact of Primary Care: A Focused Review," *Scientifica* 2012 (December 31, 2012): 432892, https://doi.org/10.6064/2012/432892.

4. Michael Dill, "We Already Needed More Doctors. Then COVID-19 Hit," AAMC, June 17, 2021, https://www.aamc.org/news-insights/we-already-needed-more-doctors-then-covid-19-hit.

5. Sanjay Basu et al., "Estimated Effect on Life Expectancy of Alleviating Primary Care Shortages in the United States," *Annals of Internal Medicine* 174, no. 7 (July 20, 2021): 920–26, https://doi.org/10.7326/M20-7381.

6. IHS Markit Ltd., "The Complexities of Physician Supply and Demand: Projections from 2019 to 2034," AAMC, June 2021, https://www.aamc.org/media/54681/download?attachment.

7. Brad N. Greenwood et al., "Physician–Patient Racial Concordance and Disparities in Birthing Mortality for Newborns," *PNAS* 117, no. 35 (September 1, 2020): 21194–200, https://doi.org/10.1073/pnas.1913405117.

8. Elizabeth Hlavinka, "Racial Bias in Flexner Report Permeates Medical Education Today," *MedPage Today*, June 18, 2020, https://www.medpagetoday.com/publichealthpolicy/medicaleducation/87171.

9. Devin B. Morris et al., "Diversity of the National Medical Student Body: Four Decades of Inequities," *New England Journal of Medicine* 384, no. 17 (April 29, 2021): 1661–68, https://doi.org/10.1056/NEJMsr2028487.

10. Heather Hollingsworth and Grant Schulte, "Health Workers Once Saluted as Heroes Now Get Threats," *AP News*, September 29, 2021, sec. Coronavirus pandemic, https://apnews.com/article/coronavirus-pandemic-business-health-missouri-omaha-b73e167eba4987cab9e58fdc92ce0b72.

11. Rayna M. Letourneau, "Amid a Raging Pandemic, the US Faces a Nursing Shortage. Can We Close the Gap?" *The Conversation*, November 20, 2020, http://theconversation.com/amid-a-raging-pandemic-the-us-faces-a-nursing-shortage-can-we-close-the-gap-149030.

12. Leslie Brody, "Medical Schools Are Getting Flooded with Applicants," *Wall Street Journal*, April 30, 2021, sec. US, https://www.wsj.com/articles/medical-schools-are-getting-flooded-with-applicants-11619795836.

13. John Eisenberg, "Samuel Preston Martin III," *Proceedings of the Association of American Physicians* 110, no. 4 (August 1998): 371–72.

14. Eric Moskowitz et al., "Development and Evaluation of a 1-Day Interclerkship Program for Medical Students on Medical Errors and Patient Safety," *American Journal of Medical Quality: The Official Journal of the American College of Medical Quality* 22, no. 1 (February 2007): 13–17, https://doi.org/10.1177/1062860606296669.

15. Ibid.

16. Abraham Flexner, *Medical Education in the United States and Canada* (New York: Carnegie Foundation, 1910), http://archive.carnegiefoundation.org/publications/pdfs/elibrary/Carnegie_Flexner_Report.pdf.

17. Thomas P. Duffy, "The Flexner Report—100 Years Later," *Yale Journal of Biology and Medicine* 84, no. 3 (September 2011): 269–76, https://www.ncbi.nlm.nih.gov/pmc/articles/PMC3178858/.

18. Ibid.

19. Marc J. Kahn and Ernest J. Sneed, "Promoting the Affordability of Medical Education to Groups Underrepresented in the Profession: The Other

Side of the Equation," *AMA Journal of Ethics* 17, no. 2 (February 1, 2015): 172–75, https://doi.org/10.1001/virtualmentor.2015.17.2.oped1-1502.

20. Ryan Syrek, "The Horror of Medical School Captured on Film," *Medscape*, October 16, 2020, http://www.medscape.com/viewarticle/939045.

21. William A. Schambra, "Eugenics as Philanthropic 'Best Practice,'" *Hudson Institute*, November 14, 2011, http://www.hudson.org/research/8496-eugenics-as-philanthropic-best-practice-.

22. Duffy, "The Flexner Report—100 Years Later."

23. Flexner, *Medical Education in the United States and Canada*, 180–81.

24. Hlavinka, "Racial Bias in Flexner Report."

25. Harriet A. Washington, "Apology Shines Light on Racial Schism in Medicine," *New York Times*, July 29, 2008, sec. Health, https://www.nytimes.com/2008/07/29/health/views/29essa.html.

26. Association of American Medical Colleges, "Diversity in Medicine: Facts and Figures 2019," https://www.aamc.org/data-reports/workforce/data/table-6-us-medical-schools-150-or-more-black-or-african-american-graduates-alone-or-combination-2009.

27. Duffy, "The Flexner Report—100 Years Later."

28. Molly Worthen, "A Once-in-a-Century Crisis Can Help Educate Doctors," *New York Times*, April 10, 2021, sec. Opinion, https://www.nytimes.com/2021/04/10/opinion/sunday/covid-medical-school-humanities.html.

29. Steven Scheinman, interview by Charles Wohlforth, September 13, 2021.

30. Mark Schuster, interview by Charles Wohlforth, October 1, 2021.

31. William Mobley, interview by Charles Wohlforth, November 9, 2021.

32. Josh Moody, "10 Most Expensive Private Medical Schools," *US News & World Report*, May 25, 2021, https://www.usnews.com/education/best-graduate-schools/the-short-list-grad-school/articles/most-expensive-private-medical-schools.

33. Hlavinka, "Racial Bias in Flexner Report."

34. Abigail Johnson Hess, "Princeton University Costs $73,450 per Year—but Here's How Much Students Actually Pay," CNBC, May 4, 2019, https://www.cnbc.com/2019/05/03/it-costs-73450-to-go-to-princetonheres-how-much-students-pay.html.

35. Gregor Aisch et al., "Economic Diversity and Student Outcomes at Princeton," *New York Times*, January 18, 2017, sec. The Upshot, https://www.nytimes.com/interactive/projects/college-mobility/princeton-university.

36. Kristen Moon, "This Medical School Has an Admission Rate of Less Than 1%: Here's How to Get In," *Forbes*, June 21, 2021, https://www.forbes.com/sites/kristenmoon/2021/06/21/this-medical-school-has-an-admission-rate-of-less-than-1-heres-how-to-get-in/.

37. Christopher Cannavino, interview by Charles Wohlforth, November 9, 2021.

38. Lisa Eyler, interview by Charles Wohlforth, November 9, 2021.

39. Kaiser Family Foundation, "Total Number of Medical School Graduates," *KFF*, May 7, 2021, https://www.kff.org/other/state-indicator/total-medical-school-graduates/.

40. "MD Brochure 2020," Geisinger, 2020, https://issuu.com/geisingercommonwealth/docs/gcsommd2020.

41. Nina Feldman, "Black Doctors COVID-19 Consortium to Open Clinic Offering Primary Care," *WHYY*, September 22, 2021, https://whyy.org/articles/black-doctors-covid-19-consortium-to-open-clinic-offering-primary-care/.

42. Khadeeja Safdar et al., "Young Doctors Struggle to Treat Coronavirus Patients: 'We Are Horrified and Scared,'" *Wall Street Journal*, April 29, 2020, sec. US, https://www.wsj.com/articles/young-doctors-struggle-to-treat-coronavirus-patients-we-are-horrified-and-scared-11588171553.

43. Ibid.

44. Ibid.

45. OpenSecrets, "Association of American Medical Colleges," https://www.opensecrets.org/orgs/association-of-american-medical-colleges/summary?id=D000047379.

46. Eric J. Warm et al., "A Dynamic Risk Management Approach for Reducing Harm from Invasive Bedside Procedures Performed during Residency," *Academic Medicine: Journal of the Association of American Medical Colleges* 96, no. 9 (September 1, 2021): 1268–75, https://doi.org/10.1097/ACM.0000000000004066.

47. Ibid.

48. Mary Ellen J. Goldhamer et al., "Can Covid Catalyze an Educational Transformation? Competency-Based Advancement in a Crisis," *New England Journal of Medicine* 383, no. 11 (September 10, 2020): 1003–5, https://doi.org/10.1056/NEJMp2018570.

49. Warm et al., "A Dynamic Risk Management Approach."

50. Goldhamer et al., "Can Covid Catalyze an Educational Transformation?"

51. Accreditation Council for Graduate Medical Education, "Milestones," https://acgme.org/what-we-do/accreditation/milestones/overview/.

52. Joseph Fins, Joan Leiman, and Herbet Pardes, "Primum Non Nocere: Daniel Patrick Moynihan and the Defense of Academic Medicine," *Alpha Omega Alpha*, 2017, https://www.alphaomegaalpha.org/wp-content/uploads/2021/03/2017-2-Fins.pdf.

53. Barbara O. Wynn, Robert Smalley, and Kristina M. Cordasco, *Does It Cost More to Train Residents or to Replace Them? A Look at the Costs and Benefits of Operating Graduate Medical Education Programs* (Santa Monica, CA: RAND Corporation, 2013), https://www.rand.org/content/dam/rand/pubs/research_reports/RR300/RR324/RAND_RR324.pdf.

54. Kristina Fiore, "Is a Residency Program an Asset to Be Sold?" *MedPage Today*, September 20, 2019, https://www.medpagetoday.com/special-reports/exclusives/82292.

55. David Lenihan, "The Covid-19 Relief Bill Created 1,000 More Residency Slots for New Doctors: Wealthy Hospitals Should Be Last in Line to Get Them," *STAT*, June 25, 2021, https://www.statnews.com/2021/06/25/new-residency-slots-wealthy-hospitals-last-in-line/.

56. David Brooks, "How to Get Really Rich!" *New York Times*, February 26, 2021, sec. Opinion, https://www.nytimes.com/2021/02/25/opinion/inequality-medicine-law.html.

57. Quoctrung Bui, "The Most Common Jobs for the Rich, Middle Class and Poor," NPR, October 16, 2014, sec. Jobs, https://www.npr.org/sections/money/2014/10/16/356176018/the-most-popular-jobs-for-the-rich-middle-class-and-poor.

CHAPTER 9

1. Melanie Evans and Alexandra Berzon, "Why Hospitals Can't Handle Covid Surges: They're Flying Blind," *Wall Street Journal*, September 30, 2020, sec. US, https://www.wsj.com/articles/hospitals-covid-surge-data-11601478409; Annie Gowen, "48 Hours to Live: An Oklahoma Hospital's Rush to Find an ICU Bed for a Covid Patient," *Washington Post*, October 15, 2021, sec. Coronavirus, https://www.washingtonpost.com/nation/interactive/2021/hospital-covid-patient/.

2. Evans and Berzon, "Why Hospitals Can't Handle Covid Surges."

3. Elizabeth A. Regan, "COVID-19 Revealed How Sick the US Health Care Delivery System Really Is," *The Conversation*, March 2, 2021, http://theconversation.com/covid-19-revealed-how-sick-the-us-health-care-delivery-system-really-is-153614.

4. Michael A. Cusumano, "Boeing's 737 MAX: A Failure of Management, Not Just Technology," *Communications of the ACM* 64, no. 1 (January 2021): 22–25, https://cacm.acm.org/magazines/2021/1/249448-boeings-737-max/fulltext.

5. Andrew Tangel, "Boeing Board to Face 737 MAX Lawsuit," *Wall Street Journal*, September 8, 2021, sec. Business, https://www.wsj.com/articles/boeing-board-to-face-737-max-oversight-lawsuit-11631114438.

6. David B. Nash, "Technology Tackles a Persistent Clinical Problem: Unwarranted Variation," *MedPage Today*, August 30, 2021, https://www.medpagetoday.com/opinion/focusonpolicy/94284; G. Alexander Fleming et al., "Diabetes Digital App Technology: Benefits, Challenges, and Recommendations. A Consensus Report by the European Association for the Study of Diabetes

(EASD) and the American Diabetes Association (ADA) Diabetes Technology Working Group," *Diabetes Care* 43, no. 1 (January 1, 2020): 250–60, https://doi.org/10.2337/dci19-0062; Julie Appleby, "Is Your Living Room the Future of Hospital Care?" *Kaiser Health News*, May 24, 2021, https://khn.org/news/article/is-your-living-room-the-future-of-hospital-care/.

7. R. S. Evans, "Electronic Health Records: Then, Now, and in the Future," *Yearbook of Medical Informatics*, Suppl 1 (May 20, 2016): S48–61, https://doi.org/10.15265/IYS-2016-s006.

8. Karen DeSalvo, interview by Charles Wohlforth, April 16, 2021.

9. Danielle Ofri, "The Business of Health Care Depends on Exploiting Doctors and Nurses," *New York Times*, June 8, 2019, sec. Opinion, https://www.nytimes.com/2019/06/08/opinion/sunday/hospitals-doctors-nurses-burnout.html.

10. Evans, "Electronic Health Records."

11. "Healthcare Data Breach Statistics," *HIPAA Journal*, 2021, https://www.hipaajournal.com/healthcare-data-breach-statistics/.

12. Judd Hollander, interview by Charles Wohlforth, September 21, 2021.

13. Judd E. Hollander and Brendan G. Carr, "Virtually Perfect? Telemedicine for Covid-19," *New England Journal of Medicine* 382, no. 18 (April 30, 2020): 1679–81, https://doi.org/10.1056/NEJMp2003539.

14. Ibid.

15. AJMC Staff, "A Timeline of COVID-19 Developments in 2020," *American Journal of Managed Care*, January 1, 2021, https://www.ajmc.com/view/a-timeline-of-covid19-developments-in-2020.

16. Julie Appleby, "Telehealth's Limits: Battle over State Lines and Licensing Threatens Patients' Options," *Kaiser Health News*, August 31, 2021, https://khn.org/news/article/state-medical-licensing-rules-threatens-telehealth-patient-options/.

17. Judd E. Hollander and Aaron Neinstein, "Maturation from Adoption-Based to Quality-Based Telehealth Metrics," *NEJM Catalyst Innovations in Care Delivery*, September 9, 2020, https://catalyst.nejm.org/doi/full/10.1056/CAT.20.0408.

18. Citation numbers downloaded from Google Scholar, December 18, 2021, https://scholar.google.com/.

19. Hollander and Carr, "Virtually Perfect?"

20. Marshall H. Chin, "Uncomfortable Truths—What Covid-19 Has Revealed about Chronic-Disease Care in America," *New England Journal of Medicine* 385, no. 18 (October 28, 2021): 1633–36, https://doi.org/10.1056/NEJMp2112063.

21. Sarah Krouse, "Covid-19 Patients Put Remote Care to the Test," *Wall Street Journal*, October 16, 2020, sec. Business, https://www.wsj.com/articles/covid-19-patients-put-remote-care-to-the-test-11602840627.

22. Hollander and Neinstein, "Maturation from Adoption-Based."

23. Judd Hollander interview, 2021.

24. Steven Scheinman, interview by Charles Wohlforth, September 13, 2021.

25. Oleg Bestsennyy et al., "Telehealth: A Quarter-Trillion-Dollar Post-COVID-19 Reality?" *McKinsey & Company*, July 9, 2021, https://www.mckinsey.com/industries/healthcare-systems-and-services/our-insights/telehealth-a-quarter-trillion-dollar-post-covid-19-reality.

26. Judd Hollander interview, 2021.

27. Yan-Ya Chen et al., "Effect of Telehealth Intervention on Breast Cancer Patients' Quality of Life and Psychological Outcomes: A Meta-Analysis," *Journal of Telemedicine and Telecare* 24, no. 3 (April 1, 2018): 157–67, https://doi.org/10.1177/1357633X16686777.

28. Sue Romanick-Schmiedl and Ganesh Raghu, "Telemedicine: Maintaining Quality during Times of Transition," *Nature Reviews Disease Primers* 6, no. 1 (June 1, 2020): 1–2, https://doi.org/10.1038/s41572-020-0185-x.

29. Zaz Hollander, "Investigation Finds Dozens of Unqualified Florida Doctors Tried to Get Emergency Licenses in Alaska," *Anchorage Daily News*, October 30, 2021, sec. Alaska News, https://www.adn.com/alaska-news/2021/10/29/investigation-finds-dozens-of-unqualified-florida-doctors-tried-to-get-emergency-licenses-in-alaska/; Stephanie Armour and Robbie Whelan, "Telehealth Rollbacks Leave Patients Stranded, Some Doctors Say," *Wall Street Journal*, November 22, 2021, sec. Health, https://www.wsj.com/articles/telehealth-rollbacks-leave-patients-stranded-some-doctors-say-11637577001.

30. Appleby, "Is Your Living Room the Future of Hospital Care?"

31. Ibid.

32. Appleby, "Telehealth's Limits."

33. Armour and Whelan, "Telehealth Rollbacks."

34. Ibid.

35. Marty Lupinetti, interview by Charles Wohlforth, May 10, 2021.

36. US Department of Health and Human Services, "State Health Information Exchange," *HealthIT.gov*, April 29, 2019, https://www.healthit.gov/topic/onc-hitech-programs/state-health-information-exchange.

37. Marty Lupinetti interview, 2021.

38. Christopher Jason, "Exploring 3 Levels of Health Information Exchange, Data Access," *EHRIntelligence*, October 12, 2020, https://ehrintelligence.com/news/exploring-3-levels-of-health-information-exchange-data-access.

39. Regan, "COVID-19 Revealed."

40. Karen DeSalvo, interview by Charles Wohlforth, April 16, 2021.

41. Jackie Drees, "EHR Market Share 2021: 10 Things to Know about Major Players Epic, Cerner, Meditech & Allscripts," *Becker's Health IT*, May 21, 2021, https://www.beckershospitalreview.com/ehrs/ehr-market-share-2021-10-things-to-know-about-major-players-epic-cerner-meditech-allscripts.html.

42. Regan, "COVID-19 Revealed."

43. Jeff Zucker, interview by Charles Wohlforth, September 29, 2021.

44. Jordan Rau, "A Digital Tool Promised to Help Patients Manage Their Diabetes. Then the Hospital behind It Pulled the Plug," *Washington Post*, August 17, 2021, sec. Business, https://www.washingtonpost.com/business/2021/08/17/hospitals-venture-capitalists-diabetes-app/.

45. Ibid.

46. Geoffrey A. Fowler and Heather Kelly, "Amazon's New Health Band Is the Most Invasive Tech We've Ever Tested," *Washington Post*, December 10, 2020, sec. Consumer Tech, https://www.washingtonpost.com/technology/2020/12/10/amazon-halo-band-review/.

47. Natasha Singer, "The Hot New Covid Tech Is Wearable and Constantly Tracks You," *New York Times*, November 15, 2020, sec. Technology, https://www.nytimes.com/2020/11/15/technology/virus-wearable-tracker-privacy.html.

48. David B. Nash, "Google's Rise in Healthcare," *MedPage Today*, June 30, 2021, https://www.medpagetoday.com/opinion/focusonpolicy/93368.

49. Apple, "Healthcare—Health Records," https://www.apple.com/healthcare/health-records/.

50. Trever B. Burgon et al., "Engaging Primary Care Providers to Reduce Unwanted Clinical Variation and Support ACO Cost and Quality Goals: A Unique Provider-Payer Collaboration," *Population Health Management* 22, no. 4 (August 1, 2019): 321–29, https://doi.org/10.1089/pop.2018.0111.

51. William P. Luan et al., "Large Spending Variations Found among Military HMO Enrollees: A Look Using Compulsory Patient Migration," *Institute for Defense Analyses*, January 9, 2019, http://dx.doi.org/10.13140/RG.2.2.22515.37920.

52. Nash, "Technology Tackles a Persistent Clinical Problem."

53. Burgon et al., "Engaging Primary Care Providers."

CHAPTER 10

1. Gary Claxton et al., "2021 Employer Health Benefits Survey," *KFF*, November 10, 2021, https://www.kff.org/health-costs/report/2021-employer-health-benefits-survey/.

2. Craig Palosky and Lisa Zamosky, "Vast Majority of Large Employers Surveyed Say Broader Government Role Will Be Necessary to Control Health Costs and Provide Coverage, Survey Finds," *KFF*, April 29, 2021, https://www.kff.org/health-reform/press-release/

vast-majority-of-large-employers-surveyed-say-broader-government-role-will-be-necessary-to-control-health-costs-and-provide-coverage-survey-finds/.

3. Elise Gould and Melat Kassa, "Low-Wage, Low-Hours Workers Were Hit Hardest in the COVID-19 Recession: The State of Working America 2020 Employment Report," Economic Policy Institute, May 20, 2021, https://www.epi.org/publication/swa-2020-employment-report/.

4. Byron Scott, interview by Charles Wohlforth, September 23, 2021.

5. L. Hannah Gould et al., "Contributing Factors in Restaurant-Associated Foodborne Disease Outbreaks, FoodNet Sites, 2006 and 2007," *Journal of Food Protection* 76, no. 11 (November 2013): 1824–28, https://doi.org/10.4315/0362-028X.JFP-13-037.

6. Steven Sumner et al., "Factors Associated with Food Workers Working while Experiencing Vomiting or Diarrhea," *Journal of Food Protection* 74, no. 2 (February 1, 2011): 215–20, https://doi.org/10.4315/0362-028X.JFP-10-108.

7. Tara Nurin, "The Fight for Paid Leave Could Benefit Restaurant Workers More Than Most," *Forbes*, July 23, 2021, sec. Food & Drink, https://www.forbes.com/sites/taranurin/2021/07/23/the-fight-for-paid-leave-could-benefit-restaurant-workers-more-than-most/.

8. Julia R. Raifman et al., "Paid Leave Policies Can Help Keep Businesses Open and Food on Workers' Tables," *Health Affairs*, October 25, 2021, https://www.healthaffairs.org/do/10.1377/hblog20211021.197121/full/.

9. Tara Nurin, 2021.

10. Logan Ray et al., "Decreased Incidence of Infections Caused by Pathogens Transmitted Commonly through Food during the COVID-19 Pandemic—Foodborne Diseases Active Surveillance Network, 10 U.S. Sites, 2017–2020," *Morbidity and Mortality Weekly Report* 70, no. 38 (September 24, 2021): 1332–36, https://doi.org/10.15585/mmwr.mm7038a4.

11. Centers for Disease Control and Prevention, "2020–2021 Flu Season Summary," October 25, 2021, https://www.cdc.gov/flu/season/faq-flu-season-2020-2021.htm.

12. Lauren Garrow, Lavanya Marla, and John-Paul Clarke, "Airline Response to COVID-19," *ORMS Today*, February 2, 2021, https://pubsonline.informs.org/do/10.1287/orms.2021.01.20/full/.

13. Niraj Chokshi and Noam Scheiber, "Inside United Airlines' Decision to Mandate Coronavirus Vaccines," *New York Times*, October 2, 2021, sec. Business, https://www.nytimes.com/2021/10/02/business/united-airlines-coronavirus-vaccine-mandate.html.

14. Chip Cutter and Thomas Gryta, "Covid-19 Vaccine Mandates Turn into Religious Tests at GE, Disney—Some Longer Than Others," *Wall Street Journal*, October 31, 2021, sec. Business, https://www.wsj.com/articles/covid-19-vaccine-mandates-turn-into-religious-tests-at-ge-disneysome-longer-than-others-11635688800.

15. Zeynep Tufekci, "The Unvaccinated May Not Be Who You Think," *New York Times*, October 15, 2021, sec. Opinion, https://www.nytimes.com/2021/10/15/opinion/covid-vaccines-unvaccinated.html.

16. Ibid.

17. Spencer Kimball, "White House Tells Businesses to Proceed with Vaccine Mandate Despite Court-Ordered Pause," CNBC, November 8, 2021, sec. Health and Science, https://www.cnbc.com/2021/11/08/biden-vaccine-mandate-white-house-tells-business-to-go-ahead-despite-court-pause.html.

18. Omar Abdel-Baqui, "Amtrak, Changing Course, Suspends Covid-19 Vaccine Mandate for Workers," *Wall Street Journal*, December 14, 2021, https://www.wsj.com/articles/amtrak-changing-course-suspends-covid-19-vaccine-mandate-for-workers-11639521984; Paul Ziobro, "GE, Union Pacific Suspend Covid-19 Vaccination Mandates after Injunction on Biden Order," *Wall Street Journal*, December 9, 2021, https://www.wsj.com/articles/ge-union-pacific-suspend-covid-19-vaccination-mandates-after-injunction-on-biden-order-11639089010.

19. Kimball, "White House Tells Businesses to Proceed with Vaccine Mandate Despite Court-Ordered Pause."

20. Katherine Keisler-Starkey and Lisa N. Bunch, "Health Insurance Coverage in the United States: 2020," U.S. Census Bureau, September 14, 2021, https://www.census.gov/library/publications/2021/demo/p60-274.html.

21. Palosky and Zamosky, "Vast Majority of Large Employers Surveyed."

22. Anjalee Khemlani, "Buffett on Failed Health Care Venture Haven: 'We Were Fighting a Tapeworm in the American Economy. And the Tapeworm Won,'" *Yahoo Finance*, May 1, 2021, https://finance.yahoo.com/news/buffett-on-failed-health-care-venture-haven-we-were-fighting-a-tapeworm-in-the-american-economy-and-the-tapeworm-won-220812439.html.

23. Anjalee Khemlani, "It's No Surprise That Amazon, Berkshire, JPM Health Venture Haven Is Disbanding: Experts," *Yahoo Finance*, January 5, 2021, https://finance.yahoo.com/news/its-no-surprise-that-amazon-berkshire-jpm-health-venture-haven-is-disbanding-experts-213818212.html.

24. Heather Long, "It's Not a 'Labor Shortage.' It's a Great Reassessment of Work in America," *Washington Post*, May 7, 2021, sec. Economy, https://www.washingtonpost.com/business/2021/05/07/jobs-report-labor-shortage-analysis/.

25. Kim Parker, Ruth Igielnik, and Rakesh Kochhar, "Unemployed Americans Are Feeling the Emotional Strain of Job Loss; Most Have Considered Changing Occupations," *Pew Research Center*, February 10, 2021, https://www.pewresearch.org/fact-tank/2021/02/10/unemployed-americans-are-feeling-the-emotional-strain-of-job-loss-most-have-considered-changing-occupations/.

26. Josh Mitchell, Lauren Weber, and Sarah Chaney Cambon, "4.3 Million Workers Are Missing. Where Did They Go?" *Wall Street*

Journal, October 14, 2021, sec. Economy, https://www.wsj.com/articles/labor-shortage-missing-workers-jobs-pay-raises-economy-11634224519.

27. Amara Omeokwe, "Covid-19 Pushed Many Americans to Retire: The Economy Needs Them Back," *Wall Street Journal*, October 31, 2021, sec. Economy, https://www.wsj.com/articles/covid-19-pushed-many-americans-to-retire-the-economy-needs-them-back-11635691340.

28. Vanessa Fuhrmans and Lauren Weber, "Burned Out and Restless from the Pandemic, Women Redefine Their Career Ambitions," *Wall Street Journal*, September 27, 2021, sec. Business, https://www.wsj.com/articles/womens-careers-covid-19-toll-11632506362.

29. Kim Parker, Ruth Igielnik, and Rakesh Kochhar, 2021.

30. Rachel Thomas et al., *Women in the Workplace 2021*, McKinsey & Company, 2021, https://wiw-report.s3.amazonaws.com/Women_in_the_Workplace_2021.pdf.

31. Rachel Minkin, "COVID-19 Pandemic Saw an Increase in the Share of U.S. Mothers Who Would Prefer Not to Work for Pay," Pew Research Center, August 31, 2021, https://www.pewresearch.org/fact-tank/2021/08/31/covid-19-pandemic-saw-an-increase-in-the-share-of-u-s-mothers-who-would-prefer-not-to-work-for-pay/.

32. Eli Rosenberg, "Hotel Industry Emerges from Pandemic with New Business Model, Possibly Fewer Workers," *Washington Post*, June 11, 2021, sec. Business, https://www.washingtonpost.com/business/2021/06/11/hotel-workers-reduced-cleaning/.

33. Mitchell, Weber, and Cambon, "4.3 Million Workers Are Missing."

34. Eduardo Porter, "Low-Wage Workers Now Have Options, Which Could Mean a Raise," *New York Times*, July 20, 2021, sec. Business, https://www.nytimes.com/2021/07/20/business/economy/workers-wages-mobility.html.

35. Claxton et al., "2021 Employer Health Benefits Survey."

36. McDonald's, "McDonald's USA to Raise Wages at Company-Owned Restaurants across the Country," May 13, 2021, https://corporate.mcdonalds.com/corpmcd/en-us/our-stories/article/.mcopco-wage-raise.html.

37. US House of Representatives, "Coronavirus Infections and Deaths among Meatpacking Workers at Top Five Companies Were Nearly Three Times Higher Than Previous Estimates," US House of Representatives, October 27, 2021, https://coronavirus.house.gov/sites/democrats.coronavirus.house.gov/files/2021.10.27%20Meatpacking%20Report.Final_.pdf.

38. Ana Swanson, David Yaffe-Bellany, and Michael Corkery, "Pork Chops vs. People: Battling Coronavirus in an Iowa Meat Plant," *New York Times*, May 10, 2020, sec. Business, https://www.nytimes.com/2020/05/10/business/economy/coronavirus-tyson-plant-iowa.html.

39. Lauren Hirsch and Michael Corkery, "How Tyson Foods Got 60,500 Workers to Get the Coronavirus Vaccine Quickly," *New York Times*, November

4, 2021, sec. Business, https://www.nytimes.com/2021/11/04/business/tyson-vaccine-mandate.html.

40. BP, "BP Wellbeing Program," BP Life Benefits, 2021, https://hr.bpglobal. com/LifeBenefits/Sites/inpat/BP-Life-benefits/Employee-benefits-handbook/ BP-Medical-Program/How-the-BP-Medical-Program-works/BP-Wellness-Program.aspx.

41. Soeren Mattke et al., "Workplace Wellness Programs Study," *Rand Health Quarterly* 3, no. 2 (June 1, 2013), https://www.rand.org/pubs/research_reports/RR254.html.

42. Stefano DellaVigna and Ulrike Malmendier, "Paying Not to Go to the Gym," *American Economic Review* 96, no. 3 (June 2006): 694–719, https://doi.org/10.1257/aer.96.3.694.

43. William Park, "The Lifelong Exercise That Keeps Japan Moving," BBC, June 19, 2020, https://www.bbc.com/worklife/article/20200609-the-life-long-exercise-that-keeps-japan-moving.

44. Hannah Ritchie, "Which Countries Eat the Most Meat?" BBC, February 4, 2019, sec. Health, https://www.bbc.com/news/health-47057341.

45. Jean Marie Abraham, "Employer Wellness Programs—A Work in Progress," *JAMA* 321, no. 15 (April 16, 2019): 1462–63, https://doi.org/10.1001/jama.2019.3376.

46. Claxton et al., "2021 Employer Health Benefits Survey," 11–12.

47. Zirui Song and Katherine Baicker, "Effect of a Workplace Wellness Program on Employee Health and Economic Outcomes," *JAMA* 321, no. 15 (April 16, 2019): 1491–1501, https://doi.org/10.1001/jama.2019.3307.

48. Ibid.

49. Alyssa Schroer, "Wearable Technology in Healthcare: 11 Companies to Know 2021," Built In, July 17, 2019, https://builtin.com/healthcare-technology/wearable-technology-in-healthcare; Rolfe Winkler, "Apple Studying Potential of AirPods as Health Device," *Wall Street Journal*, October 13, 2021, sec. Tech, https://www.wsj.com/articles/apple-studying-potential-of-airpods-as-health-device-11634122800; Sarah Silbert, "Smart Shoes: The Latest Wearable Phenomenon," *Lifewire*, December 2, 2020, https://www.lifewire.com/smart-shoes-latest-wearable-phenomenon-3946235.

50. Karen DeSalvo, "Comments at the 20th Population Health Colloquium" (20th Population Health Colloquium, Thomas Jefferson University, October 5, 2020).

51. Elizabeth A. Brown, "COVID-19 Employee Health Checks Create New Privacy Risks," in *Work Law Under COVID-19*, ed. Sachin S. Pandya and Jeffrey M. Hirsch (published online, 2021), https://worklawcovid19book.netlify.app/privacyrisks.html.

52. Elizabeth A. Brown, "Workplace Wellness: Social Injustice," *New York University Journal of Legislation and Public Policy* 20, no. 191 (2017):

191–246, https://nyujlpp.org/wp-content/uploads/2017/04/Brown-Workplace-Wellness-Social-Injustice-20nyujlpp191.pdf.

53. Elizabeth A. Brown, "The Femtech Paradox: How Workplace Monitoring Threatens Women's Equity," *Jurimetrics* 61, no. 3 (2021): 289–329, https://www.proquest.com/docview/2568314630?pq-origsite=gscholar&fromopenview=true.

54. Brown, "COVID-19 Employee Health Checks."

55. Brown, "Workplace Wellness."

56. Brown, "COVID-19 Employee Health Checks."

57. Claxton et al., "2021 Employer Health Benefits Survey," 13.

58. Ron Z. Goetzel et al., *Seven Ways Businesses Can Align with Public Health for Bold Action and Innovation*, de Beaumont Foundation, February 23, 2021, https://debeaumont.org/wp-content/uploads/2021/02/Seven-Ways-Businesses-Can-Align-with-Public-Health.pdf.

CHAPTER 11

1. Mary Cooper interview by Charles Wohlforth, September 2, 2021.

2. Andy Pasztor, "Can Hospitals Learn about Safety from Airlines?" *Wall Street Journal*, September 2, 2021, sec. Life & Work, https://www.wsj.com/articles/can-hospitals-learn-about-safety-from-airlines-11630598112.

3. Kriti Prasad et al., "Prevalence and Correlates of Stress and Burnout among U.S. Healthcare Workers during the COVID-19 Pandemic: A National Cross-Sectional Survey Study," *EClinicalMedicine* 35 (May 16, 2021), https://doi.org/10.1016/j.eclinm.2021.100879.

4. Tait D. Shanafelt et al., "Suicidal Ideation and Attitudes Regarding Help Seeking in US Physicians Relative to the US Working Population," *Mayo Clinic Proceedings* 96, no. 8 (August 1, 2021): 2067–80, https://doi.org/10.1016/j.mayocp.2021.01.033.

5. Pauline Anderson, "Physicians Experience Highest Suicide Rate of Any Profession," *Medscape*, May 7, 2018, http://www.medscape.com/viewarticle/896257.

6. Nikitha K. Menon et al., "Association of Physician Burnout with Suicidal Ideation and Medical Errors," *JAMA Network Open* 3, no. 12 (December 9, 2020): e2028780, https://doi.org/10.1001/jamanetworkopen.2020.28780.

7. J. Matthew Austin and Allen Kachalia, "The State of Health Care Quality Measurement in the Era of COVID-19: The Importance of Doing Better," *JAMA* 324, no. 4 (July 28, 2020): 333–34, https://doi.org/10.1001/jama.2020.11461.

8. Lindsey M. Weiner-Lastinger et al., "The Impact of Coronavirus Disease 2019 (COVID-19) on Healthcare-Associated Infections in 2020: A Summary of

Data Reported to the National Healthcare Safety Network," *Infection Control & Hospital Epidemiology*, September 3, 2021, 1–14, https://doi.org/10.1017/ice.2021.362.

9. Tara N. Palmore and David K. Henderson, "Healthcare-Associated Infections during the Coronavirus Disease 2019 (COVID-19) Pandemic," *Infection Control & Hospital Epidemiology* 42, no. 11 (November 2021): 1372–73, https://doi.org/10.1017/ice.2021.377.

10. Martin A. Makary and Michael Daniel, "Medical Error—the Third Leading Cause of Death in the US," *BMJ* 353 (May 3, 2016): 2139, https://doi.org/10.1136/bmj.i2139.

11. Michael L. Millenson, "How the US News Media Made Patient Safety a Priority," *BMJ* 324, no. 7344 (April 27, 2002): 1044, https://www.ncbi.nlm.nih.gov/pmc/articles/PMC1122982/.

12. Lawrence K. Altman, "Big Doses of Chemotherapy Drug Killed Patient, Hurt 2d," *New York Times*, March 24, 1995, sec. U.S., https://www.nytimes.com/1995/03/24/us/big-doses-of-chemotherapy-drug-killed-patient-hurt-2d.html.

13. Institute of Medicine Committee on Quality of Health Care in America, Linda T. Kohn, Janet M. Corrigan, and Molla S. Donaldson, eds., *To Err Is Human: Building a Safer Health System* (Washington, DC: National Academies Press, 2000), https://www.ncbi.nlm.nih.gov/books/NBK225179/.

14. Atul Gawande, *The Checklist Manifesto: How to Get Things Right* (New York: Metropolitan Books, 2009).

15. Joseph A. Simonetti, "Checklists to Improve Patient Safety Have Mixed Results," *The Hospitalist*, January 25, 2018, sec. Practice Management, https://www.the-hospitalist.org/hospitalist/article/157054/critical-care; Rachel E White et al., "Checking It Twice: An Evaluation of Checklists for Detecting Medication Errors at the Bedside Using a Chemotherapy Model," *Quality & Safety in Health Care* 19, no. 6 (December 2010): 562–67, https://doi.org/10.1136/qshc.2009.032862.

16. Robert Wears and Kathleen Sutcliffe, *Still Not Safe: Patient Safety and the Middle-Managing of American Medicine* (Oxford University Press, 2019), https://doi.org/10.1093/oso/9780190271268.001.0001.

17. Oren Guttman interview by Charles Wohlforth, December 17, 2020.

18. National Alert Network, "Age-Related COVID-19 Vaccine Mix-Ups," National Coordinating Council for Medication Error Reporting and Prevention, December 6, 2021, https://www.nccmerp.org/sites/default/files/nan-alert-dec-6-21-covid-19-vaccine-mixups.pdf.

19. David W. Chen, "Boy, 6, Dies of Skull Injury during M.R.I.," *New York Times*, July 31, 2001, sec. New York, https://www.nytimes.com/2001/07/31/nyregion/boy-6-dies-of-skull-injury-during-mri.html.

20. Jonathan Gleason interview by Charles Wohlforth, November 22, 2021.

21. Pasztor, "Can Hospitals Learn about Safety from Airlines?"

22. David Meyers, "CANDOR: An Evolving Approach to Patient Harm," *Relias Media*, May 1, 2017, sec. Emergency, https://www.reliasmedia.com/articles/140522-candor-an-evolving-approach-to-patient-harm.

23. Ibid.

24. Michelle M. Mello et al., "Malpractice Liability and Health Care Quality: A Review," *JAMA* 323, no. 4 (January 28, 2020): 352–66, https://doi.org/10.1001/jama.2019.21411.

25. Meyers, "CANDOR."

26. David B. Nash, "'Sunshine Is the Best Disinfectant,'" *American Health & Drug Benefits* 10, no. 4 (June 2017): 163–64, https://www.ncbi.nlm.nih.gov/pmc/articles/PMC5536192/.

27. Sankey V. Williams, David B. Nash, and Neil Goldfarb, "Differences in Mortality from Coronary Artery Bypass Graft Surgery at Five Teaching Hospitals," *JAMA* 266, no. 6 (August 14, 1991): 810–15, https://doi.org/10.1001/jama.1991.03470060072029.

28. Lucian L. Leape, *Making Healthcare Safe: The Story of the Patient Safety Movement* (New York: Springer, 2021).

29. Cooper interview; David Meyers, 2017.

30. "Communication and Optimal Resolution (CANDOR)," Agency for Healthcare Research and Quality, April 2018, https://www.ahrq.gov/patient-safety/capacity/candor/index.html.

31. Altman, "Big Doses of Chemotherapy."

32. Institute of Medicine Committee on Quality of Health Care in America, *Crossing the Quality Chasm: A New Health System for the 21st Century* (Washington, DC: National Academies Press, 2001), 79–80, http://www.ncbi.nlm.nih.gov/books/NBK222274/.

33. Jessica Jensen and Steven Thompson, "The Incident Command System: A Literature Review," *Disasters* 40, no. 1 (January 2016): 158–82, https://doi.org/10.1111/disa.12135.

34. National Research Council, *Facing Hazards and Disasters: Understanding Human Dimensions* (Washington, DC: National Academies Press, 2006), 141, https://doi.org/10.17226/11671.

35. Cooper noted that, at this writing, proning had not been shown to be effective in randomized clinical trials, but academic research on the technique is in early stages.

36. Paul E. Plsek and Trisha Greenhalgh, "The Challenge of Complexity in Health Care," *BMJ: British Medical Journal* 323, no. 7313 (September 15, 2001): 625–28, https://www.ncbi.nlm.nih.gov/pmc/articles/PMC1121189/.

CHAPTER 12

1. National Transportation Safety Board, "The Investigative Process," National Transportation Safety Board, accessed December 21, 2021, https://www.ntsb.gov/investigations/process/Pages/default.aspx.

2. Gallup and West Health, *West Health-Gallup 2021 Healthcare in America Report*, Gallup, December 2021, https://www.gallup.com/analytics/357932/healthcare-in-america-2021.aspx.

3. Ibid.

4. David Murrell, "Inside the Ridiculously Vicious and Increasingly Nasty Local Elections in Bucks County," *Philadelphia*, December 18, 2021, https://www.phillymag.com/news/2021/12/18/bucks-county-school-board-elections/; TaRhonda Thomas, "Central Bucks School Board Accused of Allowing Hate Speech during Public Comment," 6 Action News, WPVI, Philadelphia, November 11, 2021, https://6abc.com/central-bucks-school-district-hate-speech-freedom-of-transgender-slur/11220859/.

5. Ibid.

6. Matt Stevens, "At Late-Night Rally, Trump Suggests He May Fire Fauci 'after the Election,'" *New York Times*, November 2, 2020, https://www.nytimes.com/2020/11/02/us/politics/at-late-night-rally-trump-suggests-he-may-fire-fauci-after-the-election.html.

7. Emma Newburger, "Dr. Fauci Says His Daughters Need Security as Family Continues to Get Death Threats," CNBC, August 5, 2020, https://www.cnbc.com/2020/08/05/dr-fauci-says-his-daughters-need-security-as-family-continues-to-get-death-threats.html.

8. Hailey Fuchs, "Trump Attack on Diversity Training Has a Quick and Chilling Effect," *New York Times*, October 13, 2020, https://www.nytimes.com/2020/10/13/us/politics/trump-diversity-training-race.html.

9. Liz Hamel et al., "KFF COVID-19 Vaccine Monitor: September 2021," *KFF*, September 28, 2021, https://www.kff.org/coronavirus-covid-19/poll-finding/kff-covid-19-vaccine-monitor-september-2021/.

10. Philip Bump, "Trump's Message on Vaccines Isn't as Powerful as Trumpism's Message," *Washington Post*, December 21, 2021, https://www.washingtonpost.com/politics/2021/12/21/trumps-message-vaccines-isnt-powerful-trumpisms-message/.

11. Daniel Wood and Geoff Brumfiel, "Pro-Trump Counties Now Have Far Higher COVID Death Rates. Misinformation Is to Blame," NPR, *Morning Edition*, December 5, 2021, https://www.npr.org/sections/health-shots/2021/12/05/1059828993/data-vaccine-misinformation-trump-counties-covid-death-rate.

12. Melissa Block, "Biden Aims to Help Hospitals by Sending Military Doctors and Nurses to Help," NPR, *Morning Edition*, December 22, 2021,

https://www.npr.org/2021/12/22/1066642286/biden-aims-to-help-hospitals-by-
is-sending-military-doctors-and-nurses-to-help.

13. Ibid.

14. Mensah M. Dean, "Philly to Pay $2.5 Million to Walter Wallace Jr.'s
Family to Settle Claims over His Killing by Police," *Philadelphia Inquirer*,
October 28, 2021, https://www.inquirer.com/news/walter-wallace-death-
police-shooting-philadelphia-lawsuit-settlement-20211028.html.

15. Jonathan Tamari, "Sen. Bob Casey Cites Shooting of Walter Wallace Jr.
in Pushing Bills to Divert 911 Calls for Mental Health Crises," *Philadelphia
Inquirer*, December 9, 2020, https://www.inquirer.com/politics/nation/bob-
casey-police-reform-walter-wallace-jr-20201209.html.

16. Lorna Collier, "Incarceration Nation," *Monitor on Psychology, American
Psychological Association* 5, no. 9 (October 2014): 56, https://www.apa.org/
monitor/2014/10/incarceration.

17. Dean, "Philly to Pay $2.5 Million."

18. Mike Newell and Chris Palmer, "Overnight Curfew Lifted in Philly as
Tensions over the Police Killing of Walter Wallace Jr. Continue," *Philadelphia
Inquirer*, October 29, 2020, https://www.inquirer.com/news/philadelphia-
police-shooting-walter-wallace-jr-protests-unrest-20201028.html.

19. Dean, "Philly to Pay $2.5 Million."

20. Washington Post, "Fatal Force," online database, *Washington Post*,
reviewed December 21, 2021, https://www.washingtonpost.com/graphics/
investigations/police-shootings-database/.

21. Chris Mai and Ram Subramanian, "The Price of Prisons," Vera Center
on Sentencing and Corrections, May 2017, https://www.vera.org/publications/
price-of-prisons-2015-state-spending-trends/.

22. Donald M. Berwick, "The Moral Determinants of Health," *JAMA* 324,
no. 3 (2020): 225–226. doi:10.1001/jama.2020.11129.

23. Philadelphia Department of Public Health, and Drexel University
Urban Health Collaborative, *Close to Home: The Health of Philadelphia's
Neighborhoods*, Philadelphia Department of Public Health, July 31,
2019, https://www.phila.gov/media/20190801133844/Neighborhood-
Rankings_7_31_19.pdf.

24. Ibid.

25. Kerry Dooley Young, "Patient-Safety Leader Challenges Hospital
Nationwide to Establish 10 Crucial Teams," Association of Health Care
Journalists, Center for Excellence in Health Care Journalism, December
14, 2021, https://healthjournalism.org/blog/2021/12/patient-safety-leader-
challenges-hospitals-nationwide-to-establish-10-teams-to-reverse-the-flow-of-
health-care-resources/.

26. Berwick, "The Moral Determinants of Health." This paper also gave us the idea of comparing life expectancies in different neighborhoods to the potential life expectancy improvement of curing heart disease.

27. Anna Wilde Mathews, "The Pandemic Didn't Unfold How Dr. Christine Hancock Expected," *Wall Street Journal*, December 16, 2021, https://www.wsj.com/articles/pandemic-struggle-patients-who-dont-have-covid-11639668552.

28. Ibid.

29. Kelly Gooch, "Healthcare Has Lost Half a Million Workers since 2020," *Becker's Hospital Review*, October 12, 2021, beckershospitalreview.com/workforce/healthcare-has-lost-half-a-million-workers-since-2020.html.

30. Deborah D. Stine, *The Manhattan Project, the Apollo Program, and Federal Energy Technology R&D Programs: A Comparative Analysis* (Washington, DC: Congressional Research Service, June 30, 2009), https://sgp.fas.org/crs/misc/RL34645.pdf.

31. Centers for Medicare and Medicaid Services, "National Health Expenditure Data," https://www.cms.gov/Research-Statistics-Data-and-Systems/Statistics-Trends-and-Reports/NationalHealthExpendData, accessed December 22, 2021.

32. National Association of Home Builders, "Housing's Contribution to Gross Domestic Product," https://www.nahb.org/news-and-economics/housing-economics/housings-economic-impact/housings-contribution-to-gross-domestic-product, accessed December 22, 2021.

33. Kelly Gooch, "18 Healthcare Organization Suspending COVID-19 Vaccination Mandates," *Becker's Hospital Review*, December 20, 2021, https://www.beckershospitalreview.com/workforce/5-health-systems-suspending-vaccination-mandates.html.

34. Mary Ann Peberdy et al., "Survival from In-Hospital Cardiac Arrest during Nights and Weekends," *JAMA* 299, no. 7 (2008): 785–92, https://jamanetwork.com/journals/jama/fullarticle/181485.

35. Ian W. Toll, *Twilight of the Gods: War in the Western Pacific, 1944–1945* (New York: W.W. Norton, 2020), 791.

Bibliography

Abdalla, Salma M., Nason Maani, Catherine K. Ettman, and Sandro Galea. "Claiming Health as a Public Good in the Post-COVID-19 Era." *Development* 63, no. 2 (December 1, 2020): 200–204. https://doi.org/10.1057/s41301-020-00255-z.

Abdel-Baqui, Omar. "Amtrak, Changing Course, Suspends Covid-19 Vaccine Mandate for Workers." *Wall Street Journal*, December 14, 2021, sec. US. https://www.wsj.com/articles/amtrak-changing-course-suspends-covid-19-vaccine-mandate-for-workers-11639521984.

Abelson, Reed. "In Bid for Better Care, Surgery with a Warranty." *New York Times*, May 17, 2007, sec. Business. https://www.nytimes.com/2007/05/17/business/17quality.html.

Abraham, Jean Marie. "Employer Wellness Programs—A Work in Progress." *JAMA* 321, no. 15 (April 16, 2019): 1462–63. https://doi.org/10.1001/jama.2019.3376.

Accreditation Council for Graduate Medical Education. "Milestones." https://acgme.org/what-we-do/accreditation/milestones/overview/.

Adams, Faith, and William Willsea. *The US Health Insurers Customer Experience Index, 2018*. Forrester, June 19, 2018. https://www.forrester.com/report/The-US-Health-Insurers-Customer-Experience-Index-2018/RES142622.

Advocacy Department. "Facts: Bridging the Gap, CVD and Health Equity." American Heart Association, 2015.

Agarwal, Rajender, Joshua M. Liao, Ashutosh Gupta, and Amol S. Navathe. "The Impact of Bundled Payment on Health Care Spending, Utilization, and Quality: A Systematic Review." *Health Affairs* 39, no. 1 (January 1, 2020): 50–57. https://doi.org/10.1377/hlthaff.2019.00784.

Agarwal, Rajender, Olena Mazurenko, and Nir Menachemi. "High-Deductible Health Plans Reduce Health Care Cost and Utilization, Including Use of Needed Preventive Services." *Health Affairs* 36, no. 10 (October 1, 2017): 1762–68. https://doi.org/10.1377/hlthaff.2017.0610.

Agency for Healthcare Research and Quality. "Communication and Optimal Resolution (CANDOR)." Agency for Healthcare Research and Quality, April 2018. https://www.ahrq.gov/patient-safety/capacity/candor/index.html.

Ahmad, Farida B., Jodi Cisewski, Arialdi Miniño, and Robert Anderson. "Provisional Mortality Data—United States, 2020." *MMWR. Morbidity and Mortality Weekly Report* 70 (April 9, 2021): 519–22. https://doi.org/10.15585/mmwr.mm7014e1.

Aisch, Gregor, Larry Buchanan, Amanda Cox, and Kevin Quealy. "Economic Diversity and Student Outcomes at Princeton." *New York Times*, January 18, 2017, sec. The Upshot. https://www.nytimes.com/interactive/projects/college-mobility/princeton-university.

AJMC Staff. "A Timeline of COVID-19 Developments in 2020." *American Journal of Managed Care*, January 1, 2021. https://www.ajmc.com/view/a-timeline-of-covid19-developments-in-2020.

Alkire, Michael J., Doug Miller, and Beth Cloyd. "PINC AI Data Shows Hospitals Paying $24B More for Labor amid COVID-19." *Premier*, October 6, 2021. https://www.premierinc.com/newsroom/blog/pinc-ai-data-shows-hospitals-paying-24b-more-for-labor-amid-covid-19-pandemic.

Alter, Alexandra, and Elizabeth A. Harris. "'A Publisher's Worst Nightmare': How Cuomo's Book Became a Cautionary Tale." *New York Times*, August 10, 2021, sec. Books. https://www.nytimes.com/2021/08/10/books/cuomo-book-penguin-random-house.html.

Althoff, Keri N., David J. Schlueter, Hoda Anton-Culver, James Cherry, Joshua C. Denny, Isaac Thomsen, Elizabeth W. Karlson, et al. "Antibodies to SARS-CoV-2 in All of Us Research Program Participants, January 2–March 18, 2020." *Clinical Infectious Diseases*, no. ciab519 (June 15, 2021). https://doi.org/10.1093/cid/ciab519.

Altman, Lawrence K. "Big Doses of Chemotherapy Drug Killed Patient, Hurt 2d." *New York Times*, March 24, 1995, sec. U.S. https://www.nytimes.com/1995/03/24/us/big-doses-of-chemotherapy-drug-killed-patient-hurt-2d.html.

Anderson, Pauline. "Physicians Experience Highest Suicide Rate of Any Profession." *Medscape*, May 7, 2018. http://www.medscape.com/viewarticle/896257.

Ansell, David A. *The Death Gap: How Inequality Kills*. Chicago University of Chicago Press, 2021. https://press.uchicago.edu/ucp/books/book/chicago/D/bo113685153.html.

Ansell, David A., Darlene Oliver-Hightower, Larry J. Goodman, Omar B. Lateef, and Tricia J. Johnson. "Health Equity as a System Strategy: The Rush University Medical Center Framework." *NEJM Catalyst* 2, no. 5. Accessed May 20, 2021. https://doi.org/10.1056/CAT.20.0674.

Antman, Elliott M., and Eugene Braunwald. "Managing Stable Ischemic Heart Disease." *New England Journal of Medicine* 382, no. 15 (April 9, 2020): 1468–70. https://doi.org/10.1056/NEJMe2000239.

Apple. "Healthcare—Health Records." https://www.apple.com/healthcare/health-records/.

Appleby, Julie. "Is Your Living Room the Future of Hospital Care?" *Kaiser Health News* (blog), May 24, 2021. https://khn.org/news/article/is-your-living-room-the-future-of-hospital-care/.

———. "Telehealth's Limits: Battle over State Lines and Licensing Threatens Patients' Options." *Kaiser Health News* (blog), August 31, 2021. https://khn.org/news/article/state-medical-licensing-rules-threatens-telehealth-patient-options/.

Arias, Elizabeth, Betzaida Tejada-Vera, Farida Ahmad, and Kenneth Kochanek. "Provisional Life Expectancy Estimates for 2020." Centers for Disease Control and Prevention, July 2021. https://doi.org/10.15620/cdc:100392.

Armour, Stephanie, and Robbie Whelan. "Telehealth Rollbacks Leave Patients Stranded, Some Doctors Say." *Wall Street Journal*, November 22, 2021, sec. Business. https://www.wsj.com/articles/telehealth-rollbacks-leave-patients-stranded-some-doctors-say-11637577001.

Asch, David A., MD Nazmul Islam, Natalie E. Sheils, Yong Chen, Jalpa A. Doshi, John Buresh, and Rachel M. Werner. "Patient and Hospital Factors Associated with Differences in Mortality Rates among Black and White US Medicare Beneficiaries Hospitalized with COVID-19 Infection." *JAMA Network Open* 4, no. 6 (June 17, 2021): e2112842–e2112842. https://doi.org/10.1001/jamanetworkopen.2021.12842.

Associated Press. "Warp-Speed Spending and Other Surreal Stats of COVID Times." *US News & World Report*, March 13, 2021, sec. Health News. https://www.usnews.com/news/health-news/articles/2021-03-13/warp-speed-spending-and-other-surreal-stats-of-covid-times.

Association of American Medical Colleges. "Diversity in Medicine: Facts and Figures 2019." https://www.aamc.org/data-reports/workforce/data/table-6-us-medical-schools-150-or-more-black-or-african-american-graduates-alone-or-combination-2009.

Association of State and Territorial Health Officials. "New Data on State Health Agencies Shows Shrinking Workforce and Decreased Funding Leading up to the COVID-19 Pandemic." Association of State and Territorial Health Officials, September 24, 2020. https://astho.org/Press-Room/

New-Data-on-State-Health-Agencies-Shows-Shrinking-Workforce-and-Decreased-Funding-Leading-up-to-the-COVID-19-Pandemic/09-24-20/.

Atsma, Femke, Glyn Elwyn, and Gert Westert. "Understanding Unwarranted Variation in Clinical Practice: A Focus on Network Effects, Reflective Medicine and Learning Health Systems." *International Journal for Quality in Health Care* 32, no. 4 (June 2020): 271–74. https://doi.org/10.1093/intqhc/mzaa023.

Austin, J. Matthew, and Allen Kachalia. "The State of Health Care Quality Measurement in the Era of COVID-19: The Importance of Doing Better." *JAMA* 324, no. 4 (July 28, 2020): 333–34. https://doi.org/10.1001/jama.2020.11461.

Baer, Tamara, Matthew Isaacs, Alex Mandel, and Pradeep Prabhala. "How Healthcare Payers Can Expand Nutrition Support for the Food Insecure." McKinsey & Company, November 24, 2021. https://www.mckinsey.com/featured-insights/food-security/how-healthcare-payers-can-expand-nutrition-support-for-the-food-insecure?cid=other-eml%E2%80%A6.

Barry, Dan, and Caitlin Dickerson. "The Killer Flu of 1918: A Philadelphia Story." *New York Times*, April 4, 2020. https://www.nytimes.com/2020/04/04/us/coronavirus-spanish-flu-philadelphia-pennsylvania.html.

Barry-Jester, Anna Maria, Hannah Recht, Michelle R. Smith, and Lauren Weber. "Pandemic Backlash Jeopardizes Public Health Powers, Leaders." *Kaiser Health News*, December 15, 2020. https://khn.org/news/article/pandemic-backlash-jeopardizes-public-health-powers-leaders/.

Basen, Ryan. "COVID Patients' Crackpot Theories Take Toll on Healthcare Workers." *MedPage Today*, November 19, 2020. https://www.medpagetoday.com/infectiousdisease/covid19/89796.

Basu, Sanjay, Russell S. Phillips, Seth A. Berkowitz, Bruce E. Landon, Asaf Bitton, and Robert L. Phillips. "Estimated Effect on Life Expectancy of Alleviating Primary Care Shortages in the United States." *Annals of Internal Medicine* 174, no. 7 (July 20, 2021): 920–26. https://doi.org/10.7326/M20-7381.

Beaulieu, Nancy D., Leemore S. Dafny, Bruce E. Landon, Jesse B. Dalton, Ifedayo Kuye, and J. Michael McWilliams. "Changes in Quality of Care after Hospital Mergers and Acquisitions." *New England Journal of Medicine* 382, no. 1 (January 2, 2020): 51–59. https://doi.org/10.1056/NEJMsa1901383.

Beiriger, Jason, and David B. Nash. "Testing Testimonial." *Population Health Management*, April 16, 2021. https://doi.org/10.1089/pop.2021.0056.

Bender, Michael C., and Rebecca Ballhaus. "How Trump Sowed Covid Supply Chaos. 'Try Getting It Yourselves.'" *Wall Street Journal*, August 31, 2020, sec. US. https://www.wsj.com/articles/how-trump-sowed-covid-supply-chaos-try-getting-it-yourselves-11598893051.

Berkowitz, Seth A., Jean Terranova, Liisa Randall, Kevin Cranston, David B. Waters, and John Hsu. "Association between Receipt of a Medically Tailored Meal Program and Health Care Use." *JAMA Internal Medicine* 179, no. 6 (June 1, 2019): 786–93. https://doi.org/10.1001/jamainternmed.2019.0198.

Berry, Leonard L., Sunjay Letchuman, Nandini Ramani, and Paul Barach. "The High Stakes of Outsourcing in Health Care." *Mayo Clinic Proceedings* 96(11):2879–90 (August 16, 2021). https://doi.org/10.1016/j.mayocp.2021.07.003.

Berwick, Donald M. "The Moral Determinants of Health." *JAMA* 324, no. 3 (July 21, 2020): 225–26. https://doi.org/10.1001/jama.2020.11129.

Bestsennyy, Oleg, Greg Gilbert, Alex Harris, and Jennifer Rost. "Telehealth: A Quarter-Trillion-Dollar Post-COVID-19 Reality?" McKinsey & Company, July 9, 2021. https://www.mckinsey.com/industries/healthcare-systems-and-services/our-insights/telehealth-a-quarter-trillion-dollar-post-covid-19-reality.

Biniek, Jeannie Fuglesten, Meredith Freed, Anthony Damico, and Tricia Neuman. "Medicare Advantage in 2021: Star Ratings and Bonuses." *KFF*, June 21, 2021. https://www.kff.org/medicare/issue-brief/medicare-advantage-in-2021-star-ratings-and-bonuses/.

Birkmeyer, John D., Amber Barnato, Nancy Birkmeyer, Robert Bessler, and Jonathan Skinner. "The Impact of the COVID-19 Pandemic on Hospital Admissions in the United States." *Health Affairs* 39, no. 11 (November 1, 2020): 2010–17. https://doi.org/10.1377/hlthaff.2020.00980.

Blake, Aaron. "The Most-Vaccinated Big Counties in America Are Beating the Worst of the Coronavirus." *Washington Post*, December 4, 2021. https://www.washingtonpost.com/politics/2021/12/04/big-counties-are-proving-how-vaccination-works/.

Block, Melissa. "Biden Aims to Help Hospitals by Sending Military Doctors and Nurses to Help." NPR, *Morning Edition*, December 22, 2021, sec. Health. https://www.npr.org/2021/12/22/1066642286/biden-aims-to-help-hospitals-by-is-sending-military-doctors-and-nurses-to-help.

Boburg, Shawn, Robert O'Harrow, Neena Satija, and Amy Goldstein. "Inside the Coronavirus Testing Failure: Alarm and Dismay among the Scientists Who Sought to Help." *Washington Post*, April 3, 2020. https://www.washingtonpost.com/investigations/2020/04/03/coronavirus-cdc-test-kits-public-health-labs/.

Boots, Michelle Theriault, and Emily Goodykoontz. "Jewish Leaders Decry Use of Holocaust Symbolism to Protest Anchorage Mask Ordinance." *Anchorage Daily News*, September 30, 2021, sec. Anchorage. https://www.adn.com/alaska-news/anchorage/2021/09/30/a-direct-disrespect-jewish-leaders-decry-use-of-holocaust-symbolism-to-protest-anchorage-mask-ordinance/.

BP. "BP Wellbeing Program." BP Life Benefits, 2021. https://hr.bpglobal.com/ LifeBenefits/Sites/inpat/BP-Life-benefits/Employee-benefits-handbook/ BP-Medical-Program/How-the-BP-Medical-Program-works/BP-Wellness-Program.aspx.

Bressman, Eric. "Safety Net: Reflections on the Elmhurst Experience." *NEJM Journal Watch*, May 19, 2020. https://blogs.jwatch.org/general-medicine/ index.php/2020/05/safety-net-reflections-on-the-elmhurst-experience/.

Brody, Leslie. "Medical Schools Are Getting Flooded with Applicants." *Wall Street Journal*, April 30, 2021, sec. US. https://www.wsj.com/articles/ medical-schools-are-getting-flooded-with-applicants-11619795836.

Brooks, David. "How to Get Really Rich!" *New York Times*, February 26, 2021, sec. Opinion. https://www.nytimes.com/2021/02/25/opinion/inequality-medicine-law.html.

Brown, Elizabeth A. "COVID-19 Employee Health Checks Create New Privacy Risks." In *Work Law Under COVID-19*, edited by Sachin S. Pandya and Jeffrey M. Hirsch, 2021. Published online. https://worklawcovid19book. netlify.app/privacyrisks.html.

———. "The Femtech Paradox: How Workplace Monitoring Threatens Women's Equity." *Jurimetrics* 61, no. 3 (2021): 289–329.

———. "Workplace Wellness: Social Injustice." *New York University Journal of Legislation and Public Policy* 20, no. 191 (2017): 191–246.

Brown, Timothy T. "Returns on Investment in California County Departments of Public Health." *American Journal of Public Health* 106, no. 8 (August 1, 2016): 1477–82. https://doi.org/10.2105/AJPH.2016.303233.

Brubaker, Harold. "Jefferson Completes Acquisition of Health Partners Insurer from Temple Health." *Philadelphia Inquirer*, November 1, 2021, sec. Healthcare. https://www.inquirer.com/business/health/jefferson-completes-acquisition-health-partners-hpp-temple-20211101.html.

Buchanan, Larry, Quoctrung Bui, and Jugal K. Patel. "Black Lives Matter May Be the Largest Movement in U.S. History." *New York Times*, July 3, 2020, sec. U.S. https://www.nytimes.com/interactive/2020/07/03/us/george-floyd-protests-crowd-size.html.

Buchanan, Tom. "Why Do People Spread False Information Online? The Effects of Message and Viewer Characteristics on Self-Reported Likelihood of Sharing Social Media Disinformation." *PLOS ONE* 15, no. 10 (October 7, 2020): e0239666. https://doi.org/10.1371/journal.pone.0239666.

Bui, Quoctrung. "The Most Common Jobs for the Rich, Middle Class and Poor." NPR, October 16, 2014, sec. Jobs. https://www.npr.org/sections/money/2014/10/16/356176018/the-most-popular-jobs-for-the-rich-middle-class-and-poor.

Bump, Philip. "Trump's Message on Vaccines Isn't as Powerful as Trumpism's Message." *Washington Post*, December 21, 2021, sec.

Politics.   https://www.washingtonpost.com/politics/2021/12/21/
trumps-message-vaccines-isnt-powerful-trumpisms-message/.

———. "The Two Halves of the Pandemic." *Washington Post*, December 1,
2021, sec. Politics. https://www.washingtonpost.com/politics/2021/12/01/
two-halves-pandemic/.

Burgon, Trever B., James Cox-Chapman, Catherine Czarnecki, Robert Kropp,
Richard Guerriere, David Paculdo, and John W. Peabody. "Engaging
Primary Care Providers to Reduce Unwanted Clinical Variation and Support
ACO Cost and Quality Goals: A Unique Provider-Payer Collaboration."
Population Health Management 22, no. 4 (August 1, 2019): 321–29. https://
doi.org/10.1089/pop.2018.0111.

Business Roundtable. "Business Roundtable Redefines the Purpose of a
Corporation to Promote 'An Economy That Serves All Americans.'" August
19, 2019. https://www.businessroundtable.org/business-roundtable-rede-
fines-the-purpose-of-a-corporation-to-promote-an-economy-that-serves-all-
americans.

BusinessWire. "Amazon Hiring 75,000 Employees across Fulfillment and
Transportation, with Average Starting Pay of Over $17 per Hour and Sign-On
Bonuses of Up to $1,000." May 13, 2021. https://www.businesswire.
com/news/home/20210513005366/en/Amazon-Hiring-75000-Employees-
Across-Fulfillment-and-Transportation-With-Average-Starting-Pay-of-
Over-17-Per-Hour-and-Sign-On-Bonuses-of-Up-To-1000.

Buxbaum, Jason D., Michael E. Chernew, A. Mark Fendrick, and David M.
Cutler. "Contributions of Public Health, Pharmaceuticals, and Other Medical
Care to US Life Expectancy Changes, 1990–2015." *Health Affairs* 39, no. 9
(September 1, 2020): 1546–56. https://doi.org/10.1377/hlthaff.2020.00284.

Carpentier, Megan. "No Child Left Behind Has Been Unsuccessful,
Says Bipartisan Report." *The Guardian*, August 9, 2016, sec.
Education.   https://www.theguardian.com/education/2016/aug/09/
no-child-left-behind-bill-unsuccessful-report-us-schools.

Center for Countering Digital Hate. *The Disinformation Dozen*. London:
CCDH, 2021. https://www.counterhate.com/disinformationdozen.

Center for Rural Pennsylvania. "Demographics—County Profiles." https://
www.rural.palegislature.us/county_profiles.cfm.

Centers for Disease Control and Prevention. "Drug Overdose Deaths in the
U.S. Top 100,000 Annually." Centers for Disease Control and Prevention,
November 17, 2021. https://www.cdc.gov/nchs/pressroom/nchs_press_
releases/2021/20211117.htm.

———. "First Travel-Related Case of 2019 Novel Coronavirus Detected in
United States." Centers for Disease Control and Prevention, February 18,
2020. https://www.cdc.gov/media/releases/2020/p0121-novel-coronavirus-
travel-case.html.

————. "In-Hospital Mortality among Hospital Confirmed COVID-19 Encounters by Week from Selected Hospitals." Centers for Disease Control and Prevention, May 17, 2021. https://www.cdc.gov/nchs/covid19/nhcs/hospital-mortality-by-week.htm.

————. *Interim Pre-Pandemic Planning Guidance: Community Strategy for Pandemic Influenza Mitigation in the United States—Early, Targeted, Layered Use of Nonpharmaceutical Interventions.* Atlanta, GA: Centers for Disease Control and Prevention, February 2007. https://www.cdc.gov/flu/pandemic-resources/pdf/community_mitigation-sm.pdf.

————. "New CDC Data Finds Adult Obesity Is Increasing." Centers for Disease Control and Prevention, September 17, 2020. https://www.cdc.gov/media/releases/2020/s0917-adult-obesity-increasing.html.

————. "1918 Pandemic (H1N1 Virus)." Centers for Disease Control and Prevention, June 16, 2020. https://www.cdc.gov/flu/pandemic-resources/1918-pandemic-h1n1.html.

————. "2020–2021 Flu Season Summary." Centers for Disease Control and Prevention, October 25, 2021. https://www.cdc.gov/flu/season/faq-flu-season-2020-2021.htm.

Centers for Medicare and Medicaid Services. "Medicare and Medicaid Programs; Policy and Regulatory Revisions in Response to the COVID-19 Public Health Emergency." Federal Register, April 6, 2020. https://www.federalregister.gov/documents/2020/04/06/2020-06990/medicare-and-medicaid-programs-policy-and-regulatory-revisions-in-response-to-the-covid-19-public.

————. "Medicare Participating Heart Bypass Center Demonstration." May 4, 2021. https://innovation.cms.gov/medicare-demonstrations/medicare-participating-heart-bypass-center-demonstration.

————. "National Health Expenditure Data." December 1, 2021. https://www.cms.gov/Research-Statistics-Data-and-Systems/Statistics-Trends-and-Reports/NationalHealthExpendData.

————. "National Health Expenditure Data Fact Sheet." December 16, 2020. https://www.cms.gov/Research-Statistics-Data-and-Systems/Statistics-Trends-and-Reports/NationalHealthExpendData/NHE-Fact-Sheet.

Chang, Alisa, and Eric Klinenberg. "What a 1995 Heat Wave May Teach Us about Responding to the Coronavirus Outbreak." NPR, March 31, 2020. https://www.npr.org/2020/03/31/824730922/what-a-1995-heat-wave-may-teach-us-about-responding-to-the-coronavirus-outbreak.

Chang, Serina, Emma Pierson, Pang Wei Koh, Jaline Gerardin, Beth Redbird, David Grusky, and Jure Leskovec. "Mobility Network Models of COVID-19 Explain Inequities and Inform Reopening." *Nature* 589, no. 7840 (January 2021): 82–87. https://doi.org/10.1038/s41586-020-2923-3.

Chaudry, Ajay, Christopher Wimer, Suzanne Macartney, Lauren Frohlich, Colin Campbell, Kendall Swenson, Don Oellerich, and Susan Hauan. "Poverty in the United States: 50-Year Trends and Safety Net Impacts." Office of the Assistant Secretary for Planning and Evaluation, US Department of Health and Human Services, March 2016. https://aspe.hhs.gov/sites/default/files/private/pdf/154286/50YearTrends.pdf.

Chen, David W. "Boy, 6, Dies of Skull Injury during M.R.I." *New York Times*, July 31, 2001, sec. New York. https://www.nytimes.com/2001/07/31/nyregion/boy-6-dies-of-skull-injury-during-mri.html.

Chen, Pauline W. "Where Have All the Hospital Patients Gone?" *New York Times*, October 20, 2020, sec. Well. https://www.nytimes.com/2020/10/20/well/where-have-all-the-hospital-patients-gone.html.

Chen, Yan-Ya, Bing-Sheng Guan, Ze-Kai Li, and Xing-Yi Li. "Effect of Telehealth Intervention on Breast Cancer Patients' Quality of Life and Psychological Outcomes: A Meta-Analysis." *Journal of Telemedicine and Telecare* 24, no. 3 (April 1, 2018): 157–67. https://doi.org/10.1177/1357633X16686777.

Chen, Yea-Hung, Maria Glymour, Alicia Riley, John Balmes, Kate Duchowny, Robert Harrison, Ellicott Matthay, and Kirsten Bibbins-Domingo. "Excess Mortality Associated with the COVID-19 Pandemic among Californians 18–65 Years of Age, by Occupational Sector and Occupation: March through November 2020." *PLOS ONE* 16, no. 6 (June 4, 2021): e0252454. https://doi.org/10.1371/journal.pone.0252454.

Chernew, Michael, Zack Cooper, Eugene Larsen-Hallock, and Fiona Scott Morton. "Are Health Care Services Shoppable? Evidence from the Consumption of Lower-Limb MRI Scans." Working Paper. Working Paper Series. National Bureau of Economic Research, July 2018. https://doi.org/10.3386/w24869.

Chetty, Raj, Michael Stepner, Sarah Abraham, Shelby Lin, Benjamin Scuderi, Nicholas Turner, Augustin Bergeron, and David Cutler. "The Association between Income and Life Expectancy in the United States, 2001–2014." *JAMA* 315, no. 16 (April 26, 2016): 1750–66. https://doi.org/10.1001/jama.2016.4226.

Chidambaram, Priya, Rachel Garfield, Tricia Neuman, and Larry Levitt. "Is the End of the Long-Term Care Crisis within Sight? New COVID-19 Cases and Deaths in Long-Term Care Facilities Are Dropping." *KFF*, February 24, 2021. https://www.kff.org/policy-watch/is-the-end-of-the-long-term-care-crisis-within-sight-new-covid-19-cases-and-deaths-in-long-term-care-facilities-are-dropping/.

Chin, Marshall H. "Uncomfortable Truths: What Covid-19 Has Revealed about Chronic-Disease Care in America." *New England Journal of Medicine* 385, no. 18 (October 28, 2021): 1633–36. https://doi.org/10.1056/NEJMp2112063.

Choi, Ann, Olivia Winslow, and Arthur Browne. "Long Island Divided." *Newsday*, November 17, 2019, sec. Long Island. https://projects.newsday.com/long-island/real-estate-agents-investigation/.

Chokshi, Niraj, and Noam Scheiber. "Inside United Airlines' Decision to Mandate Coronavirus Vaccines." *New York Times*, October 2, 2021, sec. Business. https://www.nytimes.com/2021/10/02/business/united-airlines-coronavirus-vaccine-mandate.html.

City of New York. "Top Languages Spoken at Home" online factsheet, 2015. https://www1.nyc.gov/assets/planning/download/pdf/data-maps/nyc-population/acs/top_lang_2015pums5yr_nyc.pdf.

Clark, Emily, Jennifer Rost, and Anna Stolyarovna. "What Payer-Led Managed Care Models May Look Like." McKinsey & Company, December 2, 2021. https://www.mckinsey.com/industries/healthcare-systems-and-services/our-insights/innovation-and-value-what-payer-led-managed-care-models-may-look-like.

Claxton, Gary, Matthew Rae, Gregory Young, and Nisha Kurani. "2021 Employer Health Benefits Survey." *KFF*, November 10, 2021. https://www.kff.org/health-costs/report/2021-employer-health-benefits-survey/.

Clymer, Adam. "The Health Care Debate: The Overview; National Health Program, President's Greatest Goal, Declared Dead in Congress." *New York Times*, September 27, 1994, sec. U.S. https://www.nytimes.com/1994/09/27/us/health-care-debate-overview-national-health-program-president-s-greatest-goal.html.

CNN. "CNN's Facts First Searchable Database." https://www.cnn.com/factsfirst/politics/factcheck_e58c20c6-8735-4022-a1f5-1580bc732c45.

Cobb, Tyson K. "Wrong Site Surgery—Where Are We and What Is the Next Step?" *Hand* 7, no. 2 (June 2012): 229–32. https://doi.org/10.1007/s11552-012-9405-5.

Cohn, D'vera, Paul Taylor, Mark Hugo Lopez, Catherine a Gallagher, Kim Parker, and Kevin T. Maass. "Gun Homicide Rate Down 49% Since 1993 Peak; Public Unaware." Pew Research Center, May 7, 2013. https://www.pewresearch.org/social-trends/2013/05/07/gun-homicide-rate-down-49-since-1993-peak-public-unaware/.

Collier, Lorna. "Incarceration Nation." *Monitor on Psychology, American Psychological Association* 45, no. 9 (October 2014): 56.

Conway, Earl, and Paul Batalden. "Like Magic? ('Every System Is Perfectly Designed . . .')." Institute for Healthcare Improvement, August 21, 2015. http://www.ihi.org/communities/blogs/origin-of-every-system-is-perfectly-designed-quote.

Costa, Dora. "Health and the Economy in the United States, from 1750 to the Present." *Journal of Economic Literature* 53, no. 3 (September 2015): 503–70. https://doi.org/10.1257/jel.53.3.503.

Costa, Robert, and Philip Rucker. "Woodward Book: Trump Says He Knew Coronavirus Was 'Deadly' and Worse Than the Flu While Intentionally Misleading Americans." *Washington Post*, September 9, 2020. https://www.washingtonpost.com/politics/bob-woodward-rage-book-trump/2020/09/09/0368fe3c-efd2-11ea-b4bc-3a2098fc73d4_story.html.

Cramer, Maria. "Philadelphia Hospital to Stay Closed after Owner Requests Nearly $1 Million a Month." *New York Times*, March 27, 2020, sec. U.S. https://www.nytimes.com/2020/03/27/us/coronavirus-philadelphia-hahne-mann-hospital.html.

Cusumano, Michael A. "Boeing's 737 MAX: A Failure of Management, Not Just Technology." *Communications of the ACM* 64, no. 1 (January 2021): 22–25.

Cutler, David M., Edward L. Glaeser, and Jesse M. Shapiro. "Why Have Americans Become More Obese?" *Journal of Economic Perspectives* 17, no. 3 (September 2003): 93–118. https://doi.org/10.1257/089533003769204371.

Cutter, Chip, and Thomas Gryta. "Covid-19 Vaccine Mandates Turn into Religious Tests at GE, Disney—Some Longer Than Others." *Wall Street Journal*, October 31, 2021, sec. Business. https://www.wsj.com/articles/covid-19-vaccine-mandates-turn-into-religious-tests-at-ge-disneysome-lon-ger-than-others-11635688800.

Dean, Mensah M. "Philly to Pay $2.5 Million to Walter Wallace Jr.'s Family to Settle Claims over His Killing by Police." *Philadelphia Inquirer*, October 28, 2021, sec. News, news, news. https://www.inquirer.com/news/walter-wallace-death-police-shooting-philadelphia-lawsuit-settlement-20211028.html.

DellaVigna, Stefano, and Ulrike Malmendier. "Paying Not to Go to the Gym." *American Economic Review* 96, no. 3 (June 2006): 694–719. https://doi.org/10.1257/aer.96.3.694.

DeSalvo, Karen. "Comments at the 20th Population Health Colloquium." Presented at the 20th Population Health Colloquium, Thomas Jefferson University, October 5, 2020.

DeSalvo, Karen, Bob Hughes, Mary Bassett, Georges Benjamin, Michael Fraser, Sandro Galea, J. Nadine Gracia, and and Jeffrey Howard. "Public Health COVID-19 Impact Assessment: Lessons Learned and Compelling Needs." *NAM Perspectives*, April 7, 2021. https://doi.org/10.31478/202104c.

Diamond, Dan. "Feuds, Fibs and Finger-Pointing: Trump Officials Say Coronavirus Response Was Worse Than Known." *Washington Post*, March 29, 2021. https://www.washingtonpost.com/health/2021/03/29/trump-officials-tell-all-coronavirus-response/.

Digital Scholarship Lab, University of Richmond. "Mapping Inequality: Redlining in New Deal America." *American Panorama*, 2021. https://dsl.richmond.edu/panorama/redlining/.

Dill, Michael. "We Already Needed More Doctors. Then COVID-19 Hit." AAMC, June 17, 2021. https://www.aamc.org/news-insights/we-already-needed-more-doctors-then-covid-19-hit.

District Performance Office. "District Scorecard." School District of Philadelphia, June 4, 2021. https://www.philasd.org/performance/programsservices/school-progress-reports/district-scorecard/.

Drees, Jackie. "EHR Market Share 2021: 10 Things to Know about Major Players Epic, Cerner, Meditech & Allscripts." *Becker's Health IT*, May 21, 2021. https://www.beckershospitalreview.com/ehrs/ehr-market-share-2021-10-things-to-know-about-major-players-epic-cerner-meditech-allscripts.html.

Du Bois, W. E. Burghardt. *The Philadelphia Negro: A Social Study.* University of Pennsylvania, 1899.

Duffy, Thomas P. "The Flexner Report—100 Years Later." *Yale Journal of Biology and Medicine* 84, no. 3 (September 2011): 269–76.

DuGoff, Eva, Ruth Tabak, Tyler Diduch, and Viviane Garth. "Quality, Health, and Spending in Medicare Advantage and Traditional Medicare." *American Journal of Managed Care* 27, no. 9 (September 2021): 395–400. https://doi.org/10.37765/ajmc.2021.88641.

Duncan, Ian, Tamim Ahmed, Henry Dove, and Terri L. Maxwell. "Medicare Cost at End of Life." *American Journal of Hospice & Palliative Care* 36, no. 8 (August 2019): 705–10. https://doi.org/10.1177/1049909119836204.

Dyrda, Laura. "70% of Physicians Are Now Employed by Hospitals or Corporations." *Becker's ASC Review*, July 1, 2021. https://www.becker-sasc.com/asc-transactions-and-valuation-issues/70-of-physicians-are-now-employed-by-hospitals-or-corporations.html.

Editors of *NEJM*. "Dying in a Leadership Vacuum." *New England Journal of Medicine*, October 7, 2020. https://doi.org/10.1056/NEJMe2029812.

Ehrenreich, Barbara, and John Ehrenreich. *American Health Empire: Power, Profits, and Politics.* New York: Vintage Books, 1970.

Eisenberg, John. "Samuel Preston Martin III." *Proceedings of the Association of American Physicians* 110, no. 4 (August 1998): 371–72.

Elesh, David. "Deindustrialization." *The Encyclopedia of Greater Philadelphia*, 2017. https://philadelphiaencyclopedia.org/archive/deindustrialization/.

Ellerbeck, Alexandra. "The Health 202: Here's How the U.S. Compares to Other Countries on the Coronavirus Pandemic." *Washington Post*, April 12, 2021. https://www.washingtonpost.com/politics/2021/04/12/health-202-here-how-us-compares-other-countries-coronavirus-pandemic/.

Emanuel, Ezekiel J., Emily Gudbranson, Jessica Van Parys, Mette Gørtz, Jon Helgeland, and Jonathan Skinner. "Comparing Health Outcomes of Privileged US Citizens with Those of Average Residents of Other Developed

Countries." *JAMA Internal Medicine* 181, no. 3 (March 1, 2021): 339–44. https://doi.org/10.1001/jamainternmed.2020.7484.

Englund, Will, and Joel Jacobs. "How Government Incentives Shaped the Nursing Home Business—and Left It Vulnerable to a Pandemic." *Washington Post*, November 27, 2020. https://www.washingtonpost.com/business/2020/11/27/nursing-home-incentives/.

Evans, Melanie, and Alexandra Berzon. "Why Hospitals Can't Handle Covid Surges: They're Flying Blind." *Wall Street Journal*, September 30, 2020, sec. US. https://www.wsj.com/articles/hospitals-covid-surge-data-11601478409.

Evans, Melanie, Alexandra Berzon, and Daniela Hernandez. "Some California Hospitals Refused Covid-19 Transfers for Financial Reasons, State Emails Show." *Wall Street Journal*, October 19, 2020, sec. Investigations. https://www.wsj.com/articles/some-california-hospitals-refused-covid-19-transfers-for-financial-reasons-state-emails-show-11603108814.

Evans, Melanie, and Michael Siconolfi. "U.S. Strategic Stockpile of Medical Supplies Is Outmatched by Coronavirus." *Wall Street Journal*, March 23, 2020, sec. US, https://www.wsj.com/articles/u-s-strategic-stockpile-of-medical-supplies-is-outmatched-by-coronavirus-11584990542.

Evans, R. S. "Electronic Health Records: Then, Now, and in the Future." *Yearbook of Medical Informatics*, no. Suppl 1 (May 20, 2016): S48–61. https://doi.org/10.15265/IYS-2016-s006.

Fair, Kathyrn R., Vadim A. Karatayev, Madhur Anand, and Chris T. Bauch. "Estimating COVID-19 Cases and Deaths Prevented by Non-Pharmaceutical Interventions, and the Impact of Individual Actions: A Retrospective Model-Based Analysis." *MedRxiv*, June 24, 2021, 2021.03.26.21254421. https://doi.org/10.1101/2021.03.26.21254421.

Feldman, Nina. "Black Doctors COVID-19 Consortium to Open Clinic Offering Primary Care." *WHYY*, September 22, 2021. https://whyy.org/articles/black-doctors-covid-19-consortium-to-open-clinic-offering-primary-care/.

———. "Why the Head of the Black Doctors COVID-19 Consortium Decided to Get Vaccinated." *WHYY*, December 16, 2020. https://whyy.org/articles/why-the-head-of-the-black-doctors-covid-19-consortium-decided-to-get-vaccinated/.

Fine, Marshall. "Hollywood's Newest Villain: HMOs." *Los Angeles Times*, July 3, 1998. https://www.latimes.com/archives/la-xpm-1998-jul-03-ca-264-story.html.

Fineout, Gary. "Poll Shows DeSantis on Solid Ground as Democrats Try to Find Openings." *Politico*, May 12, 2021, sec. Politico Florida. https://politi.co/3uKdt1Z.

Fins, Joseph, Joan Leiman, and Herbet Pardes. "Primum Non Nocere: Daniel Patrick Moynihan and the Defense of Academic Medicine." *Alpha*

Omega Alpha, 2017. https://www.alphaomegaalpha.org/wp-content/uploads/2021/03/2017-2-Fins.pdf.

Fiore, Kristina. "Is a Residency Program an Asset to Be Sold?" *MedPage Today*, September 20, 2019. https://www.medpagetoday.com/special-reports/exclusives/82292.

Fiorillo, Victor, and Gabby Houck. "*Good Morning America* Told Ala Stanford the City Named a Street After Her. It Didn't." *Philadelphia Magazine*, April 14, 2021. https://www.phillymag.com/news/2021/04/14/ala-stanford-street-philadelphia/.

Fischer, Claude. "Paradoxes of American Individualism." *Sociological Forum* 23, no. 2 (June 2008). https://doi.org/10.1111/j.1573-7861.2008.00066.x.

Fiscus, Michelle. "Tennessee's Former Top Vaccine Official: 'I Am Afraid for My State.'" *The Tennessean*, July 12, 2021, sec. Health. https://www.tennessean.com/story/news/health/2021/07/12/covid-19-tennessee-fired-vaccine-official-michelle-fiscus-fears-state/7945291002/.

Fleming, G. Alexander, John R. Petrie, Richard M. Bergenstal, Reinhard W. Holl, Anne L. Peters, and Lutz Heinemann. "Diabetes Digital App Technology: Benefits, Challenges, and Recommendations. A Consensus Report by the European Association for the Study of Diabetes (EASD) and the American Diabetes Association (ADA) Diabetes Technology Working Group." *Diabetes Care* 43, no. 1 (January 1, 2020): 250–60. https://doi.org/10.2337/dci19-0062.

Flexner, Abraham. *Medical Education in the United States and Canada*. New York: Carnegie Foundation, 1910. http://archive.carnegiefoundation.org/publications/pdfs/elibrary/Carnegie_Flexner_Report.pdf.

Flynn, Maggie. "48 States Saw Nursing Home Occupancy of 80% or Worse as 2021 Dawned—With Census as Low as 56%." *Skilled Nursing News*, January 25, 2021. https://skillednursingnews.com/2021/01/48-states-saw-nursing-home-occupancy-of-80-or-worse-as-2021-dawned-with-census-as-low-as-56/.

Fortune. "UnitedHealth Group." June 2, 2021. https://fortune.com/company/unitedhealth-group/fortune500/.

Fowler, Geoffrey A., and Heather Kelly. "Amazon's New Health Band Is the Most Invasive Tech We've Ever Tested." *Washington Post*, December 10, 2020, sec. Consumer Tech. https://www.washingtonpost.com/technology/2020/12/10/amazon-halo-band-review/.

Freed, Meredith, Jeannie Fuglesten Biniek, Anthony Damico, and Tricia Neuman. "Medicare Advantage in 2021: Enrollment Update and Key Trends." *KFF*, June 21, 2021. https://www.kff.org/medicare/issue-brief/medicare-advantage-in-2021-enrollment-update-and-key-trends/.

Freudenheim, Milt. "Humana Bets All on Managed Care." *New York Times*, May 20, 1993, sec. Business. https://www.nytimes.com/1993/05/20/business/humana-bets-all-on-managed-care.html.

Fuchs, Hailey. "Trump Attack on Diversity Training Has a Quick and Chilling Effect." *New York Times*, October 13, 2020, sec. U.S. https://www.nytimes.com/2020/10/13/us/politics/trump-diversity-training-race.html.

Fuhrmans, Vanessa, and Lauren Weber. "Burned Out and Restless from the Pandemic, Women Redefine Their Career Ambitions." *Wall Street Journal*, September 27, 2021, sec. Business. https://www.wsj.com/articles/womens-careers-covid-19-toll-11632506362.

Galea, Sandro. *The Contagion Next Time*. Oxford, New York: Oxford University Press, 2021.

———. *Well: What We Need to Talk about When We Talk about Health*. Oxford, New York: Oxford University Press, 2019.

Gallup, and West Health. *West Health-Gallup 2021 Healthcare in America Report*. Gallup, December 2021. https://www.gallup.com/analytics/357932/healthcare-in-america-2021.aspx.

García, Lily E., and Otha Thornton. "'No Child' Has Failed." *Washington Post*, February 13, 2015, sec. Opinions. https://www.washingtonpost.com/opinions/no-child-has-failed/2015/02/13/8d619026-b2f8-11e4-827f-93f454140e2b_story.html.

Garrow, Lauren, Lavanya Marla, and John-Paul Clarke. "Airline Response to COVID-19." *ORMS Today*, February 2, 2021. https://pubsonline.informs.org/do/10.1287/orms.2021.01.20/full/.

Gawande, Atul. *The Checklist Manifesto: How to Get Things Right*. New York: Metropolitan Books, 2009.

Geisinger. "Fresh Food Farmacy." https://www.geisinger.org/freshfoodfarmacy/learn-more.

———. "Geisinger: An Evolution of Caring." https://www.geisinger.org/about-geisinger.

———. "Leadership Team." https://www.geisinger.org/about-geisinger/leadership/leadership-team/jaewon-ryu.

———. "Lifetime Hip and Knee Guarantee." https://www.geisinger.org/patient-care/conditions-treatments-specialty/lifetime-hip-and-knee.

———. "MD Brochure 2020." https://issuu.com/geisingercommonwealth/docs/gcsommd2020.

Gleason, Jonathan, Wendy Ross, Alexander Fossi, Heather Blonsky, Jane Tobias, and Mary Stephens. "The Devastating Impact of Covid-19 on Individuals with Intellectual Disabilities in the United States." *NEJM Catalyst Innovations in Care Delivery*, March 5, 2021. https://catalyst.nejm.org/doi/full/10.1056/CAT.21.0051.

Bibliography

Glover, Richard. "10 Reasons for Australia's Covid-19 Success Story." *Washington Post*, March 15, 2021. https://www.washingtonpost.com/opinions/2021/03/15/10-reasons-australias-covid-19-success-story/.

Goetzel, Ron Z., Enid Chung Roemer, Karen B. Kent, Inge Myburgh, Brian C. Castrucci, Emily Yu, and Abbey Johnson. "Seven Ways Businesses Can Align with Public Health for Bold Action and Innovation." The de Beaumont Foundation, February 23, 2021. https://debeaumont.org/wp-content/uploads/2021/02/Seven-Ways-Businesses-Can-Align-with-Public-Health.pdf.

Gold, Russell, and Melanie Evans. "Why Did Covid Overwhelm Hospitals? A Yearslong Drive for Efficiency." *Wall Street Journal*, September 17, 2020, sec. US. https://www.wsj.com/articles/hospitals-for-years-banked-on-lean-staffing-the-pandemic-overwhelmed-them-11600351907.

Goldberg, Zachary N. and David B. Nash. "The Payvider: An Evolving Model." *Population Health Management*, October 2021, 528–30. http://doi.org/10.1089/pop.2021.0164.

Goldhamer, Mary Ellen J., Martin V. Pusic, John Patrick T. Co, and Debra F. Weinstein. "Can Covid Catalyze an Educational Transformation? Competency-Based Advancement in a Crisis." *New England Journal of Medicine* 383, no. 11 (September 10, 2020): 1003–5. https://doi.org/10.1056/NEJMp2018570.

Gooch, Kelly. "18 Healthcare Organizations Suspending COVID-19 Vaccination Mandates." *Becker's Hospital Review*, December 20, 2021. https://www.beckershospitalreview.com/workforce/5-health-systems-suspending-vaccination-mandates.html.

———. "Healthcare Has Lost Half a Million Workers since 2020." *Becker's Hospital Review*, October 12, 2021. https://www.beckershospitalreview.com/workforce/healthcare-has-lost-half-a-million-workers-since-2020.html.

Gorges, Rebecca J., and R. Tamara Konetzka. "Factors Associated with Racial Differences in Deaths among Nursing Home Residents with COVID-19 Infection in the US." *JAMA Network Open* 4, no. 2 (February 10, 2021): e2037431\. https://doi.org/10.1001/jamanetworkopen.2020.37431.

Gould, Elise, and Melat Kassa. "Low-Wage, Low-Hours Workers Were Hit Hardest in the COVID-19 Recession: The State of Working America 2020 Employment Report." Economic Policy Institute, May 20, 2021. https://www.epi.org/publication/swa-2020-employment-report/.

Gould, L. Hannah, Ida Rosenblum, David Nicholas, Qyuen Phan, and Timothy F. Jones. "Contributing Factors in Restaurant-Associated Foodborne Disease Outbreaks, FoodNet Sites, 2006 and 2007." *Journal of Food Protection* 76, no. 11 (November 2013): 1824–28. https://doi.org/10.4315/0362-028X.JFP-13-037.

Gowen, Annie. "48 Hours to Live: An Oklahoma Hospital's Rush to Find an ICU Bed for a Covid Patient." *Washington Post*, October 15, 2021, sec. Coronavirus. https://www.washingtonpost.com/nation/interactive/2021/hospital-covid-patient/.

Graham, David A. "It's Not Vaccine Hesitancy. It's COVID-19 Denialism." *The Atlantic*, April 27, 2021, sec. Ideas. https://www.theatlantic.com/ideas/archive/2021/04/its-not-vaccine-hesitancy-its-covid-denialism/618724/.

Greenwood, Brad N., Rachel R. Hardeman, Laura Huang, and Aaron Sojourner. "Physician–Patient Racial Concordance and Disparities in Birthing Mortality for Newborns." *Proceedings of the National Academy of Sciences* 117, no. 35 (September 1, 2020): 21194–200. https://doi.org/10.1073/pnas.1913405117.

Hall, Kellie, Nathalie Robin, and Kari O'Donnell. "The 2018 Forces of Change in America's Local Public Health System." National Association of County and City Health Officials. *NACCHO Voice*, November 20, 2018. https://www.naccho.org/blog/articles/the-2018-forces-of-change-in-americas-local-public-health-system.

Hamel, Liz, Lunna Lopes, Grace Sparks, Ashley Kirzinger, Audrey Kearney, Mellisha Stokes, and Mollyann Brodie. "KFF COVID-19 Vaccine Monitor: September 2021." *KFF*, September 28, 2021. https://www.kff.org/coronavirus-covid-19/poll-finding/kff-covid-19-vaccine-monitor-september-2021/.

The Harris Poll. "Harris Poll: Only Nine Percent of U.S. Consumers Believe Pharma and Biotechnology Put Patients over Profits; Only 16 Percent Believe Health Insurers Do." January 17, 2017. https://theharrispoll.com/only-nine-percent-of-u-s-consumers-believe-pharmaceutical-and-biotechnology-companies-put-patients-over-profits-while-only-16-percent-believe-health-insurance-companies-do-according-to-a-harris-pol/.

Hasco, Linda. "Here Are Pa.'s 20 Largest Employers, and the Biggest Employers in Each County." *PennLive*, April 20, 2018, sec. Pennsylvania Real-Time News. https://www.pennlive.com/news/erry-2018/04/eb7d0c4952761/pas_top_20_employers_and_the_t.html.

"Healthcare Data Breach Statistics." *HIPAA Journal*, 2021. https://www.hipaajournal.com/healthcare-data-breach-statistics/.

Hess, Abigail Johnson. "Princeton University Costs $73,450 per Year—but Here's How Much Students Actually Pay." *CNBC*, May 4, 2019. https://www.cnbc.com/2019/05/03/it-costs-73450-to-go-to-princetonheres-how-much-students-pay.html.

Hirsch, Lauren, and Michael Corkery. "How Tyson Foods Got 60,500 Workers to Get the Coronavirus Vaccine Quickly." *New York Times*, November 4, 2021, sec. Business. https://www.nytimes.com/2021/11/04/business/tyson-vaccine-mandate.html.

Hlavinka, Elizabeth. "Racial Bias in Flexner Report Permeates Medical Education Today." *MedPage Today*, June 18, 2020. https://www.medpageto-day.com/publichealthpolicy/medicaleducation/87171.

Hofstede, Geert. "Dimensionalizing Cultures: The Hofstede Model in Context." *Online Readings in Psychology and Culture* 2, no. 1 (December 1, 2011). https://doi.org/10.9707/2307-0919.1014.

———. "The 6 Dimensions Model of National Culture." 2021. https://geer-thofstede.com/culture-geert-hofstede-gert-jan-hofstede/6d-model-of-natio-nal-culture/.

Hojat, Mohammadreza, Michael J. Vergare, Kaye Maxwell, George Brainard, Steven K. Herrine, Gerald A. Isenberg, Jon Veloski, and Joseph S. Gonnella. "The Devil Is in the Third Year: A Longitudinal Study of Erosion of Empathy in Medical School." *Academic Medicine: Journal of the Association of American Medical Colleges* 84, no. 9 (September 2009): 1182–91. https://doi.org/10.1097/ACM.0b013e3181b17e55.

Holford, Theodore R., Rafael Meza, Kenneth E. Warner, Clare Meernik, Jihyoun Jeon, Suresh H. Moolgavkar, and David T. Levy. "Tobacco Control and the Reduction in Smoking-Related Premature Deaths in the United States, 1964–2012." *JAMA: The Journal of the American Medical Association* 311, no. 2 (January 8, 2014): 164–71. https://doi.org/10.1001/jama.2013.285112.

Hollander, Judd E., and Brendan G. Carr. "Virtually Perfect? Telemedicine for Covid-19." *New England Journal of Medicine* 382, no. 18 (April 30, 2020): 1679–81. https://doi.org/10.1056/NEJMp2003539.

Hollander, Judd E., and Aaron Neinstein. "Maturation from Adoption-Based to Quality-Based Telehealth Metrics." *NEJM Catalyst Innovations in Care Delivery*, September 9, 2020. https://catalyst.nejm.org/doi/full/10.1056/CAT.20.0408.

Hollander, Zaz. "Impossible Choices inside Alaska's Inundated Hospitals." *Anchorage Daily News*, September 17, 2021, sec. Alaska News. https://www.adn.com/alaska-news/2021/09/17/impossible-choices-inside-alaskas-inundated-hospitals/.

———. "Investigation Finds Dozens of Unqualified Florida Doctors Tried to Get Emergency Licenses in Alaska." *Anchorage Daily News*, October 30, 2021, sec. Alaska News. https://www.adn.com/alaska-news/2021/10/29/investigation-finds-dozens-of-unqualified-florida-doctors-tried-to-get-emer-gency-licenses-in-alaska/.

Hollingsworth, Heather, and Grant Schulte. "Health Workers Once Saluted as Heroes Now Get Threats." *AP NEWS*, September 29, 2021, sec. Coronavirus pandemic. https://apnews.com/article/coronavirus-pandemic-business-health-missouri-omaha-b73e167eba4987cab9e58fdc92ce0b72.

Hunter, David J. "The Complementarity of Public Health and Medicine: Achieving 'the Highest Attainable Standard of Health.'" *New England Journal of Medicine* 385, no. 6 (August 5, 2021): 481–84. https://doi.org/10.1056/NEJMp2102550.

IHS Markit Ltd. "The Complexities of Physician Supply and Demand: Projections from 2019 to 2034." AAMC, June 2021. https://www.aamc.org/media/54681/download?attachment.

Institute of Medicine Committee for the Study of the Future of Public Health. *The Future of Public Health.* Washington, DC: National Academies Press, 1988. https://www.ncbi.nlm.nih.gov/books/NBK218224/.

Institute of Medicine Committee on Quality of Health Care in America. *Crossing the Quality Chasm: A New Health System for the 21st Century.* Washington, DC: National Academies Press, 2001. http://www.ncbi.nlm.nih.gov/books/NBK222274/.

Institute of Medicine Committee on Quality of Health Care in America, Linda T. Kohn, Janet M. Corrigan, and Molla S. Donaldson, eds. *To Err Is Human: Building a Safer Health System.* Washington, DC: National Academies Press, 2000. https://www.ncbi.nlm.nih.gov/books/NBK225179/.

Iscol, Zachary. "What I Saw at the Javits Center's Covid-19 Hospital." CNN, May 8, 2020. https://www.cnn.com/2020/05/08/opinions/javits-centers-covid-19-hospital-iscol/index.html.

Jain, Sachin. "Medicare for All? The Better Route to Universal Coverage Would Be Medicare Advantage for All." *Modern Healthcare*, January 7, 2021. https://www.modernhealthcare.com/opinion-editorial/medicare-all-better-route-universal-coverage-would-be-medicare-advantage-all.

Jason, Christopher. "Exploring 3 Levels of Health Information Exchange, Data Access." *EHRIntelligence*, October 12, 2020. https://ehrintelligence.com/news/exploring-3-levels-of-health-information-exchange-data-access.

Jensen, Jessica, and Steven Thompson. "The Incident Command System: A Literature Review." *Disasters* 40, no. 1 (January 2016): 158–82. https://doi.org/10.1111/disa.12135.

Jiwani, Aliya, David Himmelstein, Steffie Woolhandler, and James G. Kahn. "Billing and Insurance-Related Administrative Costs in United States' Health Care: Synthesis of Micro-Costing Evidence." *BMC Health Services Research* 14, no. 1 (November 13, 2014): 556. https://doi.org/10.1186/s12913-014-0556-7.

Johns Hopkins University. "Coronavirus Resource Center." Johns Hopkins Coronavirus Resource Center, December 2021. https://coronavirus.jhu.edu/.

Johns Hopkins University and Medicine. "Mortality Analyses." Johns Hopkins Coronavirus Resource Center, 2021. https://coronavirus.jhu.edu/data/mortality.

Johnson, Garret, Zoe M. Lyon, and Austin Frakt. "Provider-Offered Medicare Advantage Plans: Recent Growth and Care Quality." *Health Affairs* 36, no. 3 (March 1, 2017): 539–47. https://doi.org/10.1377/hlthaff.2016.0722.

Jordan, Edwin O. *Epidemic Influenza: A Survey.* Chicago: American Medical Association, 1927. http://hdl.handle.net/2027/spo.8580flu.0016.858.

Kahn, Marc J., and Ernest J. Sneed. "Promoting the Affordability of Medical Education to Groups Underrepresented in the Profession: The Other Side of the Equation." *AMA Journal of Ethics* 17, no. 2 (February 1, 2015): 172–75. https://doi.org/10.1001/virtualmentor.2015.17.2.oped1-1502.

Kaiser Family Foundation. "Total Number of Medical School Graduates." *KFF*, May 7, 2021. https://www.kff.org/other/state-indicator/total-medical-school-graduates/.

Kaiser Permanente. "Kaiser Permanente 2019 Annual Report." https://healthy.kaiserpermanente.org/static/health/annual_reports/kp_annualreport_2019/.

Kamp, John, Robbie Whelan, and Anthony DeBarros. "U.S. Covid-19 Deaths in 2021 Surpass 2020s." *Wall Street Journal*, November 20, 2021, sec. US. https://www.wsj.com/articles/u-s-covid-19-deaths-in-2021-surpass-2020-11637426356.

Kanthor, Rebecca. "Revisiting Wuhan a Year after the Coronavirus Hit the City." *The World from PRX*, January 21, 2021. https://www.pri.org/stories/2021-01-21/revisiting-wuhan-year-after-coronavirus-hit-city.

Kaplan, Robert M., and Arnold Milstein. "Contributions of Health Care to Longevity: A Review of 4 Estimation Methods." *The Annals of Family Medicine* 17, no. 3 (May 1, 2019): 267–72. https://doi.org/10.1370/afm.2362.

Kassel, Kathleen, and Anikka Martin. "Ag and Food Sectors and the Economy." USDA Economic Research Service, October 12, 2021. https://www.ers.usda.gov/data-products/ag-and-food-statistics-charting-the-essentials/ag-and-food-sectors-and-the-economy/.

Kavanagh, Nolan M., Rishi R. Goel, and Atheendar S. Venkataramani. "County-Level Socioeconomic and Political Predictors of Distancing for COVID-19." *American Journal of Preventive Medicine* 61, no. 1 (July 2021): 13–19. https://doi.org/10.1016/j.amepre.2021.01.040.

Keisler-Starkey, Katherine, and Lisa N. Bunch. "Health Insurance Coverage in the United States: 2020." US Census Bureau, September 14, 2021. https://www.census.gov/library/publications/2021/demo/p60-274.html.

Kellner, Hans. "Heat Vulnerability Index Highlights City Hot Spots." City of Philadelphia, July 16, 2019. https://www.phila.gov/2019-07-16-heat-vulnerability-index-highlights-city-hot-spots/.

Kern, Howard. "So You Want to Start a Health Plan? A Look at Sentara's Integrated Model—and President and CEO Howard Kern's Advice." *Becker's Hospital Review*, November 9, 2020. https://www.beckershospitalreview.

com/strategy/so-you-want-to-start-a-health-plan-a-look-at-sentara-s-inte-grated-model-and-president-ceo-howard-kern-s-advice.html.

Khamsi, Roxanne. "A Lack of Transparency Is Undermining Pandemic Policy." *Wired*, November 16, 2020. https://www.wired.com/story/a-lack-of-transparency-is-undermining-pandemic-policy/.

Khanna, Gunjan, Ebben Smith, and Saum Sutaria. "Provider-Led Health Plans: The Next Frontier—or the 1990s All Over Again?" McKinsey & Company, 2015. https://healthcare.mckinsey.com/sites/default/files/Provider-led%20 health%20plans.pdf.

Khemlani, Anjalee. "Buffett on Failed Health Care Venture Haven: 'We Were Fighting a Tapeworm in the American Economy. And the Tapeworm Won.'" Yahoo Finance, May 1, 2021. https://finance.yahoo.com/news/buffett-on-failed-health-care-venture-haven-we-were-fighting-a-tapeworm-in-the-american-economy-and-the-tapeworm-won-220812439.html.

———. "It's No Surprise That Amazon, Berkshire, JPM Health Venture Haven Is Disbanding: Experts." Yahoo Finance, January 5, 2021. https://finance.yahoo.com/news/its-no-surprise-that-amazon-berkshire-jpm-health-venture-haven-is-disbanding-experts-213818212.html.

Kim, Jerome H., Peter Hotez, Carolina Batista, Onder Ergonul, J. Peter Figueroa, Sarah Gilbert, Mayda Gursel, et al. "Operation Warp Speed: Implications for Global Vaccine Security." *The Lancet Global Health* 9, no. 7 (July 1, 2021): e1017–21. https://doi.org/10.1016/S2214-109X(21)00140-6.

Kimball, Spencer. "White House Tells Businesses to Proceed with Vaccine Mandate Despite Court-Ordered Pause." CNBC, November 8, 2021, sec. Health and Science. https://www.cnbc.com/2021/11/08/biden-vaccine-man-date-white-house-tells-business-to-go-ahead-despite-court-pause.html.

King, Martin Luther, Jr. *Letter from Birmingham Jail.* London: Penguin Classics, 2018.

Kliff, Sarah, Josh Katz, and Rumsey Taylor. "Hospitals and Insurers Didn't Want You to See These Prices. Here's Why." *New York Times*, August 22, 2021, sec. The Upshot. https://www.nytimes.com/interactive/2021/08/22/upshot/hospital-prices.html.

Klinenberg, Eric. *Heat Wave: A Social Autopsy of Disaster in Chicago.* Second edition. Chicago: University of Chicago Press, 2015.

———. "We Need Social Solidarity, Not Just Social Distancing." *New York Times*, March 14, 2020, sec. Opinion. https://www.nytimes.com/2020/03/14/opinion/coronavirus-social-distancing.html.

Kolata, Gina. "In a First, *New England Journal of Medicine* Joins Never-Trumpers." *New York Times*, October 7, 2020, sec. Health. https://www.nytimes.com/2020/10/07/health/new-england-journal-trump.html.

Krakow, Morgan, and Annie Berman. "Alaska Used to Lead the Nation in COVID-19 Vaccinations. Six Months in, the State Has Fallen Behind."

Anchorage Daily News, June 11, 2021, sec. Alaska News. https://www.adn.com/alaska-news/2021/06/10/alaska-used-to-lead-the-nation-in-covid-19-vaccinations-six-months-later-the-state-has-fallen-behind/.

Krouse, Sarah. "Covid-19 Patients Put Remote Care to the Test." *Wall Street Journal*, October 16, 2020, sec. Business. https://www.wsj.com/articles/covid-19-patients-put-remote-care-to-the-test-11602840627.

Kumar, Sanjaya, and David Nash. *Demand Better! Revive Our Broken Healthcare System*. Bozeman, MT: Second River Healthcare Press, 2011.

Kurtz, Alec, Kenneth Grant, Rachel Marano, Antonio Arrieta, Kenneth Grant, William Feaster, Caroline Steele, and Louis Ehwerhemuepha. "Long-Term Effects of Malnutrition on Severity of COVID-19." *Scientific Reports* 11, no. 1 (July 22, 2021). https://doi.org/10.1038/s41598-021-94138-z.

Law, Sylvia A. *Blue Cross: What Went Wrong?* New Haven, CT: Yale University Press, 1976.

Leape, Lucian L. *Making Healthcare Safe: The Story of the Patient Safety Movement*. New York: Springer, 2021.

Lenihan, David. "The Covid-19 Relief Bill Created 1,000 More Residency Slots for New Doctors: Wealthy Hospitals Should Be Last in Line to Get Them." *STAT*, June 25, 2021. https://www.statnews.com/2021/06/25/new-residency-slots-wealthy-hospitals-last-in-line/.

Leonhardt, David. "U.S. Covid Deaths Get Even Redder." *New York Times*, November 8, 2021, sec. Briefing. https://www.nytimes.com/2021/11/08/briefing/covid-death-toll-red-america.html.

Lerner, Michael. "Going Dry." National Endowment for the Humanities, September 2011. https://www.neh.gov/humanities/2011/septemberoctober/feature/going-dry.

Letourneau, Rayna M. "Amid a Raging Pandemic, the US Faces a Nursing Shortage. Can We Close the Gap?" *The Conversation*, November 20, 2020. http://theconversation.com/amid-a-raging-pandemic-the-us-faces-a-nursing-shortage-can-we-close-the-gap-149030.

Levine, James A. "Poverty and Obesity in the U.S." *Diabetes* 60, no. 11 (November 1, 2011): 2667–68. https://doi.org/10.2337/db11-1118.

Lin, Summer. "Why Did Trump Lose? His Own Top Pollster Blames COVID, More in Newly Released Report." McClatchy Washington Bureau, February 2, 2021, sec. Politics & Government. https://www.mcclatchydc.com/news/politics-government/article248943964.html.

Long, Heather. "It's Not a 'Labor Shortage.' It's a Great Reassessment of Work in America." *Washington Post*, May 7, 2021, sec. Economy. https://www.washingtonpost.com/business/2021/05/07/jobs-report-labor-shortage-analysis/.

Long, Heather, and Amy Goldstein. "Poverty Fell Overall in 2020 as Result of Massive Stimulus Checks and Unemployment Aid, Census Bureau Says." *Washington Post*, September 14, 2021, sec.

Economy. https://www.washingtonpost.com/business/2021/09/14/
us-census-poverty-health-insurance-2020/.

Luan, William P., Todd C. Leroux, Cara Olsen, Douglas Robb, Jonathan
Skinner, and Patrick Richard. "Large Spending Variations Found among
Military HMO Enrollees: A Look Using Compulsory Patient Migration."
Institute for Defense Analyses, January 9, 2019. http://dx.doi.org/10.13140/
RG.2.2.22515.37920.

MacGillis, Alec. "What Philadelphia Reveals about America's Homicide
Surge." ProPublica, July 30, 2021. https://www.propublica.org/article/
philadelphia-homicide-surge?token=tg74b8VQrqWdM-PFRUNWBD84Z-
paGuM3h.

Mai, Chris, and Ram Subramanian. "The Price of Prisons." Vera
Institute of Justice, May 2017. https://www.vera.org/publications/
price-of-prisons-2015-state-spending-trends.

Makary, Martin A., and Michael Daniel. "Medical Error—the Third Leading
Cause of Death in the US." *BMJ* 353 (May 3, 2016): i2139. https://doi.
org/10.1136/bmj.i2139.

Mandavilli, Apoorva. "Editor of *JAMA* Leaves after Outcry over Colleague's
Remarks on Racism." *New York Times*, June 1, 2021. https://www.nytimes.
com/2021/06/01/health/jama-bauchner-racism.html.

Markel, Howard, Harvey B. Lipman, J. Alexander Navarro, Alexandra Sloan,
Joseph R. Michalsen, Alexandra Minna Stern, and Martin S. Cetron.
"Nonpharmaceutical Interventions Implemented by US Cities During the
1918–1919 Influenza Pandemic." *JAMA* 298, no. 6 (August 8, 2007): 644.
https://doi.org/10.1001/jama.298.6.644.

Markel, Howard, Alexandra Stern, J. Alexander Navarro, and Joseph R.
Michalsen. *A Historical Assessment of Nonpharmaceutical Disease
Containment Strategies Employed by Selected U.S. Communities during
the Second Wave of the 1918–1920 Influenza Pandemic.* Washington, DC:
US Department of Defense/Defense Threat Reduction Agency, January 31,
2006.

Marshall, Thomas R. "The 1964 Surgeon General's Report and Americans'
Beliefs about Smoking." *Journal of the History of Medicine and Allied
Sciences* 70, no. 2 (April 2015): 250–78. https://doi.org/10.1093/jhmas/
jrt057.

Masters, Rebecca, Elspeth Anwar, Brendan Collins, Richard Cookson, and
Simon Capewell. "Return on Investment of Public Health Interventions: A
Systematic Review." *Journal of Epidemiology and Community Health* 71,
no. 8 (August 1, 2017): 827–34. https://doi.org/10.1136/jech-2016-208141.

Mathews, Anna Wilde. "The Pandemic Didn't Unfold How
Dr. Christine Hancock Expected." *Wall Street Journal,*

December 16, 2021, sec. US. https://www.wsj.com/articles/
pandemic-struggle-patients-who-dont-have-covid-11639668552.

Mattke, Soeren, Harry H. Liu, John P. Caloyeras, Christina Y. Huang, Kristin
R. Van Busum, Dmitry Khodyakov, and Victoria Shier. "Workplace Wellness
Programs Study." *Rand Health Quarterly* 3, no. 2 (June 1, 2013). https://
www.rand.org/pubs/research_reports/RR254.html.

Maxmen, Amy. "Inequality's Deadly Toll." *Nature* 592 (April 29, 2021):
674–80.

———. "Why Did the World's Pandemic Warning System Fail When COVID
Hit?" *Nature* 589, no. 7843 (January 23, 2021): 499–500. https://doi.
org/10.1038/d41586-021-00162-4.

McCullough, J. Mac. "Declines in Spending Despite Positive Returns on
Investment: Understanding Public Health's Wrong Pocket Problem."
Frontiers in Public Health 7 (June 18, 2019): 159. https://doi.org/10.3389/
fpubh.2019.00159.

McDonald's. "McDonald's USA to Raise Wages at Company-Owned
Restaurants across the Country." May 13, 2021. https://corporate.mcdonalds.
com/corpmcd/en-us/our-stories/article/.mcopco-wage-raise.html.

McGoldrick, Debbie. "New Memoir by Michael Dowling Matches
Angela's Ashes for Biting Truth and Insight." *Irish Central*, December
21, 2020. https://www.irishcentral.com/opinion/debbiemcgoldrick/
review-michael-dowling-after-the-roof-caved-in.

Mello, Michelle M., Michael D. Frakes, Erik Blumenkranz, and David M.
Studdert. "Malpractice Liability and Health Care Quality: A Review."
JAMA 323, no. 4 (January 28, 2020): 352–66. https://doi.org/10.1001/
jama.2019.21411.

Menon, Nikitha K., Tait D. Shanafelt, Christine A. Sinsky, Mark Linzer,
Lindsey Carlasare, Keri J. S. Brady, Martin J. Stillman, and Mickey T.
Trockel. "Association of Physician Burnout with Suicidal Ideation and
Medical Errors." *JAMA Network Open* 3, no. 12 (December 9, 2020):
e2028780. https://doi.org/10.1001/jamanetworkopen.2020.28780.

Meyers, David. "CANDOR: An Evolving Approach to Patient Harm."
Relias Media, May 1, 2017, sec. Emergency. https://www.reliasmedia.com/
articles/140522-candor-an-evolving-approach-to-patient-harm.

Millenson, Michael L. "How the US News Media Made Patient Safety a
Priority." *BMJ* 324, no. 7344 (April 27, 2002): 1044.

Miller, Sarah, Laura R. Wherry, and Bhashkar Mazumder. "Estimated Mortality
Increases during the COVID-19 Pandemic by Socioeconomic Status, Race,
and Ethnicity." *Health Affairs* 40, no. 8 (August 1, 2021): 1252–60. https://
doi.org/10.1377/hlthaff.2021.00414.

Minkin, Rachel. "COVID-19 Pandemic Saw an Increase in the Share of U.S.
Mothers Who Would Prefer Not to Work for Pay." Pew Research Center,

August 31, 2021. https://www.pewresearch.org/fact-tank/2021/08/31/covid-19-pandemic-saw-an-increase-in-the-share-of-u-s-mothers-who-would-prefer-not-to-work-for-pay/.

Mitchell, Josh, Lauren Weber, and Sarah Chaney Cambon. "4.3 Million Workers Are Missing. Where Did They Go?" *Wall Street Journal*, October 14, 2021, sec. Economy. https://www.wsj.com/articles/labor-shortage-missing-workers-jobs-pay-raises-economy-11634224519.

Moody, Josh. "10 Most Expensive Private Medical Schools." *US News & World Report*, May 25, 2021. https://www.usnews.com/education/best-graduate-schools/the-short-list-grad-school/articles/most-expensive-private-medical-schools.

Moon, Kristen. "This Medical School Has an Admission Rate of Less Than 1%: Here's How to Get In." *Forbes*, June 21, 2021. https://www.forbes.com/sites/kristenmoon/2021/06/21/this-medical-school-has-an-admission-rate-of-less-than-1-heres-how-to-get-in/.

Morales, Christina, Allyson Waller, and Marie Fazio. "A Timeline of Trump's Symptoms and Treatments." *New York Times*, October 4, 2020, sec. U.S. https://www.nytimes.com/2020/10/04/us/trump-covid-symptoms-timeline.html.

Morris, Devin B., Philip A. Gruppuso, Heather A. McGee, Anarina L. Murillo, Atul Grover, and Eli Y. Adashi. "Diversity of the National Medical Student Body—Four Decades of Inequities." *New England Journal of Medicine* 384, no. 17 (April 29, 2021): 1661–68. https://doi.org/10.1056/NEJMsr2028487.

Moseley, George B. "The U.S. Health Care Non-System, 1908–2008." *AMA Journal of Ethics* 10, no. 5 (May 1, 2008): 324–31. https://doi.org/10.1001/virtualmentor.2008.10.5.mhst1-0805.

Moskowitz, Eric, J. Jon Veloski, Sylvia K. Fields, and David B. Nash. "Development and Evaluation of a 1-Day Interclerkship Program for Medical Students on Medical Errors and Patient Safety." *American Journal of Medical Quality: The Official Journal of the American College of Medical Quality* 22, no. 1 (February 2007): 13–17. https://doi.org/10.1177/1062860606296669.

Mull, Amanda. "The Logic of Pandemic Restrictions Is Falling Apart." *The Atlantic*, November 25, 2020, sec. Health. https://www.theatlantic.com/health/archive/2020/11/pandemic-restrictions-no-logic/617204/.

Murrell, David. "Inside the Ridiculously Vicious and Increasingly Nasty Local Elections in Bucks County." *Philadelphia Magazine*, December 18, 2021. https://www.phillymag.com/news/2021/12/18/bucks-county-school-board-elections/.

Muse, Queen. "How Ala Stanford Became a Champion for the Health of Black Philadelphians amid COVID." *Philadelphia Magazine*, August 8, 2020. https://www.phillymag.com/healthcare-news/2020/08/08/ala-stanford-black-doctors-covid-19-consortium/.

Mutchler, Jan. "Nearly Two-Thirds of Older Black Americans Can't Afford to Live Alone without Help—and It's Even Tougher for Latinos." *The Conversation*, November 17, 2020. http://theconversation.com/nearly-two-thirds-of-older-black-americans-cant-afford-to-live-alone-without-help-and-its-even-tougher-for-latinos-146913.

Nance, John J. *Why Hospitals Should Fly: The Ultimate Flight Plan to Patient Safety and Quality Care*. Bozeman, MT: Second River Healthcare, 2008.

Nash, David B. "Google's Rise in Healthcare." *MedPage Today*, June 30, 2021. https://www.medpagetoday.com/opinion/focusonpolicy/93368.

———. "'Sunshine Is the Best Disinfectant.'" *American Health & Drug Benefits* 10, no. 4 (June 2017): 163–64.

———. "Technology Tackles a Persistent Clinical Problem: Unwarranted Variation." *MedPage Today*, August 30, 2021. https://www.medpagetoday.com/opinion/focusonpolicy/94284.

Nash, Ira. "Big Challenges Require Large-Scale Solutions—as the COVID-19 Pandemic Is Proving." *Modern Healthcare*, April 4, 2020. https://www.modernhealthcare.com/opinion-editorial/big-challenges-require-large-scale-solutions-covid-19-pandemic-proving.

National Alert Network. "Age-Related COVID-19 Vaccine Mix-Ups." National Coordinating Council for Medication Error Reporting and Prevention, December 6, 2021. https://www.nccmerp.org/sites/default/files/nan-alert-dec-6-21-covid-19-vaccine-mixups.pdf.

National Association of Home Builders. "Housing's Contribution to Gross Domestic Product." https://www.nahb.org/news-and-economics/housing-economics/housings-economic-impact/housings-contribution-to-gross-domestic-product.

National Research Council. *Facing Hazards and Disasters: Understanding Human Dimensions*. Washington, DC: National Academies Press, 2006. https://doi.org/10.17226/11671.

National Safety Council. "Car Crash Deaths and Rates." 2021. https://injury-facts.nsc.org/motor-vehicle/historical-fatality-trends/deaths-and-rates/.

National Transportation Safety Board. "The Investigative Process." https://www.ntsb.gov/investigations/process/Pages/default.aspx.

Ndugga, Nambi, Latoya Hill, and Samantha Artiga. "Latest Data on COVID-19 Vaccinations by Race/Ethnicity." *KFF*, August 4, 2021. https://www.kff.org/coronavirus-covid-19/issue-brief/latest-data-on-covid-19-vaccinations-race-ethnicity/.

Neelon, Brian, Fedelis Mutiso, Noel T. Mueller, John L. Pearce, and Sara E. Benjamin-Neelon. "Associations between Governor Political Affiliation and COVID-19 Cases, Deaths, and Testing in the U.S." *American Journal of Preventive Medicine* 61, no. 1 (July 1, 2021): 115–19. https://doi.org/10.1016/j.amepre.2021.01.034.

New York Times. "Coronavirus in the U.S.: Latest Map and Case Count." https://www.nytimes.com/interactive/2021/us/covid-cases.html.

Newburger, Emma. "Dr. Fauci Says His Daughters Need Security as Family Continues to Get Death Threats." CNBC, August 5, 2020, sec. Health & Science. https://www.cnbc.com/2020/08/05/dr-fauci-says-his-daughters-need-security-as-family-continues-to-get-death-threats.html.

Newell, Mike, and Chris Palmer. "Overnight Curfew Lifted in Philly as Tensions over the Police Killing of Walter Wallace Jr. Continue." *Philadelphia Inquirer*, October 29, 2020, sec. News, news, news. https://www.inquirer.com/news/philadelphia-police-shooting-walter-wallace-jr-protests-unrest-20201028.html.

Newhouse, Joseph P., Alan M. Garber, Robin P. Graham, Margaret A. McCoy, Michelle Mancher, and Ashna Kibria. *Variation in Health Care Spending: Target Decision Making, Not Geography.* Washington, DC: National Academies Press, 2013. https://www.ncbi.nlm.nih.gov/books/NBK201637/.

Nirappil, Fenit. "A Black Doctor Alleged Racist Treatment before Dying of Covid-19: 'This Is How Black People Get Killed.'" *Washington Post*, December 4, 2020, sec. Health. https://www.washingtonpost.com/health/2020/12/24/covid-susan-moore-medical-racism/.

Nolen, Stephanie. "I Am Living in a Covid-Free World Just a Few Hundred Miles from Manhattan." *New York Times*, November 18, 2020, sec. Opinion. https://www.nytimes.com/2020/11/18/opinion/covid-halifax-nova-scotia-canada.html.

Northwell Health. "Fact Sheet February 2021." Northwell Health, February 2021. https://www.northwell.edu/sites/northwell.edu/files/2021-02/Fact-Sheet-February-2021.pdf.

Nurin, Tara. "The Fight for Paid Leave Could Benefit Restaurant Workers More Than Most." *Forbes*, July 23, 2021, sec. Food & Drink. https://www.forbes.com/sites/taranurin/2021/07/23/the-fight-for-paid-leave-could-benefit-restaurant-workers-more-than-most/.

Ofri, Danielle. "The Business of Health Care Depends on Exploiting Doctors and Nurses." *New York Times*, June 8, 2019, sec. Opinion. https://www.nytimes.com/2019/06/08/opinion/sunday/hospitals-doctors-nurses-burnout.html.

Oh, Sun Jung, and John Yinger. "What Have We Learned from Paired Testing in Housing Markets?" *Cityscape* 17, no. 3 (2015): 15–60.

O'Malley, Padraic, Jethro Rainford, and Alison Thompson. "Transparency during Public Health Emergencies: From Rhetoric to Reality." *Bulletin of the World Health Organization* 87 (September 1, 2009): 614–18. https://doi.org/10.2471/BLT.08.056689.

Omeokwe, Amara. "Covid-19 Pushed Many Americans to Retire: The Economy Needs Them Back." *Wall Street Journal*, October 31, 2021, sec. Economy.

https://www.wsj.com/articles/covid-19-pushed-many-americans-to-retire-the-economy-needs-them-back-11635691340.

OpenSecrets. "Association of American Medical Colleges." https://www.opensecrets.org/orgs/association-of-american-medical-colleges/summary?id=D000047379.

Orszag, Peter, and Rahul Rekhi. "The Economic Case for Vertical Integration in Health Care." *NEJM Catalyst* 1, no. 3 (June 2020). https://doi.org/10.1056/CAT.20.0119.

Otterman, Sharon. "'I Trust Science,' Says Nurse Who Is First to Get Vaccine in U.S." *New York Times*, December 14, 2020, sec. New York. https://www.nytimes.com/2020/12/14/nyregion/us-covid-vaccine-first-sandra-lindsay.html.

Outcalt, Chris. "'He Thought What He Was Doing Was Good for People.'" *The Atlantic*, August 13, 2021, sec. Politics. https://www.theatlantic.com/politics/archive/2021/08/health-care-sherman-sorensen-pfo-closures/619649/.

Pace, Eric. "Milton Roemer, H.M.O. Advocate, Dies at 84." *New York Times*, January 14, 2001, sec. U.S. https://www.nytimes.com/2001/01/14/us/milton-roemer-hmo-advocate-dies-at-84.html.

Palmore, Tara N., and David K. Henderson. "Healthcare-Associated Infections during the Coronavirus Disease 2019 (COVID-19) Pandemic." *Infection Control & Hospital Epidemiology* 42, no. 11 (November 2021): 1372–73. https://doi.org/10.1017/ice.2021.377.

Palosky, Craig, and Lisa Zamosky. "Vast Majority of Large Employers Surveyed Say Broader Government Role Will Be Necessary to Control Health Costs and Provide Coverage, Survey Finds." *KFF*, April 29, 2021. https://www.kff.org/health-reform/press-release/vast-majority-of-large-employers-surveyed-say-broader-government-role-will-be-necessary-to-control-health-costs-and-provide-coverage-survey-finds/.

Pancevski, Bojan. "Finland and Norway Avoid Covid-19 Lockdowns but Keep the Virus at Bay." *Wall Street Journal*, November 18, 2020, sec. World. https://www.wsj.com/articles/finland-and-norway-avoid-covid-19-lockdowns-but-keep-the-virus-at-bay-11605704407.

Park, William. "The Lifelong Exercise That Keeps Japan Moving." BBC, June 19, 2020. https://www.bbc.com/worklife/article/20200609-the-life-long-exercise-that-keeps-japan-moving.

Parker, Kim, Ruth Igielnik, and Rakesh Kochhar. "Unemployed Americans Are Feeling the Emotional Strain of Job Loss; Most Have Considered Changing Occupations." *Pew Research Center*, February 10, 2021. https://www.pewresearch.org/fact-tank/2021/02/10/unemployed-americans-are-feeling-the-emotional-strain-of-job-loss-most-have-considered-changing-occupations/.

Pasztor, Andy. "Can Hospitals Learn about Safety From Airlines?" *Wall Street Journal*, September 2, 2021, sec. Life & Work. https://www.wsj.com/articles/can-hospitals-learn-about-safety-from-airlines-11630598112.

Peberdy, Mary Ann, Joseph P. Ornato, G. Luke Larkin, R. Scott Braithwaite, T. Michael Kashner, Scott M. Carey, Peter A. Meaney, et al. "Survival from In-Hospital Cardiac Arrest during Nights and Weekends." *JAMA* 299, no. 7 (February 20, 2008): 785–92. https://doi.org/10.1001/jama.299.7.785.

Peeno, Linda. "Managed Care Ethics: The Close View." National Coalition of Mental Health Professionals and Consumers, May 30, 1996. https://web.archive.org/web/20080601094042/http://www.nomanagedcare.org/DrPeenotestimony.html.

Petrilli, Christopher M., Simon A. Jones, Jie Yang, Harish Rajagopalan, Luke O'Donnell, Yelena Chernyak, Katie A. Tobin, Robert J. Cerfolio, Fritz Francois, and Leora I. Horwitz. "Factors Associated with Hospital Admission and Critical Illness among 5279 People with Coronavirus Disease 2019 in New York City: Prospective Cohort Study." *BMJ* 369 (May 22, 2020): m1966. https://doi.org/10.1136/bmj.m1966.

Philadelphia Department of Public Health, and Drexel University Urban Health Collaborative. *Close to Home: The Health of Philadelphia's Neighborhoods*. Philadelphia Department of Public Health, July 31, 2019.

Pines, Jesse, Jeff Selevan, Frank McStay, Meaghan George, and Mark McClellan. "Kaiser Permanente–California: A Model for Integrated Care for the Ill and Injured." Center for Health Policy at Brookings, May 4, 2015. https://www.brookings.edu/wp-content/uploads/2015/04/050415EmerMedCaseStudyKaiser.pdf.

Plsek, Paul E, and Trisha Greenhalgh. "The Challenge of Complexity in Health Care." *BMJ: British Medical Journal* 323, no. 7313 (September 15, 2001): 625–28.

Porter, Eduardo. "Low-Wage Workers Now Have Options, Which Could Mean a Raise." *New York Times*, July 20, 2021, sec. Business. https://www.nytimes.com/2021/07/20/business/economy/workers-wages-mobility.html.

Prasad, Kriti, Colleen McLoughlin, Martin Stillman, Sara Poplau, Elizabeth Goelz, Sam Taylor, Nancy Nankivil, et al. "Prevalence and Correlates of Stress and Burnout among U.S. Healthcare Workers during the COVID-19 Pandemic: A National Cross-Sectional Survey Study." *EClinicalMedicine* 35 (May 16, 2021). https://doi.org/10.1016/j.eclinm.2021.100879.

Public Policy Institute. "COVID-19 Nursing Home Resident and Staff Deaths: AARP Nursing Home Dashboard." AARP, September 15, 2021. https://www.aarp.org/ppi/issues/caregiving/info-2020/nursing-home-covid-dashboard.html.

Quinn, Amy. "Chaos, Anxiety, Frustration—but No Appointment for a Vaccine." *NJ.Com*, January 16, 2021, sec. Opinion. https://www.nj.com/

opinion/2021/01/chaos-anxiety-frustration-but-no-appointment-for-a-vaccine-opinion.html.

Rabin, Roni Caryn. "Fever Checks Are No Safeguard Against Covid-19." *New York Times*, September 13, 2020, sec. Health. https://www.nytimes.com/2020/09/13/health/covid-fever-checks-dining.html.

Raifman, Julia R., Will Raderman, Alexandra Skinner, and Rita Hamad. "Paid Leave Policies Can Help Keep Businesses Open and Food on Workers' Tables." *Health Affairs*, October 25, 2021. https://www.healthaffairs.org/do/10.1377/hblog20211021.197121/full/.

Rau, Jordan. "A Digital Tool Promised to Help Patients Manage Their Diabetes. Then the Hospital behind It Pulled the Plug." *Washington Post*, August 17, 2021, sec. Business. https://www.washingtonpost.com/business/2021/08/17/hospitals-venture-capitalists-diabetes-app/.

Ray, Logan, Jennifer Collins, Patricia Griffin, Hazel Shah, Michelle Boyle, Paul Cieslak, John Dunn, et al. "Decreased Incidence of Infections Caused by Pathogens Transmitted Commonly through Food during the COVID-19 Pandemic—Foodborne Diseases Active Surveillance Network, 10 U.S. Sites, 2017–2020." *MMWR. Morbidity and Mortality Weekly Report* 70, no. 38 (September 24, 2021): 1332–36. https://doi.org/10.15585/mmwr.mm7038a4.

Reason, James. "Human Error: Models and Management." *BMJ: British Medical Journal* 320, no. 7237 (March 18, 2000): 768–70.

Regan, Elizabeth A. "COVID-19 Revealed How Sick the US Health Care Delivery System Really Is." *The Conversation*, March 2, 2021. http://theconversation.com/covid-19-revealed-how-sick-the-us-health-care-delivery-system-really-is-153614.

Reid, Ann H., Thomas G. Fanning, Johan V. Hultin, and Jeffery K. Taubenberger. "Origin and Evolution of the 1918 'Spanish' Influenza Virus Hemagglutinin Gene." *Proceedings of the National Academy of Sciences of the United States of America* 96, no. 4 (February 16, 1999): 1651–56.

Remes, Jaana, Katherine Linzer, Shubham Singhal, Martin Dewhurst, Penelope Dash, Jonathan Woetzel, Sven Smit, et al. "Prioritizing Health: A Prescription for Prosperity." McKinsey & Company, July 8, 2020. https://www.mckinsey.com/industries/healthcare-systems-and-services/our-insights/prioritizing-health-a-prescription-for-prosperity.

Riddle, Matthew C., and William H. Herman. "The Cost of Diabetes Care—An Elephant in the Room." *Diabetes Care* 41, no. 5 (May 1, 2018): 929–32. https://doi.org/10.2337/dci18-0012.

Rimer, Sara. "Blacks Carry Load of Care for Their Elderly." *New York Times*, March 15, 1998, sec. U.S. https://www.nytimes.com/1998/03/15/us/blacks-carry-load-of-care-for-their-elderly.html.

Ritchie, Hannah. "Which Countries Eat the Most Meat?" BBC, February 4, 2019, sec. Health. https://www.bbc.com/news/health-47057341.

Robeznieks, Andis. "Physician Survey Details Depth of Pandemic's Financial Impact." American Medical Association, October 28, 2020. https://www.ama-assn.org/practice-management/sustainability/physician-survey-details-depth-pandemic-s-financial-impact.

Rogers, Katie, Christine Hauser, Alan Yuhas, and Maggie Haberman. "Trump's Suggestion That Disinfectants Could Be Used to Treat Coronavirus Prompts Aggressive Pushback." *New York Times*, April 24, 2020, sec. U.S. https://www.nytimes.com/2020/04/24/us/politics/trump-inject-disinfectant-bleach-coronavirus.html.

Rohde, Rodney E., and Ryan McNamara. "US Is Split between the Vaccinated and Unvaccinatedand Deaths and Hospitalizations Reflect This Divide." *The Conversation*, July 22, 2021. http://theconversation.com/us-is-split-between-the-vaccinated-and-unvaccinated-and-deaths-and-hospitalizations-reflect-this-divide-164460.

Rollston, Rebekah, and Sandro Galea. "COVID-19 and the Social Determinants of Health." *American Journal of Health Promotion* 34, no. 6 (July 1, 2020): 687–89. https://doi.org/10.1177/0890117120930536b.

Romanick-Schmiedl, Sue, and Ganesh Raghu. "Telemedicine: Maintaining Quality during Times of Transition." *Nature Reviews Disease Primers* 6, no. 1 (June 1, 2020): 1–2. https://doi.org/10.1038/s41572-020-0185-x.

Rosen, Michael A., Deborah DiazGranados, Aaron S. Dietz, Lauren E. Benishek, David Thompson, Peter J. Pronovost, and Sallie J. Weaver. "Teamwork in Healthcare: Key Discoveries Enabling Safer, High-Quality Care." *American Psychologist* 73, no. 4 (2018): 433–50. https://doi.org/10.1037/amp0000298.

Rosenberg, Eli. "Hotel Industry Emerges from Pandemic with New Business Model, Possibly Fewer Workers." *Washington Post*, June 11, 2021, sec. Business. https://www.washingtonpost.com/business/2021/06/11/hotel-workers-reduced-cleaning/.

Rowland, Christopher. "Diagnosis for Family Doctors: Less Money, Greater Hardship, and Patients on Video." *Washington Post*, September 8, 2020. https://www.washingtonpost.com/business/2020/09/08/family-doctors-financial-crisis-coronavirus/.

Rudd, Rose, Noah Aleshire, Jon Zibbell, and Matthew Gladden. "Increases in Drug and Opioid Overdose Deaths—United States, 2000–2014." *Centers for Disease Control and Prevention Morbidity and Mortality Weekly Report* 64, no. 50 (January 1, 2016): 1378–82.

Ruggles, Rick. "Seven New Mexico Hospitals Swamped to Point of 'Crisis Standards' Designation." *Santa Fe New Mexican*, December 9, 2021. https://www.santafenewmexican.com/news/local_news/

seven-new-mexico-hospitals-swamped-to-point-of-crisis-standards-designa-
tion/article_a9a57e78-58fa-11ec-8dda-53fd55d95320.html.

Sabin, Janice. "How We Fail Black Patients in Pain." AAMC, January 6, 2020.
https://www.aamc.org/news-insights/how-we-fail-black-patients-pain.

Safdar, Khadeeja, Joe Palazzolo, Janet Adamy, and Shalini Ramachandran.
"Young Doctors Struggle to Treat Coronavirus Patients: 'We Are Horrified
and Scared.'" *Wall Street Journal*, April 29, 2020, sec. US. https://www.wsj.
com/articles/young-doctors-struggle-to-treat-coronavirus-patients-we-are-
horrified-and-scared-11588171553.

Safford, Monika M., Evgeniya Reshetnyak, Madeline R. Sterling, Joshua S.
Richman, Paul M. Muntner, Raegan W. Durant, John Booth, and Laura
C. Pinheiro. "Number of Social Determinants of Health and Fatal and
Nonfatal Incident Coronary Heart Disease in the REGARDS Study."
Circulation 143, no. 3 (January 19, 2021): 244–53. https://doi.org/10.1161/
CIRCULATIONAHA.120.048026.

Sampson, Hannah. "Will Business Travel Ever Be the Same?" *Washington
Post*, August 4, 2021, sec. Travel. https://www.washingtonpost.com/
travel/2021/08/04/business-travel-recovery-pandemic/.

Sarkar, Urmimala, and Christine Cassel. "Humanism Before Heroism in
Medicine." *JAMA* 326, no. 2 (July 13, 2021): 127–28. https://doi.org/10.1001/
jama.2021.9569.

Schambra, William A. "Eugenics as Philanthropic 'Best Practice.'"
Hudson Institute, November 14, 2011. http://www.hudson.org/
research/8496-eugenics-as-philanthropic-best-practice-.

Scholsberg, John, Linsey Davis, and Sabina Ghebremedhin.
"Philadelphia Doctor Takes to Streets to Help Black Communities
Get Tested for COVID-19." *ABC News*, April 29, 2020, sec.
Coronavirus Health & Science. https://abcnews.go.com/US/phil-
adelphia-doctor-takes-streets-black-communities-tested-covid/
story?id=70405257.

Schow, Diana, Elisa J. Sobo, and Stephanie McClure. "US Black and Latino
Communities Often Have Low Vaccination Rates—but Blaming Vaccine
Hesitancy Misses the Mark." *The Conversation*, July 7, 2021. http://the-
conversation.com/us-black-and-latino-communities-often-have-low-vacci-
nation-rates-but-blaming-vaccine-hesitancy-misses-the-mark-163169.

Schroer, Alyssa. "Wearable Technology in Healthcare: 11 Companies to Know
2021." Built In, July 17, 2019. https://builtin.com/healthcare-technology/
wearable-technology-in-healthcare.

Schuchat, Anne. "What I Learned in 33 Years at the C.D.C." *New York Times*,
June 10, 2021, sec. Opinion. https://www.nytimes.com/2021/06/10/opinion/
anne-schuchat-cdc-retirement.html.

Schwartz, Karyn, and Anthony Damico. "Distribution of CARES Act Funding among Hospitals." *KFF*, May 13, 2020. https://www.kff.org/coronavirus-covid-19/issue-brief/distribution-of-cares-act-funding-among-hospitals/.

Schwirtz, Michael. "The 1,000-Bed *Comfort* Was Supposed to Aid New York. It Has 20 Patients." *New York Times*, April 2, 2020, sec. New York. https://www.nytimes.com/2020/04/02/nyregion/ny-coronavirus-usns-comfort.html.

Sepkowitz, K. A., and L. Eisenberg. "Occupational Deaths among Healthcare Workers." *Emerging Infectious Diseases* 11, no. 7 (2005): 10038. doi:10.3201/eid1107.041038.

Shanafelt, Tait D., Lotte N. Dyrbye, Colin P. West, Christine Sinsky, Michael Tutty, Lindsey E. Carlasare, Hanhan Wang, and Mickey Trockel. "Suicidal Ideation and Attitudes Regarding Help Seeking in US Physicians Relative to the US Working Population." *Mayo Clinic Proceedings* 96, no. 8 (August 1, 2021): 2067–80. https://doi.org/10.1016/j.mayocp.2021.01.033.

Shi, Leiyu. "The Impact of Primary Care: A Focused Review." *Scientifica* 2012 (December 31, 2012): 432892. https://doi.org/10.6064/2012/432892.

Shindell, Drew, Yuqiang Zhang, Melissa Scott, Muye Ru, Krista Stark, and Kristie L. Ebi. "The Effects of Heat Exposure on Human Mortality throughout the United States." *GeoHealth* 4, no. 4 (2020): e2019GH000234. https://doi.org/10.1029/2019GH000234.

Shrank, William H., Teresa L. Rogstad, and Natasha Parekh. "Waste in the US Health Care System: Estimated Costs and Potential for Savings." *JAMA* 322, no. 15 (October 15, 2019): 1501. https://doi.org/10.1001/jama.2019.13978.

Shvetsova, Olga, et al., Public Health Policies as a Link between Governor Political Affiliation and COVID-19 Outcomes: Response to Neelon et al., unpublished.

Silbert, Sarah. "Smart Shoes: The Latest Wearable Phenomenon." Lifewire, December 2, 2020. https://www.lifewire.com/smart-shoes-latest-wearable-phenomenon-3946235.

Simonetti, Joseph A. "Checklists to Improve Patient Safety Have Mixed Results." *The Hospitalist*, January 25, 2018, sec. Practice Management. https://www.the-hospitalist.org/hospitalist/article/157054/critical-care.

Singer, Natasha. "The Hot New Covid Tech Is Wearable and Constantly Tracks You." *New York Times*, November 15, 2020, sec. Technology. https://www.nytimes.com/2020/11/15/technology/virus-wearable-tracker-privacy.html.

Slotkin, Jonathan R., Olivia A. Ross, M. Ruth Coleman, and Jaewon Ryu. "Why GE, Boeing, Lowe's, and Walmart Are Directly Buying Health Care for Employees." *Harvard Business Review*, June 8, 2017. https://hbr.org/2017/06/why-ge-boeing-lowes-and-walmart-are-directly-buying-health-care-for-employees.

Smith, Brad. "CMS Innovation Center at 10 Years—Progress and Lessons Learned." *New England Journal of Medicine* 384, no. 8 (February 25, 2021): 759–64. https://doi.org/10.1056/NEJMsb2031138.

Solomon, Feliz, and Wilawan Watcharasakwet. "Thailand Once Shut Out Covid-19 but Is Now Pivoting to Living with It." *Wall Street Journal*, June 19, 2021, sec. World. https://www.wsj.com/articles/thailand-once-shut-out-covid-19-but-is-now-pivoting-to-living-with-it-11624107310.

Song, Zirui, and Katherine Baicker. "Effect of a Workplace Wellness Program on Employee Health and Economic Outcomes." *JAMA* 321, no. 15 (April 16, 2019): 1491–501. https://doi.org/10.1001/jama.2019.3307.

Spanko, Alex. "Medicaid's Share of Nursing Home Revenue, Resident Days Hits Record High as Medicare Drops to Historic Low." *Skilled Nursing News*, December 11, 2019. https://skillednursingnews.com/2019/12/medicaids-share-of-nursing-home-revenue-resident-days-hits-record-high-as-medicare-drops-to-historic-low/.

Spencer, Jane, and Christina Jewett. "'Lost on the Front Line': Tracks Health Workers Who Died of COVID-19." *Kaiser Health News*, April 8, 2021. https://www.npr.org/2021/04/08/985253407/lost-on-the-front-line-tracks-health-workers-who-died-of-covid-19.

Stevens, Matt. "At Late-Night Rally, Trump Suggests He May Fire Fauci 'after the Election.'" *New York Times*, November 2, 2020, sec. U.S. https://www.nytimes.com/2020/11/02/us/politics/at-late-night-rally-trump-suggests-he-may-fire-fauci-after-the-election.html.

Stine, Deborah D. *The Manhattan Project, the Apollo Program, and Federal Energy Technology R&D Programs: A Comparative Analysis*. Washington, DC: Congressional Research Service, June 30, 2009. https://sgp.fas.org/crs/misc/RL34645.pdf.

Sumner, Steven, Laura Green Brown, Roberta Frick, Carmily Stone, Rand Carpenter, Lisa Bushnell, Dave Nicholas, et al. "Factors Associated with Food Workers Working While Experiencing Vomiting or Diarrhea." *Journal of Food Protection* 74, no. 2 (February 1, 2011): 215–20. https://doi.org/10.4315/0362-028X.JFP-10-108.

Swaim, Barton. "Politics: The Experts and the Pandemic." *Wall Street Journal*, December 18, 2020, sec. Arts. https://www.wsj.com/articles/politics-the-experts-and-the-pandemic-11608331377.

Swanson, Ana, David Yaffe-Bellany, and Michael Corkery. "Pork Chops vs. People: Battling Coronavirus in an Iowa Meat Plant." *New York Times*, May 10, 2020, sec. Business. https://www.nytimes.com/2020/05/10/business/economy/coronavirus-tyson-plant-iowa.html.

Syrek, Ryan. "The Horror of Medical School Captured on Film." *Medscape*, October 16, 2020. http://www.medscape.com/viewarticle/939045.

Tamari, Jonathan. "Sen. Bob Casey Cites Shooting of Walter Wallace Jr. in Pushing Bills to Divert 911 Calls for Mental Health Crises." *Philadelphia Inquirer*, December 9, 2021, sec. National Politics, politics, nation. https://www.inquirer.com/politics/nation/bob-casey-police-reform-walter-wallace-jr-20201209.html.

Tangel, Andrew. "Boeing Board to Face 737 MAX Lawsuit." *Wall Street Journal*, September 8, 2021, sec. Business. https://www.wsj.com/articles/boeing-board-to-face-737-max-oversight-lawsuit-11631114438.

Taylor, Charles A., Christopher Boulos, and Douglas Almond. "Livestock Plants and COVID-19 Transmission." *PNAS* 117, no. 50: 31706–15. https://doi.org/10.1073/pnas.2010115117.

Thomas, Rachel, Marianne Cooper, Kate McShane Urban, Gina Cardazone, Ali Bohrer, Sonia Mahajan, Lareina Yee, et al. *Women in the Workplace 2021*. McKinsey & Company, 2021. https://wiw-report.s3.amazonaws.com/Women_in_the_Workplace_2021.pdf.

Thomas, TaRhonda. "Central Bucks School Board Accused of Allowing Hate Speech during Public Comment." *6 Action News Philadelphia*, November 10, 2021, sec. education. https://6abc.com/central-bucks-school-district-hate-speech-freedom-of-transgender-slur/11220859/.

Toll, Ian W. *Twilight of the Gods: War in the Western Pacific, 1944–1945*. New York: W.W. Norton, 2020.

Tufekci, Zeynep. "5 Pandemic Mistakes We Keep Repeating." *The Atlantic*, February 26, 2021, sec. Ideas. https://www.theatlantic.com/ideas/archive/2021/02/how-public-health-messaging-backfired/618147/.

———. "The Unvaccinated May Not Be Who You Think." *New York Times*, October 15, 2021, sec. Opinion. https://www.nytimes.com/2021/10/15/opinion/covid-vaccines-unvaccinated.html.

———. "Why Did It Take So Long to Accept the Facts about Covid?" *New York Times*, May 7, 2021, sec. Opinion. https://www.nytimes.com/2021/05/07/opinion/coronavirus-airborne-transmission.html.

US Attorney's Office, District of New Jersey. "Opioid Manufacturer Purdue Pharma Admits Guilt in Fraud and Kickback Conspiracies." United States Department of Justice, November 24, 2020. https://www.justice.gov/usao-nj/pr/opioid-manufacturer-purdue-pharma-admits-guilt-fraud-and-kickback-conspiracies.

US Census Bureau. "U.S. Census Bureau QuickFacts: Queens County (Queens Borough), New York." U.S. Census Bureau, April 1, 2020. https://www.census.gov/quickfacts/fact/table/queenscountyqueensboroughnewyork/POP645219.

US Department of Health and Human Services. "State Health Information Exchange." HealthIT.gov, April 29, 2019. https://www.healthit.gov/topic/onc-hitech-programs/state-health-information-exchange.

US House of Representatives. "Coronavirus Infections and Deaths among Meatpacking Workers at Top Five Companies Were Nearly Three Times Higher Than Previous Estimates." US House of Representatives, October 27, 2021. https://coronavirus.house.gov/sites/democrats.coronavirus.house.gov/files/2021.10.27%20Meatpacking%20Report.Final_.pdf.

———. "Majority Changes in the House of Representatives, 1856 to Present." US House of Representatives History, Art, and Archives, 2021. https://history.house.gov/Institution/Majority-Changes/Majority-Changes/.

US Office of Management and Budget and Federal Reserve Bank of St. Louis. "Federal Net Outlays as Percent of Gross Domestic Product." Federal Reserve Bank of St. Louis. FRED, Federal Reserve Bank of St. Louis, 2021. https://fred.stlouisfed.org/series/FYONGDA188S.

VanDusky-Allen, Julie, and Olga Shvetsova. "How America's Partisan Divide over Pandemic Responses Played Out in the States." *The Conversation*, May 12, 2021. http://theconversation.com/how-americas-partisan-divide-over-pandemic-responses-played-out-in-the-states-157565.

Van Houtven, Courtney Harold, and Walter D. Dawson. "Medicare and Home Health: Taking Stock in the COVID-19 Era." Commonwealth Fund, Issues Brief, October 21, 2020. https://doi.org/10.26099/kq2n-1s19.

Venkataramani, Atheendar S., Rourke O'Brien, and Alexander C. Tsai. "Declining Life Expectancy in the United States: The Need for Social Policy as Health Policy." *JAMA* 325, no. 7 (February 16, 2021): 621–22. https://doi.org/10.1001/jama.2020.26339.

Wadman, Meredith. "Why COVID-19 Is More Deadly in People with Obesity—Even If They're Young." *Science*, September 8, 2020. https://www.science.org/content/article/why-covid-19-more-deadly-people-obesity-even-if-theyre-young.

Waldman, Hilary. "CCMC Could Lose License." *Hartford Courant*, September 17, 2005 https://www.courant.com/news/connecticut/hc-xpm-2005-09-17-0509170874-story.html.

Warm, Eric J., Yousef Ahmad, Benjamin Kinnear, Matthew Kelleher, Dana Sall, Andrew Wells, and Paul Barach. "A Dynamic Risk Management Approach for Reducing Harm from Invasive Bedside Procedures Performed during Residency." *Academic Medicine: Journal of the Association of American Medical Colleges* 96, no. 9 (September 1, 2021): 1268–75. https://doi.org/10.1097/ACM.0000000000004066.

Washington, Harriet A. "Apology Shines Light on Racial Schism in Medicine." *New York Times*, July 29, 2008, sec. Health. https://www.nytimes.com/2008/07/29/health/views/29essa.html.

Washington Post. "Fatal Force." Online database. *Washington Post*, December 21, 2021. https://www.washingtonpost.com/graphics/investigations/police-shootings-database/.

Wears, Robert, and Kathleen Sutcliffe. *Still Not Safe: Patient Safety and the Middle-Managing of American Medicine*. New York: Oxford University Press, 2019. https://doi.org/10.1093/oso/9780190271268.001.0001.

Weiner-Lastinger, Lindsey M., Vaishnavi Pattabiraman, Rebecca Y. Konnor, Prachi R. Patel, Emily Wong, Sunny Y. Xu, Brittany Smith, Jonathan R. Edwards, and Margaret A. Dudeck. "The Impact of Coronavirus Disease 2019 (COVID-19) on Healthcare-Associated Infections in 2020: A Summary of Data Reported to the National Healthcare Safety Network." *Infection Control & Hospital Epidemiology*, September 3, 2021, 1–14. https://doi.org/10.1017/ice.2021.362.

Wen, Leana S. "Opinion: The CDC Is Missing a Critical Opportunity to Get Americans Vaccinated." *Washington Post*, March 8, 2021. https://www.washingtonpost.com/opinions/cdc-recommendations-vaccinated-masks-limited/2021/03/08/a05353ac-804e-11eb-9ca6-54e187ee4939_story.html.

Werner, Rachel M., Ezekiel J. Emanuel, Hoangmai H. Pham, and Amol S. Navathe. "The Future of Value-Based Payment: A Road Map to 2030." Leonard Davis Institute of Health Economics, February 17, 2021. https://ldi.upenn.edu/our-work/research-updates/the-future-of-value-based-payment-a-road-map-to-2030/.

White, Rachel E, Patricia L Trbovich, Anthony C Easty, Pamela Savage, Katherine Trip, and Sylvia Hyland. "Checking It Twice: An Evaluation of Checklists for Detecting Medication Errors at the Bedside Using a Chemotherapy Model." *Quality & Safety in Health Care* 19, no. 6 (December 2010): 562–67. https://doi.org/10.1136/qshc.2009.032862.

Williams, Sankey V., David B. Nash, and Neil Goldfarb. "Differences in Mortality from Coronary Artery Bypass Graft Surgery at Five Teaching Hospitals." *JAMA* 266, no. 6 (August 14, 1991): 810–15. https://doi.org/10.1001/jama.1991.03470060072029.

Willman, David. "The CDC's Failed Race against Covid-19: A Threat Underestimated and a Test Overcomplicated." *Washington Post*, December 26, 2020. https://www.washingtonpost.com/investigations/cdc-covid/2020/12/25/c2b418ae-4206-11eb-8db8-395dedaaa036_story.html.

Windsor, Leah C., Gina Yannitell Reinhardt, Alistair J. Windsor, Robert Ostergard, Susan Allen, Courtney Burns, Jarod Giger, and Reed Wood. "Gender in the Time of COVID-19: Evaluating National Leadership and COVID-19 Fatalities." *PLOS ONE* 15, no. 12 (December 31, 2020): e0244531. https://doi.org/10.1371/journal.pone.0244531.

Winkler, Rolfe. "Apple Studying Potential of AirPods as Health Device." *Wall Street Journal*, October 13, 2021, sec. Tech. https://www.wsj.com/articles/apple-studying-potential-of-airpods-as-health-device-11634122800.

Wohlforth, Charles. *The Fate of Nature: Rediscovering Our Ability to Rescue the Earth*. New York: Thomas Dunne Books/St. Martin's Press, 2010.

Wood, Daniel, and Geoff Brumfiel. "Pro-Trump Counties Now Have Far Higher COVID Death Rates. Misinformation Is to Blame." NPR, December 5, 2021, sec. Untangling Disinformation. https://www.npr.org/sections/health-shots/2021/12/05/1059828993/data-vaccine-misinformation-trump-counties-covid-death-rate.

Woolf, Steven H., Derek A. Chapman, Roy T. Sabo, Daniel M. Weinberger, and Latoya Hill. "Excess Deaths from COVID-19 and Other Causes, March–April 2020." *JAMA* 324, no. 5 (August 4, 2020): 510. https://doi.org/10.1001/jama.2020.11787.

World Health Organization. "Ebola Virus Disease." WHO, February 23, 2021. https://www.who.int/news-room/fact-sheets/detail/ebola-virus-disease.

———. "Naming the Coronavirus Disease (COVID-19) and the Virus That Causes It." WHO, February 11, 2020. https://www.who.int/emergencies/diseases/novel-coronavirus-2019/technical-guidance/naming-the-coronavirus-disease-(covid-2019)-and-the-virus-that-causes-it.

———. "Weekly Epidemiological Update on COVID-19–11 May 2021." WHO, May 11, 2021. https://www.who.int/publications/m/item/weekly-epidemiological-update-on-covid-19---11-may-2021.

Worthen, Molly. "A Once-in-a-Century Crisis Can Help Educate Doctors." *New York Times*, April 10, 2021, sec. Opinion. https://www.nytimes.com/2021/04/10/opinion/sunday/covid-medical-school-humanities.html.

Wright, Aallyah. "Republican Men Are Vaccine-Hesitant, but There's Little Focus on Them." Pew Charitable Trusts, April 23, 2021. https://pew.org/3xh75RF.

Wynn, Barbara O, Robert Smalley, and Kristina M Cordasco. "Does It Cost More to Train Residents or to Replace Them? A Look at the Costs and Benefits of Operating Graduate Medical Education Programs." RAND Corporation, 2013. https://www.rand.org/content/dam/rand/pubs/research_reports/RR300/RR324/RAND_RR324.pdf.

Yeung, Caroline Au, and Robert Hest. "Exploring Public Health Indicators with State Health Compare: State Public Health Funding." State Health Access Data Assistance Center, May 2020. https://www.shadac.org/sites/default/files/State%20Public%20Health%20Funding_May%202020.pdf.

Young, Kerry Dooley. "Patient-Safety Leader Challenges Hospitals Nationwide to Establish 10 Crucial Teams." *Association of Health Care Journalists*, December 14, 2021. https://healthjournalism.org/blog/2021/12/patient-safety-leader-challenges-hospitals-nationwide-to-establish-10-teams-to-reverse-the-flow-of-health-care-resources/.

Ziobro, Paul. "GE, Union Pacific Suspend Covid-19 Vaccination Mandates after Injunction on Biden Order." *Wall Street Journal*, December 9, 2021, sec. Business. https://www.wsj.com/articles/ge-union-pacific-suspend-covid-19-vaccination-mandates-after-injunction-on-biden-order-11639089010.

Index

access to information, patients and, 198–99, 202
Accreditation Council for Graduate Medical Education, 181
addiction interventions, upstream, 59–63
admissions, 169, 171–75
advance directives, information systems and, 199–203
aerosols, 100, 123
Affordable Care Act, 52, 54, 123, 146
Agency for Healthcare Research and Quality, 232
airlines, and Covid restrictions, 207–8
Alaska, and Covid, 53–54
Amazon, 143, 209
American culture, 47–65; and failure of health care system, 14–15, 241–43; nature of, 51–59; and prevention versus cure, 15, 50, 61; recommendations in keeping with, 63–65; variations within state, 53–54

American Medical Association, 80, 224
American Rescue Plan, 182
Ansell, David, 81–83, 85–86
artificial intelligence: and continuous health monitoring, 201–2, 216, 228–29; and diagnosis, 228
Asian countries, and Covid, 48–49, 55–56
Association of American Medical Colleges, 179
Australia: and Covid, 48–49; and individualism, 58
authority gradient: and CDC test failure, 42–43; and medical errors, 10
automation, 72
autonomy, employer-led health and, 214–18
aviation safety investigation, 8; examples of, 10; and human factors engineering, 226–27; as model, 7, 25, 229–30, 252–53; pace of, 239; tools for, 222

339

About the Authors

Dr. David B. Nash is among the world's most respected experts on health care accountability, quality, and leadership. He founded the Jefferson College of Population Health in Philadelphia and remains its founding dean emeritus, continuing as full-time faculty as the Dr. Raymond C. and Doris N. Grandon Professor of Health Policy. He has held many governance positions for public- and private-sector health organizations as a trustee and board member—serving, for example, for a decade as a board member of Humana, one of the nation's largest publicly traded health care companies. He has received many awards in recognition of his achievements and is well known through his many publications and public appearances, as well as his online column on *MedPage Today*. He has authored more than one hundred peer-reviewed articles and edited twenty-five books, and he has already written widely on Covid in the academic literature. Currently, he is editor in chief of *American Journal of Medical Quality*, *Population Health Management*, and *American Health and Drug Benefits*.

Dr. Nash has been frequently cited in the *Wall Street Journal*, the *Philadelphia Inquirer*, and *Modern Healthcare Magazine*. He has been a guest on National Public Radio and the television affiliates of ABC, NBC, and CBS in the Philadelphia marketplace. For the past fourteen years, he has authored a special monthly online column on health policy for *MedPage Today*. As a result, he has an active presence on multiple social media platforms. Dr. Nash is a recognized subject matter expert for the biotech, pharma, and health information technology industries and, as such, appears regularly on advisory board webinars and national online programs. As a thought leader in physician leadership circles, his educational programs on health care quality, safety, and population health have reached more physicians, face-to-face, than any other educator in this arena nationally.

Dr. Nash received his BA in economics (Phi Beta Kappa) from Vassar College, his MD from the University of Rochester School of Medicine and Dentistry, and his MBA in Health Administration (with honors) from the Wharton School at the University of Pennsylvania. He has received honorary doctorates from Salus University in Philadelphia, Geisinger Commonwealth School of Medicine, and the University of Rochester. He lives in Ardmore, Pennsylvania, with his wife of forty years, Esther Nash, MD. They have three adult children. He enjoys tennis, jogging, biking, and yoga.

Charles Wohlforth is author of more than ten books and numerous articles and columns, a former elected official and nonprofit leader, and host of podcasts and public radio and TV shows. His work primarily explores the intersections of science and technology with culture. He has collaborated many times, most recently as lead author with Dr. Amanda Hendrix of *Beyond Earth: Our Path to a New Home in the Planets* (2016). As a solo author, his book on climate change in the Arctic won the 2004 *Los Angeles Times* Book Prize for science and technology, which was presented by astronaut Sally Ride, and he has won some three dozen other awards. Until 2019, Wohlforth wrote a newspaper column for the *Anchorage Daily News*, often investigating health care costs, and in that year was named the best columnist in the western United States by Best of the West, the region's most prestigious journalism contest.

As an author, Wohlforth has appeared on MSNBC's *Morning Joe*, NPR's *Science Friday*, and CSPAN's *Washington Journal*, as well as national public affairs interviews on ABC, Fox, and BBC, along with network affiliates in New York, Washington, DC, and other cities. His op-eds and excerpts supporting his work have been published in the *New York Times, Los Angeles Times, Scientific American, The Daily Beast*, and many other publications. He is an experienced public speaker, having given compensated lectures on his books hundreds of times across the United States and in Europe, including keynote appearances at conventions and major scientific meetings, as well as professional and public talks at many universities, including Yale, UCLA, and Cambridge.

Wohlforth graduated magna cum laude from Princeton University in 1986 with a BA degree in English. He lives in Peapack, New Jersey, and has four adult children. He enjoys cross-country skiing, biking, and boating and spends much of his summer at an off-the-grid cabin on the coast of Alaska.

CPSIA information can be obtained
at www.ICGtesting.com
Printed in the USA
BVHW082154190622
639926BV00002B/2